Fingertip Injuries

Leo M. Rozmaryn

Editor

Fingertip Injuries

Diagnosis, Management
and Reconstruction

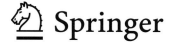 Springer

Editor
Leo M. Rozmaryn, MD
Clinical Adjunct Assistant Professor of
Orthopedics
Uniformed Services Health Sciences Center
Bethesda, MA, USA
The Orthopedic Center
Rockville, MD, USA

ISBN 978-3-319-13226-6   ISBN 978-3-319-13227-3 (eBook)
DOI 10.1007/978-3-319-13227-3

Library of Congress Control Number: 2015931212

Springer Cham Heidelberg New York Dordrecht London
© Springer International Publishing Switzerland 2015

Printed on acid-free paper

Springer International Publishing is part of Springer Science+Business Media (www.springer.com)

To "my" Sharona, who has stood by me through thick and thin.

Foreword

Perception and Execution....

The tips of our fingers are the antennae, the eyes of our upper extremity, and the tools and instruments with which we carry out our most precise and intimate functions. They are ultimate sensory organs through which we touch and perceive pressure, two-point discrimination, proprioception, temperature, shape, texture, and even danger. They are the eyes of those who have no sight.

Through the sensory organs of our fingertips, we perceive the loving touch of a soul mate and are able to caress the soft, frail, dependent trust of our newborn child. It is through this articulate sensory organ that we perceive the gentle caress of a loved one and impart sensual, protective, secure reassurance, and communication with those to whom we give our hand. Metaphorically we can leave the thumbprint of our involvement as a lasting remembrance. The skin, bones, ligaments, nail bed, sensory end organs, and even fingernails combine to form the most precise instrument of sensation and execution.

The child exploring his or her awakening universe, the musician, the artist, the sculptor creating a masterpiece of auditory, visual, or structural beauty all employ this incredible end organ in unique and creative ways. We surgeons use our fingertips to explore, diagnose, and precisely execute the maneuvers over which to perform our own art form.

Injury to the fingertip can be devastating. Loss of sensation, prehension, coordination, strength, and endurance can result when trauma or disease has affected the most distal extent of our upper extremity.

In this text, Dr. Rozmaryn has assembled the unique thoughts, experiences, and expertise of creative thought leaders in the practice of surgery of the hand to provide their individual, yet universal perspectives on this incredible, animated instrument, which combines sensory and motor precision.

The reader will be enlightened by the various perspectives on managing every component of injury to the fingertip that can occur. The creative and well-respected techniques which the authors provide will enhance the readers' ability to care for fingertip injuries and restore sensory and motor function to this extremely important instrument located at the distal extent of our hands.

It is a privilege to provide a foreword to this text which will become a staple in the library of the practicing hand surgeon.

Professor of Orthopaedic Surgery   William H. Seitz, Jr., MD
Cleveland Clinic Lerner College of Medicine
of Case Western Reserve University
Chairman, Orthopaedic Surgery, Lutheran Hospital
Cleveland Clinic Orthopaedic & Rheumatologic Institute
President, American Society for Surgery of the Hand 2014–2015

Preface

The fingertip is truly one of our windows to the world. It is our only primary sensory perception that is outside of our head and face. It is a critically important part of the hand. It is the sensory perception inherent in normal fingertip motion that gives prehension of our hands their true meaning. Without sensory perception in our fingertips, vision and hearing would have little meaning as we would be unable to interact with objects that surround us in any meaningful way.

Fingertip injuries are exceedingly common. Taken in the entirety, they constitute the largest percentage of orthopedic injuries seen in the emergency room. The scenarios in which these occur constitute the full palate of human endeavor from work, sports, home, to a simple crush in a car door. They are a leading cause of time off from work and worker's compensation claims. Children are affected as often as adults. An injury to fingertips creating anesthesia or pain severely impairs the functions of the hand. Fingertip injuries are frequently misunderstood, and thus, these are usually treated by the least skilled members of the medical team. All too frequently, these injuries end up with suboptimal results.

Mechanisms of injury vary widely from crush, avulsion, degloving, laceration, amputation, eccentric tendon overuse, hyperflexion, or extension of the distal phalanx. They can involve any and all of the structures in the finger, and injuries can be open or closed. High-pressure injection injury is a special type of fingertip injury resulting in a mini compartment syndrome in the volar pad of the finger. If it is not addressed promptly, it can result in irreversible ischemia or in gangrene or eventual amputation of the tip. Closed injuries can result in fracture of the distal phalanx, dislocation, collateral injuries of the wrist of the distal interphalangeal joints, and closed avulsions of the flexor digitorum profundus and mallet fingers. Open injuries include dorsal and volar lacerations resulting in trauma to the nail apparatus or terminal flexor and extensor tendons and digital nerve as the nail bed crush and avulsion injuries which can coexist with open fractures of the distal phalanx. Degloving injuries to the dorsal volar skin frequently accompany crush injuries to the tip. In extreme cases, the tip of the finger may be amputated by a sharp instrument leaving a deficit that is either transverse or oblique and either in the sagittal or coronal plane. The defect can be complex such as a severe crushing injury and amputations may or may not have exposed bone.

The goal of the treatment is to restore an esthetically pleasing, painless, tactile, mobile, stable fingertip that can sense pain, temperature, pressure, stereognosis, and fine touch. The fingertip must also be the terminus of the gripping mechanism of the hand. Unfortunately, all too often, these injuries are under recognized resulting in fingertip numbness, cold sensitivity, nail growth abnormalities, nail fold to volar pad deformities, hyperesthesia, and painful stiffness of the distal interphalangeal joint.

The purpose of this book is to outline the various categories of injury to the fingertip, anatomy, physiology, mechanisms of injury, treatment options and outcomes, as well as possible complications of treating these injuries. Treatment may constitute simple splinting or expectant observation to complex microvascular reconstruction, open reduction internal fixation, complex nail reconstruction, emergent decompression of high-pressure injection injuries, local and regional flap reconstructions, and free tissue transfers for finger tip coverage. Also dealt within this book are management of fingertip burns and special considerations for pediatric injuries as well as rehabilitation of the fingertip. An increased awareness of these injuries will hopefully optimize treatment of these frequently undertreated injuries and lead to better clinical care.

Leo M. Rozmaryn

Acknowledgments

I would like to acknowledge a number of people who have contributed to this textbook. First, I would like to thank my wife, Sharona, for her patience in putting up with me during the difficult task of writing and assembling all of the chapters in this book.

Additionally, I would like to thank Elizabeth Dufresne for the countless hours that she spent editing my chapters, editing and formatting the text and figures in the chapter, and interacting with my co-authors as well as the publisher and their various representatives. Without her efforts this book could never have been possible.

I would also like to thank all of the others who have gone through the texts and offered their critical evaluation of my writing as well helping me to formulate the structure of this book and its contents.

Finally, I would like to thank the stellar panel of international experts in their field who have contributed to this book, without whose vast knowledge, experience, and expertise this book could not have been possible. They not only shared their knowledge and technical expertise with us but also shared their significant wisdom which constitutes the art of medicine. Their contributions were invaluable to the quality of this book. I sincerely hope that readers will find this book to be useful in the diagnosis and management of these underdiagnosed and undertreated injuries.

Contents

Contributors

Francisco J. Aguilar C. M. Kleinert Institute for Hand and Microsurgery, Louisville, KY, USA

Sandra Lea Austin Medical College of Virginia, Fairfax, VA, USA

Alexander B. Dagum Department of Surgery, Stony Brook Medicine, Stony Brook, NY, USA

Roderick B. Jordan Department of Surgery, Division of Plastic Surgery, MetroHealth Medical Center, Cleveland, OH, USA

Bram Kaufman Department of Surgery, Division of Plastic Surgery, MetroHealth Medical Center, Cleveland, OH, USA

Matthew E. Koepplinger Department of Orthpaedic Surgery, University of Texas Health Science Center, Houston, TX, USA

Thomas P. Lehman Department of Orthopedic Surgery and Rehabilitation, University of Oklahoma, Oklahoma City, OK, USA

Kevin J. Malone Department of Orthopaedic Surgery, MetroHealth Medical Center, Case Western Reserve University School of Medicine, Cleveland, OH, USA

David T. Netscher Division of Plastic Surgery and Department of Orthopedic Surgery, Baylor College of Medicine, Cornell University, Houston, TX, USA

Weill Medical College, Cornell University, Houston, TX, USA

Fernando Simon Polo C. M. Kleinert Institute for Hand and Microsurgery, Louisville, KY, USA

Margaret A. Porembski Clinical Faculty, Oklahoma Hand Surgery Fellowship Program, OK, USA

Ghazi M. Rayan Clinical Professor Orthopedic Surgery, University of Oklahoma, OK, USA

Adjunct Professor of Anatomy / Cell Biology, University of Oklahoma, OK, USA

Director of Oklahoma Hand Surgery Fellowship Program, OK, USA

Chairman, Department of Hand Surgery, INTEGRIS Baptist Medical Center, OK, USA

Leo M. Rozmaryn Division of Uniformed Services, University Health Sciences Center, Washington, D.C, Rockville, MD, USA

M. Colin Rymer Southern Illinois University School of Medicine, Institute for Plastic Surgery, Springfield, IL, USA

Luis R. Scheker C. M. Kleinert Institute for Hand and Microsurgery, Louisville, KY, USA

Ryan W. Schmucker Southern Illinois University School of Medicine, Institute for Plastic Surgery, Springfield, IL, USA

Jaimie T. Shores Department of Plastic and Reconstructive Surgery, The Johns Hopkins University School of Medicine, Baltimore, MD, USA

Nicole Z. Sommer Southern Illinois University School of Medicine, Institute for Plastic Surgery, Springfield, IL, USA

J. B. Stephenson Hand and Microsurgery, Department of Orthopedic Surgery, Baylor College of Medicine, Houston, TX, USA

The Craniofacial & Plastic Surgery Center of Houston, Houston, TX, USA

Robert J. Strauch Department of Orthopaedic Surgery, Columbia University Medical Center, New York, NY, USA

David H. Wei Department of Orthopaedic Surgery, Columbia University Medical Center, New York, NY, USA

Anatomy and Physiology of the Fingertip

Jaimie T. Shores

Introduction

The human fingertip is a specialized structure that allows for complex digit functions that are usually not fully appreciated until the function of one or more components has been lost. An in-depth anatomical and functional knowledge of the fingertip is necessary to understand each of the components individually and how they relate as a whole.

The fingertip is composed of skeletal elements (distal phalanx, tendons, and ligamentous structures), the nail complex or *perionychium* (germinal and sterile matrices, nail plate, sheaths, and skin folds), fibrous connective tissue network with the subcutaneous tissues, vascular network, nerves with end organs, and the nonperionychial skin.

The Skeleton

The distal phalanx has a head or "tuft," a diaphysis or shaft, and a base with articular surface (Fig. 1.1). The dorsal cortex of the distal diaphysis and the tuft supports the nail plate and the underlying nail matrix. The tuft, or head, of the distal phalanx is an enlarged termination of the phalanx with a "U-shaped" tuberosity called the ungual

J. T. Shores (✉)
Department of Plastic and Reconstructive Surgery,
The Johns Hopkins University School of Medicine, 4940
Eastern Ave, Suite A512, Baltimore, MD 21224, USA
e-mail: jshores3@jhmi.edu

process. The roughened surface allows dense connective tissue attachments to anchor the skin and subcutis firmly to allow secure object manipulation. The nail bed also firmly adheres to this distal expansion of the phalanx. In addition, the nail matrix is firmly adhered to the more proximal aspect of the distal phalanx via expansive fibers from the radial and ulnar collateral ligaments that serve to anchor the matrix to the base of the distal phalanx. The terminal tendon (of the index, middle, ring, and small fingers) and extensor pollicis longus tendon (of the thumb) have terminal insertions into the dorsal base of the distal phalanx over a somewhat narrow ridge just proximal to the physis (The insertion just proximal to the physis allows for the "Seymour fracture" to occur in skeletally immature fingertips.). Injuries to these tendons, the tendonous connections, or to the dorsal base of the distal phalanx may result in "mallet deformities." On the volar aspect, the flexor digitorum longus tendon of the fingers and the flexor pollicis longus tendon of the thumb insert more broadly over the volar cortex with a larger footprint of tendon attachment. Likewise, injuries to the tendon, the tendon insertion, or fractures through this portion of the volar base of the distal phalanx can cause loss of flexion of distal interphalangeal (DIP) joint of the digit. The DIP joint itself is a "ginglymus" or hinged synovial joint stabilized by insertions of the proper and accessory collateral ligaments of the DIP joint on the tubercles of the distal phalangeal base as well as a volar plate of connective tissue that spans the joint. The phalanx tapers at the mid-

L. M. Rozmaryn (ed.), *Fingertip Injuries,* DOI 10.1007/978-3-319-13227-3_1,
© Springer International Publishing Switzerland 2015

Fig. 1.1 Skeletal anatomy of the fingertip and distal interphalangeal joint. The distal phalanx has the rough and enlarged *ungual process* (*UP*) that the radial and ulnar *lateral interosseous ligaments* (*LIL*) insert on distally and originate from proximally lateral collateral ligaments and lateral expansions of the extensor and flexor tendons. The LILs support the nail bed and help protect the neurovascular structures in the fingertip

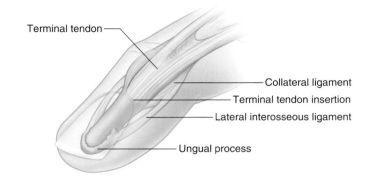

Terminal tendon

Collateral ligament

Terminal tendon insertion

Lateral interosseous ligament

Ungual process

diaphysis where the lateral interosseus ligaments span from the base to the more hypertrophied and roughened tuft and create a passageway for neurovascular structures on both the radial and ulnar aspects of the fingertip. The shape of the base itself helps confer close approximation and single vector motion by mirroring the bicondylar shape of the middle phalanx head with a central groove between the two concave articular recesses of the distal phalangeal base. These structures allow motion in the volar/dorsal plane while stabilizing the radial/ulnar and rotatory vectors [1].

The Perionychium

The perionychium, or nail complex, is a highly specialized structure that is critical to normal digit function. The nail complex allows for improved manipulation of small or fine objects, helps regulate perfusion, contributes to tactile sensation, protects the fingertip, and is possibly the most important structure of the fingertip in regards to aesthetics.

The anatomy of the perionychium includes the nail bed (sterile and germinal matrices), the paronychium, the eponychium, the nail fold, and the hyponychium. The nail plate itself is a hard, kertinaceous three-layered structure formed by contributions from multiple components [2, 3]. The perionychial components may be considered generative or formative of the nail plate, or supportive of the nail plate as structures that frame, sheath, and otherwise support the nail (Fig. 1.2).

The generative components are the nail bed epithelial structures frequently referred to as sterile and germinal matrices, though this may be an oversimplification. In reality, a dorsal, intermediate, and ventral nail matrix can be described, though this classification is debated [3–8]. What is frequently called the "germinal" or "germinative" matrix is designated the combined intermediate and dorsal matrix. The intermediate matrix consists of the matrix at the proximal aspect of the nail plate which is adherent to the deep surface of the nail plate and extends distally to the lunula. This is the primary zone of keratinization and nail plate formation. The lunula, or the distal extent of this zone, is the demarcation between the more pale-blue-gray germinal matrix and the more pink ventral matrix, frequently referred to as the sterile matrix. The germinal matrix color is thought to be distinctly different due to the light scattered by the larger nuclei of the highly synthetic cells of the intermediate/germinal matrix as it produces the majority of the nail plate and its keratin. In reality, the entire matrix is of this color, though only the distal portion is visible from beneath the eponychial fold. The intermediate matrix is thought to produce the majority of the nail plate with up to 20 % of the remaining nail plate coming from the ventral matrix, though this is controversial [3–5, 7]. The proximal aspect of the intermediate matrix transitions to the dorsal matrix, which is the deepest and most proximal portion of the proximal nail fold. This produces the most superficial layer of the nail plate and is also considered a component of the germinal matrix. The most proximal extent of the combined germinal matrix is typically less than

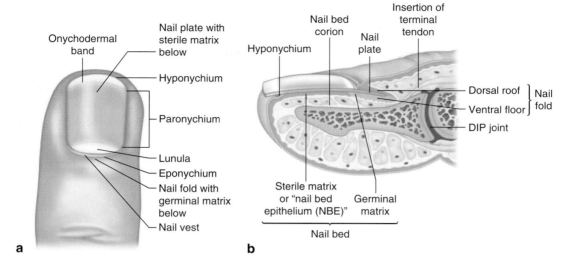

Fig. 1.2 Perionychial anatomy of the fingertip

1 mm away from the terminal fibers of the terminal tendon of the distal phalanx. At the lunula, the distal or ventral matrix begins, which has also been referred to as the "sterile" matrix, though arguments against this terminology can be made, and instead, it will be referred to as the nail bed epithelium (NBE). It is argued that this layer may contribute to approximately 20 % of the nail plate as the nail plate becomes thicker as it grows out distally over the ventral matrix/NBE. The NBE does appear to transition from a more matrix-like zone proximally to a more nonproliferative epithelial-like zone distally. The germinal matrix is thicker and has a rete pattern of attachment to the nail plate, whereas the NBE has a ridge pattern of attachment distally and is thinner. The NBE produces a thin keratinizing layer that moves distally along with the nail plate as it continuously grows to provide adherence and continued distal growth. This tight adherence contributes to the more full-thickness avulsion of NBE with nail plate avulsion than the germinal matrix, which is more typically spared a full-thickness avulsion. The ventral matrix or NBE terminates at the onychodermal band.

Histologically, the germinal matrix is distinct from NBE. Both lack a granular layer to the epithelium, but the germinal matrix is thicker and interdigitates with the nail bed fibrocollagen. Mamelons (basaloid buds) are more prominent proximally and centrally than laterally and are oriented toward the tip of the digit. The NBE is not a self-replicating structure. It is created by the matrix and moves distally with the nail plate as previously stated [7], and 81 % of the cells within the nail plate appear to be provided by the proximal 50 % of the nail matrix [2].

What is frequently referred to as the eponychial fold is more precisely called the "dorsal nail fold" or the "posterior nail fold" (PNF) which blends with the radial and ulnar (both called "lateral") nail folds. The dorsal nail fold forms a pocket called the proximal nail fold for the germinal matrix and the nail plate root. The external skin or dorsal skin of the PNF is formed by a continuation of the dorsal digit skin that is thin and lacks hair and sebaceous adnexae. The ventral component of the fold has a much thinner and flattened epithelium. This ventral component forms the roof and the matrix forms the floor of this pocket beneath the fold. These two separate epithelial layers are separated by the forming nail plate itself and are frequently stented apart from one another after PNF and/or germinal matrix injuries to prevent formation of synechiae. The proximal 75 % of the ventral epithelium of the PNF is the eponychium, which performs onycholemmal keratinization to produce a thin layer of keratin on the superficial or dorsal surface of the forming nail plate. This forms the "true cuticle" of the nail which is deep to and extends distally on the growing nail plate past the "false cuticle." The false cuticle is a softer keratin-composed structure formed mostly by the dorsal and less by the ventral surfaces of the PNF. It is not adherent to the nail plate. However, the true cuticle is adherent to the nail plate and protects the PNF pocket by sealing it off from the outside environment. If the dorsal matrix or the transition zone between the dorsal matrix and the eponychium is damaged, the nail will lose its polished appearance and appear dull and rough.

As the eponychium may be considered a transition zone from true skin to the germinal matrix component of the dorsal matrix of the nail fold, the hyponychium is a transition zone from the distal NBE to the skin of the fingertip. They both form nail/skin confluences that completely surround the nail proximally (eponychium) and laterally/distally (hyponychium) to protect the generative components of the nail. The proximal hyponychium begins where the NBE terminates and blends into epithelium of the fingertip skin. The proximal hyponychium produces the sole-horn, which functions to allow separation of the ventral or deep surface of the nail plate while still sealing the NBE. The proximal hyponychial attachment to the nail plate is visible through the nail plate as the onychodermal band, which corresponds to the most proximal point of attachment of the fingertip skin stratum corneum to the nail plate. The distal hyponychium is a narrow rim of transitional post-separation skin. The skin of the distal groove is included in this zone and the skin of this zone lacks the ridges that comprise fingerprints. This region has a deep band of connective tissue called the anterior ligament which anchors the hyponychial dermis to the periosteum of the ungual process of the rim of the distal phalanx tuft.

The nail plate is supported by the NBE and intermediate matrix, but these structures are also supported by fibrocollagenous structures termed the nail unit support system (NUSS) which lay between the matrix structures and the dorsal cortex of the distal phalanx. Though the nail bed structures are epithelial structures, there is no true dermis below them and instead the NUSS forms their supportive platform. It

directly attaches the epithelium to the deeper phalanx with ligamentous attachments made up of fascial and periosteal tissues. The tissue deep to the epithelium that attaches the matrix to the phalanx that is in the position of what would normally be dermis is termed "corium" and is made up of dense fibers created largely by modified periosteum of the dorsal distal phalanx ungual process. Proximally, the NUSS has longitudinally oriented fibers that form a fibrous sheath around the nail matrix and forms nail root ligaments. The nail root also maintains attachment to the phalanx by more oblique fibers that fuse with the fibers from the dorsal expansions of the radial and ulnar collateral ligaments and the radial and ulnar lateral interosseus ligaments (LILs) over the lateral tuberosities of the base of the distal phalanx. The proximal NUSS is somewhat loose and more delicate. In the intermediate zone beneath the NBE, large bands of collagen are arranged vertically that connect the periosteum to the NBE longitudinally. The "nail bed corium" (NBC) describes this region. The NBC has an abundance of blood vessels and glomus bodies in its longitudinally oriented framework, with its capillary bed ending at the onychodermal band. Distally, the NUSS has looser and more obliquely oriented fibers that angle distally toward the hyponychium. The anterior ligament is a crescentic band of fibers that also extends from the rim of the ungual surface to help stabilize the distal NBE and hyponychium.

The Nail Plate

The nail plate itself is a hard, durable, translucent keratinous protective shell for the dorsal fingertip that provides counterpressure to the pulp, increases the sensory abilities of the digit, increases the ability of the digits to manipulate the environment, protects the nail bed, and splints the phalangeal tuft. It has three histologic layers [2, 3]. The most dorsal or superficial layer is thin and provides its sheen and polished appearance. The middle layer is thick and the ventral or deep layer is irregular with longitudinal striations. The majority of the nail is manufactured by the germinal matrix (dorsal and intermediate matrices) with a smaller contribution by the ventral zone or NBE distal to the lunula contributing up to 20 % of its substance by some estimates. This also helps explain how the moving nail plate continues to stay attached to the nail bed. However, others believe the NBE contributes only onycholemmal substances which serve to seal the nail plate and nail bed adhesion from the outside environment without actually contributing to the nail plate itself. The nail plate of the digits of the hand is typically about 0.5 mm in thickness and is thinner and softer at its most proximal aspect, or root, within the PNF. The nail plate grows at approximately 0.1 mm per day in healthy young adults and can be affected by multiple problems and processes such as ischemia, malnutrition, smoking, cold, and cytostatic medications.

Fibrous and Ligamentous Network

The extraordinary fibrous structure provides the distal digit its significant anatomical support. The vast fibrous structure and network enables for balanced motion and stability of the distal interphalangeal (DIP) joint connection of the nail system, protection from injury, and the ability to grasp. The DIP joint is composed of both ligaments and tendons, while robust ligamentous and fascial reinforcement fastens the nail bed and skin to the concealed bone. Together, all of these different complex units of anatomy and the network they compose interrelate and contribute to the support of the joint and the unified distal digit.

LILs ("paraterminal ligaments") spread from the lateral tuberosities at the origin of the distal phalanx base to the spines of the ungual system. This ligamentous network provides reinforcement for the posterolateral nail bed fibroconnective tissue, lateral fortitude to the digit, and a guarded neurovascular network. The ligamentous network is composed of fibers which are connected with the collateral ligament and attaches to the flexor and extensor tendons.

Dense collateral ligaments spread from divots on the lateral aspect of the condyles of the middle phalangeal head to the posterior aspect of the lateral tuberosities of the distal phalanx. Acces-

sory collateral ligaments run bilaterally from the middle phalangeal head to the sides of the volar plate. These collateral ligaments send dorsal expansions that combine into the proximal nail bed connective tissue. They provide as a safeguard to the proximal matrix. Serving as an anchor, a "bone-nail" ligament develops and attaches the nail root to the lateral tuberosities.

The fibrous and connective tissues and subcutaneous fatty tissues of the tip and pad of the digit are arranged into two separate spaces referred to as the tip (distally) and the pad (proximally). The tip is organized by radially extending fascial bands from the ungual tuberosity out to the tip dermis that separate the fibrous subcutaneous fat into conical or wedge-shaped compartments. This arrangement makes the fatty and bulky padding of the fingertip very stable to pressure and shear to allow for stable manipulation of the environment by the fingertip while simultaneously allowing for dissipation of pressure or force.

The pad of the fingertip is less well organized than the tip and thus more mobile and less compact. Here, the fat lobules are more spherical in shape without the same pattern of radiating fibrous tissue as the tip. The pad contains numerous arteries, nerves, and Pacinian corpuscles. It is thought that the somewhat concave shape of the palmar surface of the distal phalanx and the ability of the pad fat to mold around objects enables this portion of the digit to be used better for gripping. In comparison to the dorsal nail complex skin, the skin of the tip and pad (collectively the "pulp") has prominent and deep eccrine glands adjacent to the fat lobules. The sweat secreted by these glands is thought to aid in grip, sensation, and manipulation of the environment.

The tip and pad have thick, glabrous skin which lacks hair follicles but has prominent eccrine glands, Meissner's corpuscles, and an adherent and complex pattern of rete ridges and papillae in its dermis. The stratum corneum is thick and the stratum lucidum is well developed. The primary epidermal ridges, or fingerprints, reflect the organizational pattern of the underlying rete ridges and papillae.

Vascular Supply

The perfusion of the fingertip is orderly and predictable with compartmentalization both by central/lateral and volar/dorsal organizations [9–11]. The arterial supply to the digit is provided through the radial and ulnar proper digital arteries volar to the mid-lateral axis of the digit. The arteries have dorsal branches at the level of each joint that perfuses the dorsal digital skin. As the proper digital arteries approach the DIP joint, a set of dorsal branches are given off at the level of the head of the middle phalanx, just proximal to the DIP joint, and then a second set of dorsal branches are given off just distal to the DIP joint at the level of the distal phalangeal base (Fig. 1.3). Both sets of these dorsal branches contribute to the superficial arcade at the base of the distal phalanx, also referred to as the "dorsal nail fold arch" or the "proximal matrix arch." The superficial arcade perfuses the dorsal skin of the fingertip and the nail complex. The redundancy of radial and ulnar contributions both proximal and distal to the DIP joint allows for preserved nail complex perfusion in the face of significant injury. The superficial arcade is located superficial or dorsal to the terminal tendon insertion just proximal to the germinal matrix and nail complex. Longitudinal branches then form from the superficial arcade that run within the NUSS deep to the germinal matrix and nail root to form the proximal subungual arcade, which spans the width of the diaphysis of the distal phalanx and sends radial and ulnar penetrating branches in between the phalanx and the LIL on both the radial and ulnar sides of the digit. The proximal subungual arcade also sends longitudinal branches within the NUSS even further distally which then unite as the next transverse arcade called the distal subungual arcade. This arcade also remains just deep to the NBE but dorsal to the distal phalanx and sends deep penetrating branches radially and ulnarly around the sides of the phalanx and medially to the LILs but also sends distal longitudinal branches that wrap around the tip of the distal phalanx and unite with branches from the volar side to perfuse the tip and pad.

Volarly, the proper digital arteries send medial branches to form the middle transverse arch

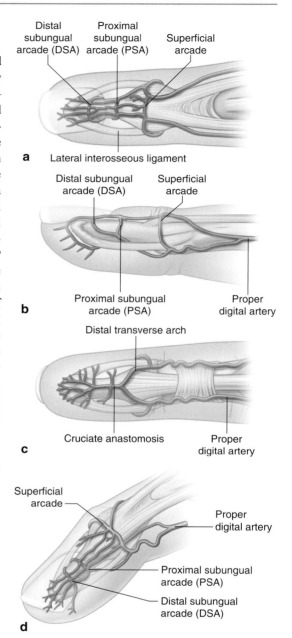

Fig. 1.3 Arterial anatomy of the fingertip. The *proper digital artery* (*PDA*) runs both radially and ulnarly and gives a dorsal branch proximal to the distal interphalangeal joint. This dorsal branch forms the *superficial arcade* (*SA*) over the dorsal base of the distal phalanx. Dorsally, longitudinal vessels run distally to the *proximal subungual arcade* (*PSA*), with more distal branches running from the *PSA* to the *distal subungual arcade* (*DSA*). Terminal distal branches then extend over the ungual process and reach volarly to anastamose with the volar arterial circulation. Volarly, the *PDA* provides dorsal branches radially and ulnarly at the level of the base of

at the level of the middle phalangeal head. This arch may provide the dorsal perforating vessels previously discussed that contribute to the superficial arch at this level. The proper digital arteries then continue across the DIP joint and form the distal transverse arch, or digital pulp arch. This arch forms on the volar aspect of the distal phalanx at the peak level of the volar concavity of the distal phalanx and is distal to the flexor tendon insertion and distal to the dorsal superficial arcade location. The distal transverse arch then forms a single longitudinal anastomosis of both its radial and ulnar components called the cruciate anastomosis. The cruciate anastomosis then forms two vessels that branch radially and ulnarly and run dorsally around the diaphysis of the distal phalanx to connect to and supply the dorsal proximal subungual arcade and the distal subungual arcades previously mentioned. Smaller branches also continue from the cruciate anastomose through the pulp volarly that anastamose with branches from the distal subungual arcade at the fingertip. These continue to form further anastomoses known as perforating arteries and anastomosing arteries to supply the pulp and tip of the digit ending in the subdermal and deep dermal plexi. This rich system of anastomoses ensures the diffusion of blood flow from multiple directions, should an injury locally interrupt one portion of the system. This rich system also explains the significant blood loss one may see from fingertip injuries.

The volar skin contains terminal capillaries which align with the epidermal ridges of the fingerprints [12].

The venous egress of blood follows both deep and superficial digital venous systems that are connected by small perforating veins (Fig. 1.4) [11, 13]. The deep system is smaller and these veins run as vena comitans to the digital arter-

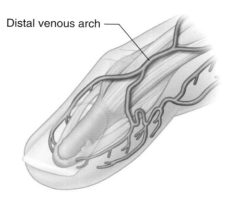

Distal venous arch

Fig. 1.4 Venous anatomy of the fingertip. The deep venous system parallels the arterial circulation while the superficial venous system creates a distal venous arch by ramifying into a single dorsal vein when it proceeds proximally over the DIP joint and then may split into two veins again proximally. The superficial and deep venous structures have volar, lateral, and dorsal contributions that form a rich network of anastomoses for venous drainage of the fingertip

ies. These make up the minority of venous return of the digit. The larger superficial or dorsal venous system is composed of dorsal, lateral, and palmar components in the fingertip that form an anastamotic network. The dorsal veins usually consist of two veins that run adjacent to the nail root that then combine to form a single mid-axial dorsal vein called the distal venous arch. This vein proceeds proximally and then divides back into two dorsal veins at the DIP joint level.

A large amount of arteriovenous anastomoses in the fingertips exists as simple shunts or the less common but more complex glomus body. A glomus body is typically an encapsulated spherical structure with a single afferent artery and efferent vein. Within it is a tortuous Sucquet–Hoyer canal surrounded by glomus cells and is densely innervated [14]. It is believed that the glomus body has thermoregulatory functions and is most numerous within the nail bed and deep dermis and subcutaneous compartment of the distal tip.

The lymphatic drainage of the fingertip roughly mirrors that of the veins. The hyponychium contains the largest density of lymphatics of any skin region of the human body, likely to aid in fighting infection in these regions which most commonly interact with the outside environment.

the proximal phalanx that forms the SA. The *PDA* then continues distally as the *distal transverse arch* (*DTA*) on the volar phalanx. Both *DSA* branches ramify into the single *cruciate anastomosis* (*CA*), which sends dorsal branches to both the *PSA* and the *DSA*. It continues distally on the volar surface as terminal branches which anastomose with the terminal dorsal branches around the ungual process. **a** Dorsal View, **b** Lateral View, **c** Volar View, **d** Oblique View

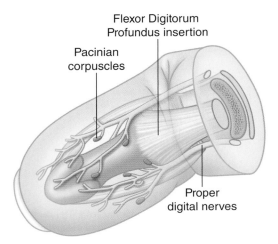

Fig. 1.5 Nervous anatomy of the fingertip. The *proper digital nerves* on the radial and ulnar side each trifurcate and send a branch to the finger pad, the dorsal skin, and the nail bed. In addition, dorsal skin and nail bed contributions may also be present from both a more proximal dorsal branch of the *proper digital nerve* and the distal branches from the superficial radial and dorsal ulnar cutaneous nerves. The nerve branches are able to innervate both dorsal and volar structures by proceeding with the arterial and venous structures medial to the LILs which help create a protected neurovascular passageway between volar and dorsal compartments. *LIL* lateral interosseous ligaments

rect dorsal collateral nerves that help supply the skin dorsally. Thus, nail beds may have sensory contributions from both the proper digital nerves and the terminal dorsal cutaneous branches of the superficial radial nerve and the dorsal ulnar cutaneous nerve.

The nerves in the fingertip have sensory and autonomic components [15–20]. Sensory nerves may end in unmyelinated free nerve endings, such as those in the dermis that sense pain and temperature, or may end in special sensory organs. Meissner's corpuscles are touch-sense organs located in dermal papillae that provide two-point sensation. Pacinian corpuscles are located in the subcutis, are large, and sense deep pressure and vibration. They measure 1–4 mm and are visible during surgery. They are most dense in the fingertip pulp and may be associated with glomus bodies. Merkel's endings are touch receptors located near basal cells of rete ridges. Typical fine touch depends on both intact skin and nerves. Two-point discrimination, usually 2–4 mm, can be broadened by dense, hyperkeratotic skin or by nerves that are damaged or displaced in a flap from another location.

Innervation

Proper digital nerves run adjacent to the proper digital arteries into the digits with a slightly more dorsal location than the arteries within the digits, though in the palm, they are more volarly positioned. At the level of the DIP joint, each of the radial and ulnar digital nerves trifurcates, with each digital nerve sending a branch to the dorsal nail bed, the fingertip, and the finger pad or pulp (Fig. 1.5) [15]. Smaller volar and dorsal collateral nerves have been described. The volar collateral nerves are thought to send oblique dorsal branches to supply the skin of the index, middle, and ring dorsal fingertip from the DIP joint to the distal nail fold and these may branch directly from the proper digital nerve as proximally as the A1 pulley of the flexor sheath [16]. The thumb and small finger may have more di-

Summary

The fingertip is a complex anatomical structure that directly interacts with the physical environment, perhaps more substantially than any other external body part, and as such, is highly specialized for this process. Rigid bony stability; specialized and dense innervation; rich perfusion with thermoregulatory functions; the complex and well-developed nail complex; and the thickened volar tip and pad skin, subcutis, and retaining ligaments all create one of our most useful tools for manipulating the world around us. Any single component that is dysfunctional can result in significant functional and/or aesthetic loss. Thus, understanding each of its components individually and as a sum of its parts is important for the hand surgeon treating fingertip conditions.

References

1. Gigis PI, Kuczynski K. The distal interphalangeal joints of human fingers. J Hand Surg Am. 1982;7(2):176–82. (Epub 1982/03/01).
2. de Berker D. Nail anatomy. Clin Dermatol. 2013;31(5):509–15. (Epub 2013/10/02).
3. Johnson M, Comaish JS, Shuster S. Nail is produced by the normal nail bed: a controversy resolved. Br J Dermatol. 1991;125(1):27–9. (Epub 1991/07/01).
4. De Berker D, Mawhinney B, Sviland L. Quantification of regional matrix nail production. Br J Dermatol. 1996;134(6):1083–6. (Epub 1996/06/01).
5. Johnson M, Shuster S. Continuous formation of nail along the bed. Br J Dermatol. 1993;128(3):277–80. (Epub 1993/03/01).
6. Lewin K. The normal finger nail. Br J Dermatol. 1965;77(8):421–30. (Epub 1965/08/01).
7. Lewis BL. Microscopic studies of fetal and mature nail and surrounding soft tissue. AMA Arch Derm Syphilol. 1954;70(6):733–47. (Epub 1954/12/01).
8. Zook EG. Anatomy and physiology of the perionychium. Clin Anat. 2003;16(1):1–8. (Epub 2002/12/18).
9. Smith DO, Oura C, Kimura C, Toshimori K. Artery anatomy and tortuosity in the distal finger. J Hand Surg Am. 1991;16(2):297–302. (Epub 1991/03/01).
10. Strauch B, de Moura W. Arterial system of the fingers. J Hand Surg Am. 1990;15(1):148–54. (Epub 1990/01/01).
11. Chaudakshetrin P, Kumar VP, Satku K, Pho RW. The arteriovenous pattern of the distal digital segment. J Hand Surg Br. 1988;13(2):164–6. (Epub 1988/05/01).
12. Inoue H. Three-dimensional observations of microvasculature of human finger skin. Hand. 1978;10(2):144–9. (Epub 1978/06/01).
13. Smith DO, Oura C, Kimura C, Toshimori K. The distal venous anatomy of the finger. J Hand Surg Am. 1991;16(2):303–7. (Epub 1991/03/01).
14. Gorgas K, Bock P, Tischendorf F, Curri SB. The fine structure of human digital arterio-venous anastomoses (Hoyer-Grosser's organs). Anat Embryol. 1977;150(3):269–89. (Epub 1977/05/12).
15. Wilgis EF, Maxwell GP. Distal digital nerve grafts: clinical and anatomical studies. J Hand Surg Am. 1979;4(5):439–43. (Epub 1979/09/01).
16. Bas H, Kleinert JM. Anatomic variations in sensory innervation of the hand and digits. J Hand Surg Am. 1999;24(6):1171–84. (Epub 1999/12/10).
17. Provitera V, Nolano M, Pagano A, Caporaso G, Stancanelli A, Santoro L. Myelinated nerve endings in human skin. Muscle Nerve. 2007;35(6):767–75. (Epub 2007/04/04).
18. Vallbo AB, Johansson RS. Properties of cutaneous mechanoreceptors in the human hand related to touch sensation. Hum Neurobiol. 1984;3(1):3–14. (Epub 1984/01/01).
19. Montagna W. Morphology of cutaneous sensory receptors. J Invest Dermatol. 1977;69(1):4–7. (Epub 1977/07/01).
20 Barron JN. The structure and function of the skin of the hand. Hand. 1970;2(2):93–6. (Epub 1970/09/01).

Closed Injuries: Bone, Ligament, and Tendon

Leo M. Rozmaryn

Mallet Deformity

Introduction

Mallet fingers are clearly far more complex to care for correctly than they appear. Patients often present to the clinic with a mallet finger, wondering why they suddenly cannot extend the tip of their finger after what appeared to be a trivial injury such as pulling up socks or tucking in a bed sheet ([1]; Fig. 2.1). Other patients describe a high-velocity sports or work impact on the finger, usually an axial load onto the fingertip or the dorsum of the fingertip [2]. Although mallet fingers may appear to be somewhat inconsequential, up to 25 % of patients miss 6 weeks of work, sports, and even activities of daily living [3].

An eccentric axial load to the tip of the finger causing the distal interphalangeal (DIP) joint to forcefully hyperflex or hyperextend can disrupt the continuity of the insertion of the conjoined lateral bands onto the dorsal aspect of the distal phalanx. This avulsion may take the form of tendon avulsion off the dorsal lip of the proximal end of the distal phalanx or an intra-articular fracture of the dorsal lip may occur with the bony fragment still attached to the terminal extensor (Fig. 2.2). The dorsal fragment's size and degree of articu-

lar involvement may vary from a fleck of bone to 70–80 % of the joint surface. Any joint involvement greater than 50 % is generally associated with volar subluxation of the DIP joint (Fig. 2.3).

With the flexor digitorum profundus (FDP) tendon unopposed, the tip of the finger will assume a flexed posture. Initially thought of as a "jammed finger" of minor importance, it is frequently ignored. The characteristically flexed posture of the distal phalanx is usually detected immediately but sometimes may only manifest after several weeks once the swelling has subsided. Patients that seek medical attention within 2–3 weeks of injury can usually be treated nonoperatively. Others may wait up to 3 or 4 months after the full extent of the disability become manifest such as DIP joint pain, erythema, skin breakdown, DIP flexion contracture, swan-neck deformity, and difficulty in navigating tight spaces such as a back pocket. While it is possible to commence nonoperative treatment, these may fail to correct the deformity and thought must be given to surgical correction [4].

Alternatively, there are patients who have undergone conservative treatment for 3–4 months only to find that the flexion deformity has persisted or recurred. In those patients, there have been weak or incomplete reattachment of the tendon end back to bone and the connection may be nothing more than a thin, transparent scar bridge with the tendon having retracted more than 3 mm ([5]; Fig. 2.4). This proximal retraction of the extensor hood causes increased tension on the central slip

L. M. Rozmaryn (✉)
Division of Uniformed Services, University Health Sciences Center, Washington, D.C, 9420 Key West Ave. Suite 300, Rockville, MD 20850, USA
e-mail: lrozmaryn@gmail.com

L. M. Rozmaryn (ed.), *Fingertip Injuries,* DOI 10.1007/978-3-319-13227-3_2,
© Springer International Publishing Switzerland 2015

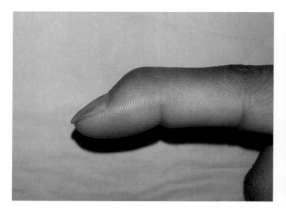

Fig. 2.1 Flexion deformity of the distal interphalangeal (DIP) joint: the mallet finger

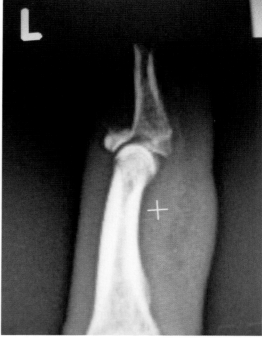

Fig. 2.3 Displaced mallet fracture involving 60 % of the articular surface. Note the volar subluxation of the distal phalanx

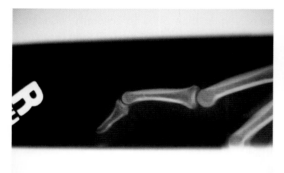

Fig. 2.2 Lateral X-ray of tendinous avulsion of the terminal extensor on the distal phalanx. Note the hyperextension of the proximal interphalangeal joint (PIP)

attachment on the middle phalanx causing proximal interphalangeal joint (PIP) hyperextension resulting in a secondary swan-neck deformity.

Epidemiology

It has been reported that the incidence of mallet finger injuries is 9.89/100,000. The peak age for the injury is young to middle-age men and older women with males outnumbering females by 3/1 [6]. Wehbe and Schneider in 1984 reported that 74 % of these injuries occurred in dominant hands and 90 % of these injuries occurred in

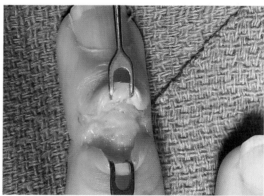

Fig. 2.4 Terminal extensor tendon. Note the loose scar bridge that connects the end of the tendon to the distal phalanx. Insufficient tension across the bridge will lead to a chronic mallet

the ulnar three digits [7]. Simpson et al. (2001), showed that mallet deformities accounted for 2 % of all sporting injuries mainly rugby, football, and basketball [8].

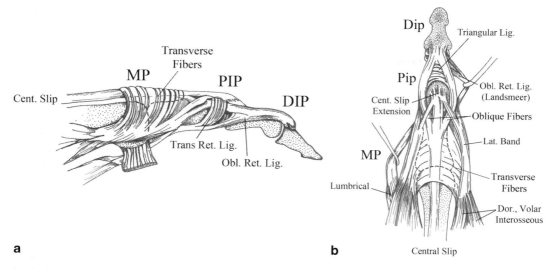

Fig. 2.5 **a** Lateral view of the extensor mechanism. Note the relationship between the central slip and the oblique retinacular ligament (ORL; With permission from Jessica Rose Waterman). **b** Coronal view of the extensor mecha-nism; note the relationship between the central slip, lateral bands, and terminal extensor (With permission from Jessica Rose Waterman)

Mechanism of Deformity

The terminal extensor tendon is a flat and thin structure measuring on the average 1.1 mm and inserts on the distal phalanx up to 1.2 mm distal to the joint margin and 1.4 mm proximal to the germinal nail matrix. The terminal extensor tendon is adherent to the underlying dorsal aspect of the DIP joint capsule. The terminal tendon is formed by the confluence of the radial and ulnar lateral bands. Just proximal to this confluence lies a thin membrane that runs transversely between the lateral bands called the triangular ligament. These prevent volar subluxation of the lateral bands. Injury to this ligament can result in the formation of a boutonniere deformity. The oblique retinacular ligaments (ORLs; Landsmeer) are thin fibers that run deep and volar to the lateral bands and they coordinate PIP and DIP flexion and extension. They originate from the lateral flexor sheath and form the outer margin of the terminal extensor tendon at the DIP joint.

The lateral bands are continuations of the interosseous and lumbrical tendons that run along the sides of the digit at the proximal phalanx. Dorsal subluxation of the lateral bands such as what is seen in swan-neck deformities is prevented by transverse retinacular ligaments that run from flexor tendon sheath dorsally to the volar rim of the lateral bands.

The central slip tendon is a continuation of the extensor digitorum communis to the finger and runs up the middle of the proximal phalanx. It connects to the lateral bands via the sagittal band fibers that run transversely and through oblique fibers that connect to the lateral bands distal to the PIP joint [5, 9] (Figs. 2.5a, b).

Schweitzer and Rayan found that the excursion of the terminal extensor tendon at the DIP joint was 1–2 mm when the joint was moved passively from full extension to full flexion [10]. They also found that PIP joint angle of flexion had significant influence on the degree of possible DIP joint flexion. If the PIP was flexed 90°, the maximal DIP flexion was 82°, whereas if the PIP was extended, the maximal DIP flexion possible was 51°. If the terminal tendon is sectioned via "Z" lengthening, it was found that 1 mm of lengthening allowed 25° of flexion. Two millimeters of lengthening allowed 36°. Three millimeters of lengthening allowed 49° and four millimeters of lengthening allowed 63° of flexion. They also found variation between each of the palmar digits with the middle finger flexing the most for each millimeter of terminal tendon lengthening. They showed that if the cut tendon end retracted more than 1 mm proximally, it was extremely difficult to approximate the tendon end to its insertion. These data illustrate what occurs when the terminal extensor tears and retracts allowing the DIP to develop an extensor lag which persists even after the gap between tendon end and bony insertion is bridged by a scar and forms the basis of the conservative treatment of these injuries.

Table 2.2 Doyle's classification of mallet finger injuries [11]

Type 1	Closed or blunt trauma with loss of tendon continuity with or without a small avulsion fracture
Type 2	Laceration at or proximal to the distal interphalangeal joint with loss of tendon continuity
Type 3	Deep abrasion with loss of skin, subcutaneous cover and tendon substance
Type 4A	Transphyseal fracture on children
Type 4B	Hyperflexion injury with fracture of the articular surface of 20–50 %
Type 4C	Hyperextension injury with fracture of the articular surface greater than 50 % with early or late volar subluxation of the distal phalanx

Classification and Diagnosis

If neglected, permanent fingertip disfigurement can result from mallet fingers, as well as dorsal DIP pain and inflammation, restricted DIP flexion, and swan-neck deformity. Prompt treatment of the injury can alleviate the risk of a scar bridge laxity of 1 mm between the terminal extensor tendon and the distal phalanx, which in turn leads to a 25° extensor lag.

To date, there have been no classification systems that refer to mallet deformities that involve tendon avulsions only. The existing ones either describe mallet "fractures" or mixed bony and tendinous injuries together ([7, 11]; see Tables 2.1 and 2.2).

Clinical Evaluation

After obtaining a history of a crush, axial load, or even a trivial fingertip "stub" on a bed sheet or a carpet surface, one observes the resting posture of the DIP and PIP joints. The extensor lag and whether it is passively correctable should be noted

Table 2.1 Webhe and Schneider's classification system of mallet fractures based on injury severity [7]

Type 1	No DIP joint subluxation
Type 2	DIP joint subluxation
Type 3	Epiphyseal and physeal injuries
Subtype 1	Less than 1/3 of the articular surface
Subtype 2	1/3–2/3 of the joint surface
Subtype 3	>2/3 of the joint surface

DIP distal interphalangeal joint

as well as any hyperextension of the PIP joint. The dorsal skin integrity should be checked for lacerations, abrasions, erythema, and tenderness (Figs. 2.6a, b). Though the injury occurs at impact, the deformity may not manifest for several days [12]. This may be due to the fact that the initial injury to the tendon may have been incomplete but with repeated stress the remaining insertion may attenuate or avulse from the distal phalanx.

X-ray assessment should include AP, lateral, and oblique views and the DIP should be evaluated for fracture, displacement of fragments, volar subluxation of the distal phalanx, and DIP joint congruity.

Nonoperative Treatment of Mallet Deformity

The goal of all closed treatment of mallet deformity whether purely tendinous or with a bony avulsion is the apposition and reattachment of the terminal extensor to the distal phalanx allowing full extension and correction of the flexion deformity. In pure tendon avulsions, this needs to be accomplished without the development of DIP flexion contracture, extensor lag from gapping between the tendon end and its insertion, and adhesions between the tendon end and the dorsal capsule of the DIP joint preventing active or passive DIP flexion. One must achieve a delicate balance between sufficient immobilization in extension and allowing careful active flexion

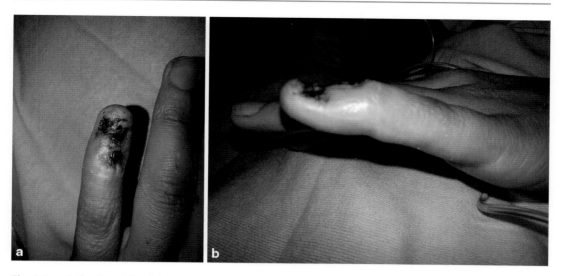

Fig. 2.6 a, b Crush avulsion injury to the tip of the fifth finger involving the terminal extensor. Note the loss of the dorsal skin and nail apparatus

to achieve gliding between the extensor tendon and joint capsule. If the immobilization period is too short, tendon rupture will occur [13].

There is some controversy whether only the DIP joint should be immobilized in extension or should DIP and PIP joints be splinted, the latter in flexion thus relaxing the terminal extensor hood and ORL [14]. Katzman in 1999 in a cadaveric study repeatedly flexed and extended the PIP and found no increased tension on a created gap at the DIP insertion. Thus, the only DIP extension needed was to preserve apposition of the extensor tendon to its insertion [15]. Others feel that it is necessary to keep the PIP flexed to allow the distal extensor mechanism to be "pulled" distally and thus relax the insertion site [16]. DIP extension alone is the more commonly used conservative approach. Typically, full-time splinting for 6 weeks followed by 2–6 weeks of part-time splinting usually at night or for strenuous activities has been accepted as the standard protocol for nonoperative treatment of mallet fingers [8].

Review of the Literature

Mason reported the first treatment of mallet finger in 1930. He advocated for quick surgical intervention of closed mallet fingers [17].

Similarly, Smillie designed a plaster splint to hold the DIP in hyperextension with the PIP joint in flexion [18]. Hallberg et al. in 1960 reported on 127 patients with mallet finger treated in a plaster cast and noted that half the patients had a poor result with a residual deformity of >20° [19]. In 1962, the Stack splint (Fig. 2.7e) was devised, which made conservative treatment of mallet fingers more popular [20]. In 1975, Pulvertaft in an address to the British hand society said that: "60% of mallet fingers had satisfactory results after splinting and that a further 20% would improve sufficiently in the course of time" [21]. Seven years later, Auchincloss compared external splinting to surgical care for acute closed mallet fingers in 41 patients [22]. He found no difference in outcome and further opined that there was no need to splint at all after a period of 6 weeks.

Today, the overall opinion in the field is that that initial treatment of closed mallet fingers should be nonoperative, in a full-time splint that keeps the DIP joint in mild hyperextension (<10°) for 6–8 weeks, followed by a 4-week period of part-time nocturnal splinting (Fig. 2.7). Evans et al. wrote that at the end of 6 weeks during the first week of immobilization, no more than 20–25° of flexion should be allowed [16]. A flexion-blocking splint would be helpful at this

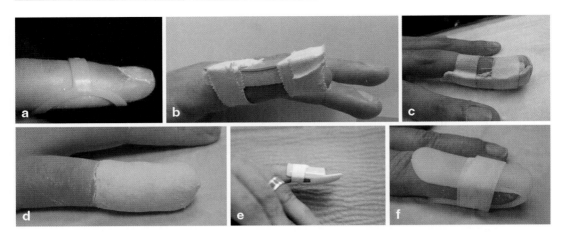

Fig. 2.7 Commonly used external splints used for the closed treatment of mallet fingers **a, b** *Top*: Oval-8 splint, dorsal AlumaFoam splint **c, d** *Middle*: Volar "cradle" splint, plaster cast **e, f** *Bottom*: Stack splint, custom coaptation splint

point. If no extensor lag develops, 35° of flexion can be permitted the following week. Patients can be allowed to flex the DIP 10–20 times, several times daily, until full flexion is allowed. If an extensor lag develops, splint again in full extension for 2 weeks then begin the process again.

Patients need to be told that conservative treatment may leave them with a residual flexion deformity of 5–10°, a mild loss of DIP flexion and the presence of a dorsal "bump" (Fig. 2.8). A second 6-week round of splinting can be tried. In the past, some advocated splinting as late as 3 months post presentation [23].

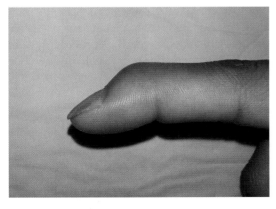

Fig. 2.8 Dorsal "lump" of the distal interphalangeal (DIP) joint from a chronic untreated mallet finger. There is a secondary swan-neck deformity of the proximal interphalangeal joint (PIP)

However, there is controversy about the best way to splint. Most of the techniques reported used the following **Crawford's criteria** to assess functional outcome of treatment [24]:

Excellent:	Full DIP extension, full flexion, no pain
Good:	0–10° of extension deficit, full flexion, no pain
Fair:	10–25° of extension deficit, any flexion loss, no pain
Poor:	>25° of extension deficit or persistent pain

Abouna and Brown's criteria [12]

Success:	Extensor lag <5°, no stiffness, normal flexion, and extension
Improved:	Extension loss 6–15°, no stiffness, normal flexion
Failure:	Extension loss >15°, DIP stiffness, impaired flexion

In 1997, Okafor et al. documented of 31 patients treated in a thermoplastic "Stack" splint for an average of 7.2 weeks [25]. They were followed for a mean of 5 years with a delay in treatment from 0 to 28 days. Of the 29 patients without fracture, or fractures less than 30 % of the joint surface, the delay in treatment had no significant effect on the outcome with regard to DIP motion or extension deficit. However, at follow-up at 6 months, 35% of the patients had and extensor lag of $>10°$ and had a flexor range of 48°. Also, 35% of those studied were mallet fractures and of those, half had degenerative changes at the DIP joint. In this series, swan-neck deformity developed far more commonly in mallet fractures than pure tendinous injuries. However, in this series, 90% were satisfied with their results and 68% noted no functional impairment in the finger. There was, however, a greater impairment of DIP joint flexion in patients with osteoarthritis (OA) though the presence of OA had no effect on extensor lag.

Garberman's study showed that with similar splinting regimens, there was no difference between early (<2 weeks) and late presentation (>4 weeks) in terms of final outcome. Both groups had $<10°$ extensor lag at final follow-up at 2–6 months [26]. There was, however, a significant positive correlation between the length of splinting and final extension deficit. Patients with an intra-articular fracture had a higher incidence of degenerative changes on X-ray than those who were purely tendinous mallets. There were no complications reported in this series.

Kinninmouth and Holburn in a randomized prospective study of 54 patients compared a custom molded perforated splint to a stack splint (Fig. 2.7). Perforated splints were better tolerated and had better results according to Crawford's criteria with less extension lag [27].

Tocco et al. in 2013 compared cast immobilization to a removable DIP orthrosis (Fig. 2.7) in 57 patients where patients were given detailed instructions in home self-care with close monitoring for compliance [28]. Follow-up was at 28 weeks. Those patients treated in a cast had an average extensor lag of 5°, whereas the orthotic group had a 9° lag. One of the factors observed was edema of the fingertip at final follow-up. Those that were edematous had a poorer outcome than those that were not. This could be due to diminished arterial, venous, and lymphatic flow to the edematous fingertip [29]. Casting allowed constant compression on the fingertip and not surprisingly had diminished edema than the other group. Colditz attributed "edema reduction" to be one of the salutary effects of plaster casting of limbs [30]. There was no difference in active flexion between the two groups at follow-up. At 6 months, there was no difference between the two groups and both had a 5° extensor lag at follow-up. Other variables such as time from injury to treatment, mallet type, or injury mechanism had no effect on the final outcome in this study.

Warren and Norris followed 116 patients, randomized to wear either a "Stack" or "Abouna" wire splint [31]. At 10 weeks, both splints were shown to be equally effective with either near or complete resolution of the mallet. Patients preferred the "Stack" splint, reporting that it was more comfortable. In a randomized trial with 60 patients, Maitra and Dorani compared the "Stack" splint with padded aluminum (Fig. 2.7) and found that, while both splints were equally effective in correcting the extensor lag, the aluminum splint was more comfortable and had less dorsal skin maceration than the "Stack" [3]. Skin maceration can be prevented by pre-wrapping the DIP joint in gauze or by padding the splint in moleskin. In 2010, Pike and Mulpuri in a prospective randomized double-blinded study investigated the following three splint types with 87 patients [32]:

- Volar-padded aluminum splint
- Dorsal-padded aluminum splint
- Custom thermoplastic splint applied to the volar side

All splint types had the DIP in "slight" hyperextension and the PIP joint free. The splints were applied full time for 6 weeks and, if there was a lag of $>20°$, to apply for an additional 4 weeks. The single, major complication was full-thickness skin ulceration from dorsal skin pressure. Additionally, there were several, minor complications with maceration and erythema. An extension lag of 5–10° in all groups was reported at follow-ups of 7, 12, and 24 weeks, but there was no statistical significance between the groups at 12 weeks.

In another randomized, controlled trial, O'Brien and Bailey compared the dorsal aluminum splints, custom circumferential thermoplastic splints, and "Stack" splints, which were followed up at 12 and 20 weeks [33]. Finger braces were worn continuously for 8 weeks. Patients wearing stack splints and aluminum splints (5/21 each) experienced skin maceration, problems with fit, pain, and splint breakage. The group that wore thermoplastic splints (22 patients) had no complications. All patients experienced excellent results by Crawford's criteria extensor lag of 6.4° and a flexion range between 59 and 64°, and there was no difference between the groups at final outcome at 20 weeks.

Additionally, Handoll and Voghella conducted a meta-analysis on splint treatment and concluded that there was "insufficient evidence to determine which splint type is best but that the splint must be stout enough to withstand everyday use [2]." There has been some discussion in the literature about the vascularity to the dorsal skin over the DIP joint relevant to blanching of that skin when the DIP is hyperextended and to potential pressure from a dorsally applied splint. Flint in 1955 described the vascularity of the dorsal skin of the DIP joint. The blood supply to the dorsal skin arises from dorsal branches arising from the volar digital arteries [34]. These dorsal terminal vessels form an arcade where the branches join. Hyperextension of the DIP joint causes blanching by stretching the volar arteries and compression of the dorsal arcades (Fig. 2.9a) by the buckling of the overlying skin (Fig. 2.9b). Rayan and Mullins in 1987 showed that skin blanching occurred when the DIP joint was hyperextended to 50% of maximum in healthy volunteers, the average normal hyperextension being 28.3° [35]. That blanching can be reproduced when a tight dorsal splint is applied.

The state of vascularity of the extensor attachment and possible healing potential may explain the apparent direct relationship between age and extensor lag seen by Pike and coauthors where patients older than 60 years had a distinctly poorer outcome than younger patients [32].

In light of the above, it is clear that when a removable thermoplastic splint is applied, it needs to be removed frequently for skin checks and cleaning at home but great care must be exercised not to allow the finger to flex during this period. Noncompliance with this program will result in failure of splinting. It is advised that the fingertip rest on a flat surface or pinch tip to tip with the thumb to prevent DIP flexion. Compliance rates have been reported to range from 50 to 70% in closely monitored studies. While no splint type has been shown to be more efficacious than another, compliance with splinting regimens appeared to be greater with custom thermoplastic splints than AlumaFoam or stack splints [36]. The most important factor in success of splint treatment is patient compliance with the regimen.

Surgical Indications

There is a whole subset of patients that cannot be treated by splinting alone. They include patients who cannot tolerate splinting either because of

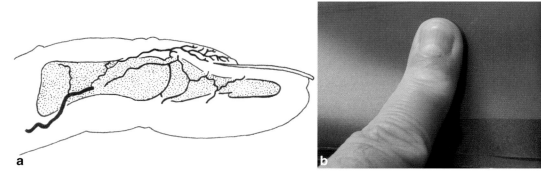

Fig. 2.9 a Lateral view of the finger with the dorsal and volar arterial distribution. Nail bed is to the right. Note the proximal and distal crossing arterial branches from the proper digital artery on the volar aspect (With permission from Jessica Rose Waterman). **b** Finger hyperextended against a firm surface. Note the blanching of the dorsal skin

repeated skin breakdown, recurrent loosening, or claustrophobia despite the type of splint chosen. Other groups such as surgeons, dentists, musicians, or competitive swimmers cannot afford to take off from their activity for 8 weeks and may opt for a percutaneous pin placed across the DIP joint in full extension and buried under the skin at the distal end of the finger. It acts as an internal splint and allows much earlier return to work activity but is prone to breakage and pin tract infection if misused. Thus, patient selection for this treatment must be made with care [37].

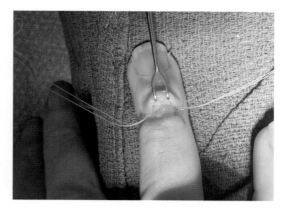

Fig. 2.10 Mitek anchors in distal phalanx securing the distal tendon and bridge drawing them both toward the distal phalanx

Open Mallet Fingers

There is little controversy in the literature about the treatment of lacerations and open avulsions at the terminus of the extensor mechanism. Zone 1 lacerations involving the terminal extensor should be directly repaired either to a terminal tendon stump with locking mattress suture which can include the skin or directly to the distal phalanx using a volar pull-out button or suture anchors [38]. Deep abrasions and skin/tendon avulsions should be first debrided and should be considered for secondary tendon repair after the wound has been rendered clean and there is adequate skin coverage. In this scenario, tendon grafting may be necessary to reestablish continuity. Postoperative regimen is similar to closed mallet fingers [39].

Complications of Treatment of Mallet Fingers

Chronic Mallet Fingers

In 2011, Makhlouf and Al-Deek reviewed the treatment of chronic mallet fingers in 11 papers. Mallet fingers are generally considered "chronic" when significant deformity (>20°) exits after 12–16 weeks of closed treatment [40].

There have been ten methods of treatment in the literature:

(1) Excision of scar and tenorrhaphy
(2) Reattachment of the tendon back to the bone

(3) Imbrication of the healed tendon (Fig. 2.10)
(4) Tenodermodesis (Fig. 2.11)
(5) Fowler central slip tenotomy
(6) Central slip tenotomy with distal repair (Figs. 2.10 and 2.12)
(7) Spiral oblique retinacular ligament reconstruction (SORL)
(8) Arthrodesis
(9) Tendon–bone graft
(10) Bridge tendon graft inserted into a bone tunnel into the distal phalanx

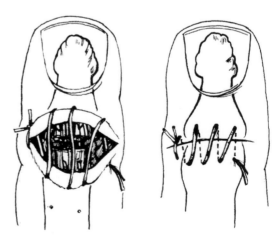

Fig. 2.11 Tenodermodesis: The tendon avulsion is sutured into extension with the overlying skin. If there is any skin redundancy, it is excised as an ellipse

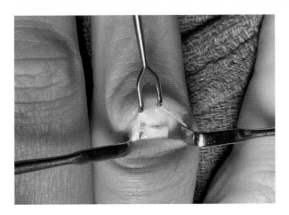

Fig. 2.12 Central slip tenotomy through a minimal dorsal approach. Great care must be exercised to avoid removing the lateral bands

Makhlouf tabulated the results of these treatments and showed the following: In the European literature, unless there is some hyperextension of the PIP joint, only the DIP joint is addressed [40]. The most frequently reported method is excising the tendon scar bridge and reattaching the tendon back to bone with an 80–100 % good to excellent result. In the US literature, Fowler releases are favored but not for extension deficits >35° [39]. If there is a significant swan-neck deformity, a SORL reconstruction is favored. They also feel that poor results are directly related to:

1. Delay in treatment >4 weeks
2. >50° extensor lag
3. Short thick fingers
4. >60-years-old
5. Poor compliance

Fowler's Central Slip Tenotomy (Fig. 2.12)

One of the simplest techniques for correction of chronic flexible tendinous mallet deformities is the central slip tenotomy. Described in 1949 by Fowler, the method is predicated on the concept that in the chronic phase of mallet deformity a scar bridge is developed between the tendon end and the distal phalanx [39]. A bridge that is a mere 3 mm too long has been shown by Schweitzer and Rayan and others can lead to a 45° extensor lag of the DIP [10]. The concept of the central slip tenotomy lies in the fact that the force

exerted by the central extrinsic tendon in the finger is dissipated by its insertion at the base of the middle phalanx. There is not enough excursion in the lateral bands and ORL to extend the DIP. Sectioning the central slip allows the whole extensor apparatus to migrate 2–3 mm proximally, thus facilitating DIP extension.

It is also seen that sectioning the central slip may lessen the hyperextension moment in the PIP that can lead to secondary swan-neck deformity often observed in chronic mallet fingers.

Fowler's central slip tenotomy is a reliable technique for reducing the degree of flexion deformity at the DIP joint but has generally not been advocated in deformities greater than 36° [39]. There have been concerns about aggressive tenotomy with subsequent injury to the triangular ligament creating a secondary extensor lag at the PIP joint and even frank boutonniere deformity. Classic papers on central tenotomy by Bowers, Hurst, and others have advocated a large mid-lateral approach, sectioning the transverse retinacular ligament lifting the extensor mechanism and releasing the central slip from below [41]. More recently, a limited approach utilizing a simple dorsal transverse incision 5 mm proximal to the PIP have been advocated [41].

Grundberg et al. reported a series of 20 patients who had their chronic mallet deformities treated with central slip tenotomies saw their extensor lag go from a pre-op average of 37–9° at final follow-up [4].

Chao and Sarwahi demonstrated in an experimental model that after sectioning the terminal extensor and creating a lengthening of about 3 mm, an extensor lag of 45° was created [42]. When a central slip tenotomy was performed in their specimens, they noted an immediate correction of 37–9°. Based on Schweitzer, that would be representing a proximal migration of 2 mm [10]. They concluded that correction greater than 36° was not possible utilizing this technique, although older clinical studies noted corrections of up to 60°. This could be due in part to remodeling of the terminal tendon. There may be no apparent correction immediately in the OR under anesthesia but correction of the DIP extensor lag can continue to improve at 1 year, something that the experimental model could not duplicate. It is clear, however, from these papers that full correction of the extensor lag was far less consistent with greater degrees of preoperative DIP flexion deformity.

Hiwatari et al. constructed an experimental cadaveric model of mallet finger in 16 fresh-frozen cadaveric fingers by sectioning and lengthening the terminal extensor so that a 45° mallet deformity was created [43]. A central slip tenotomy was created according to the technique of Bowers and Hurst [41]. The lateral bands were lifted after cutting the transverse retinacular ligaments from the center of the proximal phalanx to the center of the middle phalanx. The central slip was detached from its insertion on the dorsum of the middle phalanx and lateral band from the dorsum of the middle phalanx by one third, one half, and two thirds of the phalangeal length of the middle phalanx and the extensor lag of the PIP and DIP joints was measured. The mean pre-section DIP extensor lag was 44°. When one third was detached, the DIP lag was reduced to 19°. With one half detachment, the lag went down to 13° and when two third was cut, the lag went down to 6°. At the PIP joints, only four fingers demonstrated an extensor lag and that averaged 8° and no lag exceeded 15°. It is possible that no boutonniere deformity formed in this model because the transverse retinacular ligaments were also sectioned.

Rozmaryn described a technique where central slip tenotomy was augmented by a distal imbrication of the terminal extensor tendon and scar bridge to the distal phalanx by means of two microsuture anchors [44]. The tenotomy was performed through a minimally invasive transverse incision just proximal to the dorsal PIP crease. The fibers of the central slip were carefully separated from the lateral bands and 5 mm square of central tendon was excised. A separate transverse incision was made at the DIP joint and after two anchors were placed into the distal phalanx, the terminal extensor and scar bridge were brought up to the distal phalanx without sectioning the tendon or bridge. The DIP joint was secured in extension with a K-wire which was removed after 4 weeks and gentle active motion was

begun. Thirty-nine patients underwent the procedure. The average pre-op extensor lag was 45° and post-op average was 6.7°. There was one failure with a residual 30° extensor lag. Pre-op PIP hyperextension averaged 18° and at post-op it was 4.8°.

Tenodermodesis

Excising the scar between the tendon and the bone as well as an ellipse of the dorsal skin and repairing both together using en bloc 2.0 nylon mattress suture with pin stabilization of the DIP for 6 weeks, can have a 50–90 % excellent result at 6 months. This procedure was first described by Brooks in 1961. The technique was further refined by Graner who introduced the DIP pinning to augment the postoperative splinting that Brooks recommended. Never published by the authors, it was not until Albertoni published the results in 1988 did this procedure become popularized as the Brooks–Graner procedure. He reported a 91.6 % satisfactory result using this method [45]. In the early 1990s, the procedure became popular not only treating chronic mallet fingers but even acute mallet fingers and even in children [46].

Kardestuncer, Bae, and Waters conducted a level IV study with 10 patients with >45° ext lag. All were pinned for 6 weeks [47]. At 6.5 years follow-up, 2/10 full finger extension, 8/10 had a 20° extensor lag, and 7/10 had full DIP flexion. Iselin et al. reported on tenodermodesis in 26 patients and on final follow-up 22/26 had <10° extensor lag [48].

Similarly, Kon et al. studied 27 patients and 26 had an arc of motion of 5–60° at final follow-up [49].

Sorene and Goodwin reported on 16 patients with a chronic mallet finger deformity after a mean of 26 weeks of failed conservative treatment with an average extensor lag of 50° [50]. At surgery, all had full passive range of motion (ROM) at the DIP joint. A third of the patients had 10° hyperextension of the PIP joint. At 36 months, the mean extensor lag was 9°. However, 6/16 had a lag of 20°. Average flexion was 30°.

Kaleli et al. added an external fixator for 5 weeks to the tenodermodesis technique to secure

DIP extension while avoiding crossing the DIP [51]. At 36 months follow-up, the average extensor lag was 2° (−7 to 13°) and the flexion average was 70° (20–90°).

Excision of Scar and Tenorrhaphy

Lind et al. reported on excision of scar and tenorrhaphy in 40 patients. At final follow-up, 16/40 achieved a full ROM [52]. Another eight had good results with <8° extension lag but inability to flex more than 30°. The rest had extensor lags ranging between 30 and 60°.

Direct Reattachment of the Tendon to Bone

Ulkur in 2005 presented his results on 22 patients who had a direct reattachment of the tendon to bone via suture anchors [53]. All were diagnosed >4 weeks out. In his technique, part of the scar bridge was maintained in order to reach the distal phalanx as the terminal extensor tendon had retracted proximally. The K-wire was removed at 2.5 weeks and active ROM exercise was begun. He had 15/22 excellent results with full ROM, 5/22 good with <10° lag, and 2/22 had fair results with 10–20° extensor lag.

SORL Reconstruction (Littler)

This procedure has been recommended in the literature for swan-neck deformities that developed in the face of chronic mallet finger posture (Fig. 2.13). Originally described by Littler to regain the balance and synergy of PIP and DIP

Tendon Graft

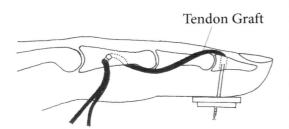

Fig. 2.13 The Thompson modification of Littler's spiral oblique retinacular ligament (SORL) reconstruction utilizing a free tendon graft anchored to the distal phalanx and passed volar to the axis of rotation of the PIP joint and anchored into the proximal phalanx. *PIP* proximal interphalangeal joint (With permission from JR Waterman)

extension by reconstructing the function of the ORL correcting the DIP flexion deficit associated with PIP hyperextension [54].

Kleinman in 1984 reported that on 12 patients having undergone an SORL, 9 regained full DIP extension and three developed hyperextension deformity at the DIP [55]. One required tenolysis and one needed graft lengthening.

Thompson–Littler 1978 described a technique where the tendon graft was connected independently into the distal phalanx via a pull-out wire and volar button and proximally threaded under Cleland's ligament between the neurovascular bundle flexor tendon sheath [54]. The graft was then passed transversely into a drill hole in the proximal phalanx mimicking the path of the lateral band described in Littler's original description.

Kanaya et al. in 2013 reviewed Thompson procedure and reported on seven patients with chronic mallet deformity and the pre-op ext lag was 42° (35–50) [56]. At final follow-up, the DIP extensor lag was 4° (0–30). Post-op DIP flexion mean was 63° (45–85). At the PIP joint, post-op flexion was 91° (85–110°) and a mean of 5° hyperextension. They also reported that the result is independent of pre-op condition of the quality of the scar bridge as no attempt was made to address that.

There is some discussion in the literature as to the correct tensioning of the tendon graft vis-à-vis PIP and DIP extension. Thompson felt that the graft should be tightened so that by passively extending the PIP joint, the DIP would go into full extension as well. Kanaya et al. felt that doing so would over tighten the graft. They therefore recommended that the DIP be allowed into 5° flexion when the PIP is held in full extension so that full simultaneous flexion of the PIP and the DIP became possible [56].

Tendon Grafting

Gu and Zhu employed the technique of free tendon grafting in 27 patients with open lacerations and 40 patients who had failed 6 weeks of conservative treatment [57]. The tendon insertion was augmented by inserting a palmaris graft into a bone tunnel in the distal phalanx and proximally into the terminal extensor leaving the DIP in full extension against gravity. All but one had less than 10° of extensor loss and had virtually full DIP flexion.

Tendon–Bone Composite Grafting

Wang et al. in 2013 reported on 28 patients with failed closed mallet fingers with an average of 34° extensor lag [58]. They created a notch at the extensor insertion on the distal phalanx and inserted a tendon–bone composite graft from the medial half of the extensor carpi radialis brevis (ECRB) insertion. The bone was fastened to the distal phalanx with a preplaced polyprophylene suture and the tendon was attached to the terminal extensor with a 1.5 cm overlap. The DIP was pinned in extension for 4 weeks.

Bone healing was achieved at a mean of 5 weeks. At 15 months follow-up, no patient reported pain and the mean extensor lag was 4° and the average DIP flexion was 65°. Eighty-six percent of the patients had achieved excellent results by Crawford's criteria.

Author's Preference

For the reconstruction of a chronic mallet finger, my preference is to perform a central slip tenotomy first and see how much correction is evident under anesthesia. Assuming the correction is minimal, I imbricate the distal phalanx insertion and pin the DIP joint in full extension for 4 weeks. Following this, one can begin full active ROM but must be very careful not to remove too much of the central slip, or an extensor lag of the middle phalanx will result.

Mallet Thumb

Mallet thumb is an exceedingly rare injury (Figs. 2.14a, b). Robb reported on 149 mallet fingers and only one was a mallet thumb [59]. Wehbe and Schneider reported on 42 mallet fingers and only one and that too was a mallet thumb [7]. This could be the extensor pollicis longus (EPL) is thicker than any of the extensor digitorum communis (EDC) tendons in the digits and the thumb is shorter and stouter than the

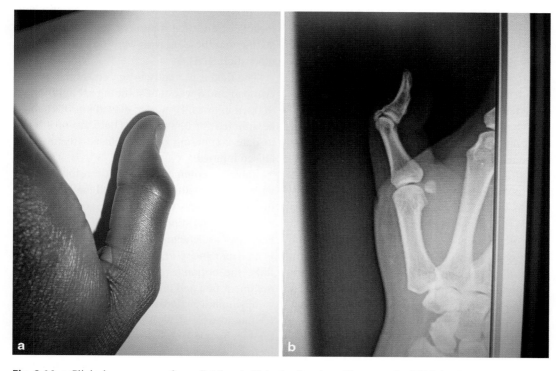

Fig. 2.14 **a** Clinical appearance of a mallet thumb. Note the dorsal swelling over the DIP joint, **b** X-ray appearance of a mallet thumb. Note the avulsion fracture of the dorsal rim of the distal phalanx. *DIP* distal interphalangeal joint

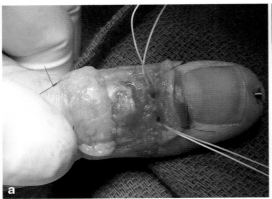
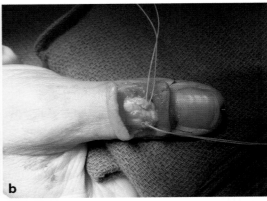

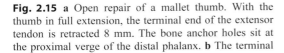

Fig. 2.15 a Open repair of a mallet thumb. With the thumb in full extension, the terminal end of the extensor tendon is retracted 8 mm. The bone anchor holes sit at the proximal verge of the distal phalanx. **b** The terminal extensor tendon has been mobilized and repaired back to the distal phalanx. There is a longitudinal 0.045 K-wire across the DIP joint. *DIP* distal interphalangeal joint

fingers which makes it more resistant to axial or hyperflexion forces.

Tabbai et al. reviewed the unique characteristics of mallet thumbs, which are anatomically based but will influence treatment [60]. Unlike the EDC in the palmar digits, the EPL lacks lateral bands, so if the insertion into the distal phalanx is interrupted, either by laceration or closed avulsion, the tendon would retract more than other digits (Figs. 2.15a, b). According to the author's report, the tendon had retracted 1.4 cm and had infolded on itself. However, this has not been reported in mallet fingers involving palmar digits.

The mechanism of closed injury is the same as other digits with acute hyperflexion force against an extended thumb. Nevertheless, Miura et al. reported that 80 % of these injuries are open, and only 20 % are closed [61]. Patients are clinically unable to extend the interphalangeal (IP) joint from a flexed position, but these are distinguished from other, more proximal EPL ruptures by the presence of pain and swelling over the dorsum of the IP joint. They did feel along with several other authors the same year that the initial treatment of closed mallet thumbs should be nonoperative with immediate surgery reserved for open lacerations. They did advocate continuous splinting of the thumb IP in full extension for 6 weeks followed by 3–6 months of 12-h/day splinting.

Din and Meggit pushed for operative treatment of closed injuries, they noted a lack of reports of successful closed treatment [62]. Splint treatment cannot compensate for the significant proximal retraction of the EPL, and the terminal extensor of the thumb is stout, lending itself to suture placement. In 1975, Verdan was the first to advocate closed treatment for these injuries, stating that these injuries were no different from other digits [63].

The field is currently in agreement that primary repair and 6 weeks of splinting are appropriate in open injuries. However, closed injuries should be splinted for 6–8 weeks. There are no studies to date comparing open to closed treatment of closed injuries.

Tabbai recommends magnetic resonance imaging (MRI) evaluation of closed mallet thumbs, in order to assess the degree of retraction ([60]; Fig. 2.16). Traditionally, 1 mm of retraction has been used as benchmark for open repair, but there is no data to support this. Of course, if treatment fails, the option exists of attempting a closed treatment first and then operating.

Nishimura et al. reported a case of a bony mallet thumb treated with an extension block pinning technique (see below) [64]. Pins were kept in for 4 weeks and splinting for 2 more weeks. At 7 months, patient's ROM at the IP joint was 16–46°.

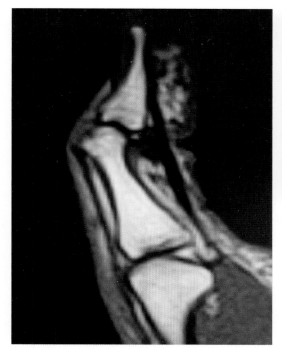

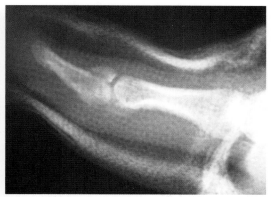

Fig. 2.17 Mallet fracture with 30% of joint involvement and no displacement. This is treated like a tendon injury with immobilization for 6–8 weeks

Fig. 2.16 MRI T-1 sagittal image of a mallet thumb. Note the degree of retraction of the extensor mechanism from the distal phalanx. There is also an oblique flexor pulley rupture in this patient. *MRI* magnetic resonance imaging

Mallet Fractures

Introduction

Most of the literature on mallet deformities written over the past 30 years combine the classification and treatment and outcome measures of tendinous mallet fingers and mallet fractures. While the clinical presentation may be similar, the mechanism of injury, treatment algorithm, and outcomes may vary. Both entities can be caused by a hyperflexion of the DIP but mallet fractures can be caused by hyperextension and axial loading which buckles the DIP joint into flexion as well. Zancolli reported that the degree of PIP flexion at the moment fingertip impact may play a role in whether the lesion at the tendon insertion is bony or tendinous [65]. He demonstrated that when the DIP joint is forcibly flexed beyond 90° when the PIP joint is in full extension, a bony avulsion occurs rather than a pure tendon avulsion.

Generally, mallet fractures whose bony components are less than 30% of the joint surface behave like and can be treated as tendinous mallet deformities (Fig. 2.17). If the articular surface of the fractured dorsal fragment is greater than 50% consideration must be given to the fact that while minimally displaced fractures will actually heal better than pure tendinous injuries with bone on bone contact (Fig. 2.18), displacement of the fragment on presentation with proximal migration of the dorsal fragment, if left untreated can be accompanied by volar subluxation of the DIP joint and if the joint surface is allowed to heal in an incongruous fashion, degenerative arthritis will in all likelihood occur (Fig. 2.19). In a

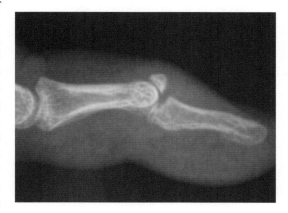

Fig. 2.18 Displaced mallet fracture involving 50% of the joint surface. The distal phalanx is subluxated volarly

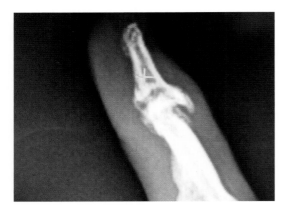

Fig. 2.19 Degenerative arthritis distal interphalangeal joint secondary to an untreated mallet fracture

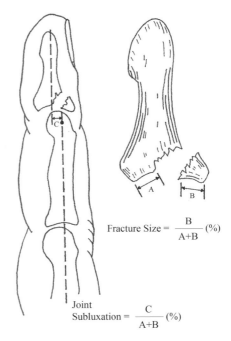

$$\text{Fracture Size} = \frac{B}{A+B}\,(\%)$$

$$\begin{array}{l}\text{Joint}\\\text{Subluxation}\end{array} = \frac{C}{A+B}\,(\%)$$

Fig. 2.20 Joint subluxation of the DIP joint defined a volar drift of the distal phalanx equal to 7% of the length of the total length of the articular surface of the distal phalanx. *DIP* distal interphalangeal joint (With permission from JR Waterman)

cadaveric study, Husain et al. demonstrated that volar joint subluxation of the distal phalanx was not observed until the joint involvement in the fracture exceeded 43 % and was consistent beyond 52 % of the joint surface [66]. It is believed that the reason why volar subluxation occurs in these larger dorsal fragments is that the joint surface cannot support contact with the proximal phalanx head and that DIP collateral ligaments may play no role in stabilizing the DIP joint. Volar subluxation was defined in this study as displacement of the long axis of the distal phalanx on the axis of the middle phalanx >7 % of the overall DIP joint surface of the distal phalanx (Fig. 2.20).

The Evidence: Review of the Literature

Nonoperative Treatment

Kalainov et al. studied the results of 21 patients who underwent nonsurgical treatment of closed displaced mallet fractures with greater than 30 % joint involvement using extension splinting for a mean of 5.5 weeks [67]. At 2 years follow-up, their patients had a high rate of satisfaction and finger function. He did note, however, that some patient developed dorsal DIP prominence, residual extension lag, DIP degenerative joint disease and swam neck deformity especially in cases of volar subluxation of the DIP joint. However, in

this study, the fracture types were not broken down according to percentage of joint involvement past 30 % [67].

Nonoperative treatment of mallet fractures include "Alumafoam" splinting, plaster finger casts, Stack and Oval-8 splints, and custom-made Thermoplast custom fit orthrosis (Fig. 2.7). All of these interventions are designed to maintain full extension of the DIP joint so that the avulsed fragment can be reasonably be opposed to the main body of the distal phalanx. An anatomic reduction of the fracture is not necessarily expected, but rather just enough continuity of the extensor mechanism to allow full DIP extension. Patients frequently remain with a tender bony "bump" on the dorsum of the DIP joint.

Complications of closed treatment also include pressure sores, maceration, and skin necrosis on the dorsum of the DIP, which can be full thickness (Fig. 2.21). This results from the tenuous blood supply to the dorsal skin overlying the

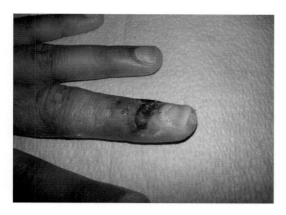

Fig. 2.21 Full-thickness necrosis of the dorsal skin over the DIP joint from a wet thermoplastic splint that was never removed for several weeks. *DIP* distal interphalangeal joint

extensor tendon insertion. Dorsal skin ischemia can result from hyperextending the DIP joint even 5° or via direct pressure placed on the dorsal skin from a tight splint. Both can occlude the tiny dorsal crossing arteriolar branches emanating from the volar digital arteries [34].

Additionally, recurrent flexion deformity and hyperextension contractures can occur. Any chronic malunions and resultant flexion deformities of more than 10° at the DIP will result in a secondary swan neck deformity and potentially degenerative changes in the DIP.

Treating mallet fractures is a highly controversial procedure. Wehbe and Schneider studied 160 patients with mallet injuries and have strongly advocated the nonoperative treatment of nearly all mallet fractures, with the exception of significant volar subluxation of the distal phalanx, on the head of the middle phalanx, and fracture involvement of >30% of the DIP articular surface [7]. The authors claim significant incidence of adverse outcomes when these injuries are treated surgically. They feel that even in the face of articular incongruity and volar subluxation, sufficient remodeling occurs to leave the patient with a pain-free functionally acceptable digit. Followed out to 3 years, however, 50% of their patients were seen to have degenerative changes and stiffness in the DIP.

Geyman et al. conducted a meta-analysis of all studies of mallet fingers from 1966 to 1998 and found that in all tendinous mallet injuries and articular fractures <30% should be treated with splinting [68]. Surgery should be reserved for large displaced fractures that cause volar subluxation of the distal phalanx.

Weber and Segmüller published a series of ten patients with >30% of the articular surface, significant displacement of the dorsal fragment but without subluxation of the DIP joint [69]. They were all treated by splinting for 4–6 weeks. All showed excellent remodeling of the joint surface, normal DIP flexion and an extension lag of <5°. Their conclusion was that secondary volar subluxation of the DIP joint only occurred if splinting was carried out incorrectly and that excellent results could be achieved by splinting alone.

Stern and Kastrup compared Kirschner (K)-wire fixation with splinting in 123 patients. In this study, all mallet deformities, bony and tendinous were included with 45 large intra-articular fractures, 37 avulsion fractures and 39 purely tendon injuries [70]. They found that splinted patients had a 45% complication rate, as compared to 53% that were operated on. In the nonoperated group, the complications included pressure sores, dorsal skin maceration, and necrosis. In the operated group, complications included nail deformity, osteomyelitis, pulp scarring/pain, nonunion or malunion, pin breakage, pin migration, and loss of reduction. They concluded that splinting was preferable to surgery. However, because surgical indications varied for each group of patients, one can call into question this chapter's conclusion as to whether surgery or conservative treatment should have been considered.

In contrast, Luhban et al. compared nonsurgical treatment with surgery in 30 patients with either joint subluxation or >30% of joint involvement [71]. They concluded that patients who had undergone surgery had cosmetically and functionally superior outcomes than nonoperative patients. They had better ROM, better DIP extension, and less deformity than the nonoperated group. In the nonoperative group, the time for healing ranged between 6 and 16 weeks. Operative fixation healed between 5 and 7 weeks.

Miura feels that by anatomically reducing the dorsal fragment, one increases the surface area for healing at the fracture site, thus speeding up healing [61].

In a 10-year prospective cohort study, Niechayev studied 150 patients with mallet deformities with pure tendon injuries in 82 patients and 68 with bony injuries. Nonoperative treatment consisted of splinting with an aluminum splint [72]. Those patients who underwent surgical treatment did so either with open K-wire fixation or a "pull-out wire" technique. They concluded that mallet fractures should be operated on if: >30 % of the joint surface was involved, displacement was greater than 3 mm or if the DIP joint was volarly subluxated [72].

Surgical Indications

Despite the favorable results reported for the closed treatment of mallet fractures, there are instances where surgical treatment is indicated.

- Open injuries
- Patients are unable to tolerate splinting
- Unstable displaced bony avulsions usually involving >50 % of the joint surface
- Displacement of the dorsal fragment >2 mm
- Volar subluxation of the distal phalanx
- Persistent DIP flexion deformity of >20° after 14 weeks of closed treatment

The goal of surgical treatment is the restoration of a stable healed congruent joint surface allowing full flexion and extension of the DIP joint.

Surgical Techniques

There have been many methods for treating mallet fractures:

Percutaneous DIP joint pinning in extension.
Tension band wiring of the avulsed fragment to the distal phalanx.
Extension block pinning to "jam" the avulsed fragment against the distal phalanx into compression.
Extension block pinning with a small external fixator.

Interfragmentary pinning/compression screw fixation of the avulsed fragment to the distal phalanx.
Suture anchor fixation of the fragment to the distal phalanx.
Pull-out wires or sutures over a volar button.
Umbrella handle technique.
Open reduction and pinning.
Open reduction—hook plate.

Technique of Extension Block Pinning

With the DIP joint flexed to 90°, a single 0.045 K-wire is introduced into the head of the middle phalanx, proximal to the avulsed fragment, through the terminal extensor tendon at an angle of 45° to the long axis of the shaft of the middle phalanx, facing proximally. One must extend the DIP until the avulsed fragment lines up with the fracture surface of the distal phalanx. It may take side-to-side and rotatory manipulation to achieve reduction. Once reduction is achieved, a pin is placed across the DIP. An interfragmentary pin can be driven across the fracture site for further stability. The pins remain in for about 6 weeks, and the finger is protected with a splint for an additional 2 weeks (Figs. 2.22a, b).

Hofmeister et al. reported their results with extension block pinning in 24 displaced closed mallet fractures whose average size was 40 % of the joint surface [73]. The average time to bony union was 35 days. At 1-year follow-up, the extension lag was 4°, and the average flexion was 77°. They noted that, according to the Crawford classification, 38 % had excellent results with no extension loss, full DIP flexion, and no residual pain. DIP flexion averaged 78°. Additionally, 54 % had good results, with up to 10° of extensor lag. There were three pin site infections and two patients had a loss of reduction.

Pegoli et al. performed extension block splint augmented by interfragmentary pinning and studied 65 patients at an average follow-up of 69 weeks [74]. They concluded that 51/65 had good to excellent results using Crawford's criteria and that the others had only a fair rating because of suboptimal initial stabilization and reduction of the fracture (Fig. 2.23).

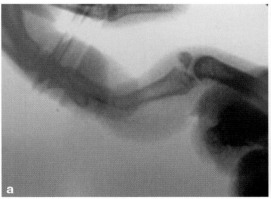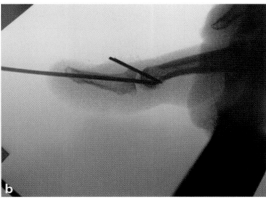

Fig. 2.22 a Extension block pinning technique. Displaced mallet fracture with the DIP flexed 45°. The K-wire(s) are inserted into the condyles of the middle phalanx at 30° to the long axis of the phalanx in a distal to proximal direction. The DIP joint is then extended allowing the dorsal fragment to reduce. Care must be taken to prevent rotation of the fragment. The DIP joint is pinned into extension. The pin must be volar to the fracture to prevent secondary displacement of the fracture, **b** Mallet fracture pinned in place with two dorsal-blocking pins and transarticular fixation. The longitudinal pin can be placed through the end of the digit or through a volar approach as long as the fracture is not breached. *DIP* distal interphalangeal joint

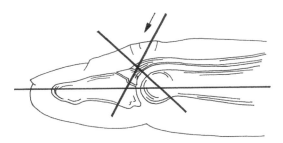

Fig. 2.23 Diagram depicting extension block fixation of a mallet fracture augmented by interfragmentary pinning. Care must be taken not to comminute the dorsal fragment during pinning (With permission from JR Waterman)

Extension Block Pinning Using a Small External Fixator

One of the problems reported with extension block pinning is dorsal rotation of the fragment once the pins are placed into the middle phalanx. Miura in 2013 reported on a technique in 12 patients where a mini external fixator is placed on the distal phalanx incorporating pins through the distal and middle phalanges and a central pin securing correct rotation of the dorsal fragment [61]. The fixator remained on for 4–7 weeks and at 4 months, the residual extensor lag was about 4° and average flexion was 74°.

Lee and Kim modified the original technique reported by Hofmeister by placing two small extension block pins (0.035") instead of one large one [73–75]. This would reduce the risk of dorsal fragment rotation. Additionally, the transarticular K-wire was placed across the DIP joint through a volar entry point, rather the fingertip. This allowed easier immobilization of the DIP joint in full extension without going through the fracture. Pins were removed at 6 weeks and full movement was permitted at 8 weeks. Pre-op, the average fragment size was 51% and the mean extensor lag was 21° and postoperatively it was 4°. DIP flexion averaged 79°. At 6 months follow-up, by Crawford's criteria 73% had excellent results, 21% had a good result, and 6% was graded as fair. Nail ridging occurred in 9%, tip parasthesias in 12%, and there was one pin site infection.

Extension Block and Intrafocal Pinning

Chung and Lee devised a modification of the extension block pinning technique to account for the fact that all too frequently when the DIP joint is extended with the extension block pin in

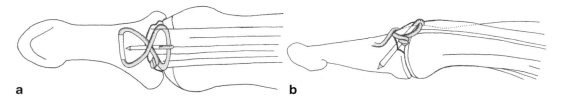

a   **b**

Fig. 2.24 a, b Tension band wiring technique. This technique has been shown to have a high complication rate (With permission from JR Waterman)

place, the dorsal fragments rotates into extension causing a joint step off and gap which can cause a persistent mallet deformity [76]. Their technique obviated this problem by placing a 0.7 mm K-wire across the distal end of the fracture from dorsal to volar in a unicortical fashion. The wire was bent proximally pushing the fragment out of extension. The wire was then driven through the volar cortex. Flexing the DIP 30° an extension block pin was inserted into the distal end of the middle phalanx. Bringing the DIP back into full extension reduced the dorsal fragment anatomically. The DIP was then secured with a longitudinal K-wire.

They studied 14 patients with an average articular involvement of 52 and 71% subluxated. Bony union was achieved in all cases in a mean of 38.4 days. There was full DIP extension and 78° of flexion. There was one pin site infection.

Technique of Tension Band Wiring (Fig. 2.24)

Jupiter et al. described a tension band wire technique. An "H" shaped incision is made over the DIP joint [77]. With the fracture exposed and debrided, 28-gauge cerclage wire is threaded transversely through a hole in the metaphysis of the distal phalanx, created by a 0.035 K-wire, 1 cm beyond the fracture site. The wire is then passed around the fragment by threading it at the point of tendon insertion on the fragment in a figure-of-eight fashion and tightened. In his review of the technique, Bischoff in 1994 reported a 45% complication rate [78]. This included wound break down, loss of reduction, avascular necrosis (AVN), extensor tendon rupture, nail growth abnormalities, and infection. These findings have been supported by other literature as well [78].

Percutaneous DIP Pinning

With the DIP in full extension or in 5° of hyperextension, a 0.045 or 0.054 K-wire is driven under X-ray control, across the DIP, into the head of the middle phalanx. The pin is either cut at the skin surface or left out with a Jurgan pin holder. Auchinloss et al. compared single pin fixation without attention to the avulsed fragment to closed treatment [22]. They found a lower complication rate with a diminished extensor lag in the pin fixation group (6 vs. 10°), and pin patients reported a better subjective outcome than the closed group.

Fritz et al. (Fig. 2.25) described a modification of the single wire technique in 24 patients [79]. The fracture was opened through a dorsal approach and debrided to a clean, cancellous surface. In DIP flexion, an antegrade 1-mm wire is drilled distally through the fracture site and through the tip of the finger, until the tip of the wire just disappears through the fracture. The DIP is extended, reducing the fragment manually, and the wire is then drilled proximally through the fragment and the DIP. The wire was removed in 4 weeks, and active ROM exercises commenced. After 43 months, fingers extended to within 2° of extension and 72° of flexion. Nineteen patients were pain-free and five had mild pain with activity.

Interfragmentary K-Wire Fixation (Fig. 2.26)

In this percutaneous technique, the dorsal fragment is reduced under fluoroscopic control and pinned with one or several K-wires passed retrograde through the fracture out of the distal phalanx. Another wire is passed through the extended DIP joint. Patients treated with this

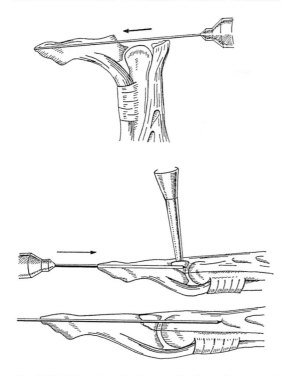

Fig. 2.25 Single longitudinal pin fixation of the dorsal fragment. It is recommended that this technique only be used with dorsal fragments that are greater than 60% of the joint surface or insufficient purchase of the dorsal fragment (With permission from JR Waterman)

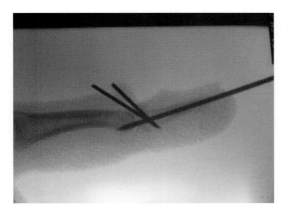

Fig. 2.26 Interfragmentary pin fixation. Acute injuries can be reduced closed and pinned but after 3 weeks post injuries, closed reduction becomes impossible and an open reduction is necessary to remove the scar and granulation tissue that has formed at the fracture site

technique in Lubahn's study had a DIP extensor lag range of 0–20°, and were able to flex the DIP joint up to 55° [71]. Complications of K-wire fixation were reported to be 52%. These included persistent pain, degenerative joint disease from residual incongruity, nail deformity, K-wire loosening or breakage and infection [38, 71].

Badia and Riano reported on their technique of reducing the volarly subluxated DIP joint with fractures encompassing 20–50% of the joint surface, with a 0.045 K-wire inserted distally and used as a joystick to facilitate reduction [80]. Once the DIP joint is reduced, the wire is advanced across the DIP joint. A second wire was placed across the fragment pinning it to the distal phalanx with the wire going through the volar pad. The wire was then bent catching the fragment and compressing the fragment against the distal phalanx and buried subcutaneously by pulling on the volar end of the wire that is allowed to protrude volarly by 2–3 mm. Wires were removed at 6 weeks. At final follow-up, the 16 patients studied had an average extensor lag of 2° (0–7°) and a flexion range of 75° (65–80°).

Kang and Lee published a series of 16 bony mallet fractures irreducible by closed techniques [81] which were opened. They included >1/3 of the joint surface, volar subluxation, and >3 mm displacement of the dorsal fragment. They passed a wire through the volar pad under the distal phalanx. After opening the DIP joint (Fig. 2.27a), two oblique wires were passed through the fracture fragments and onto the distal phalanx (Fig. 2.27b). The edges of the extensor tendon were repaired directly with 6.0 undyed nylon. At 12 months, all of the patients' fractures were united, none had residual volar subluxation or permanent nail deformity. All but two patients had <5° of extensor lag and all patients were satisfied with their function and cosmetic appearance.

Yamanaka et al. used a temporary percutaneous extension block pin to reduce and compress the fracture fragment [82]. Once this was done, K-wires were placed across the fracture site and the DIP joint was secured with another wire. The extension block pin was removed. At follow-up, their patients experienced an ROM of—1–69°.

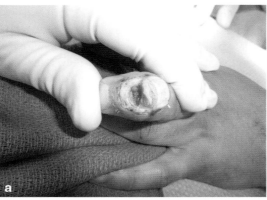

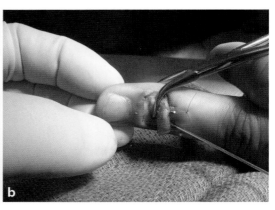

Fig. 2.27 a Dorsal view of the DIP joint with the joint "shot-gunned" open. The dorsal fragment is on the *left* and the fracture bed of the distal phalanx is on the *right*. Note the granulation tissue at the fracture site. **b** With the fracture held in reduction, two interfragmentary pins are placed across the fracture site. The fixation is completed by placement of a longitudinal K-wire across the DIP joint. *DIP* distal interphalangeal joint

Interfragmentary Screw Fixation (Fig. 2.28)

After exposing the fracture distal to the DIP through a dorsal approach, the fracture site is cleaned and held in reduction with a towel clamp. Once the reduction on X-ray is confirmed, two or three 0.5 mm drill holes are placed perpendicularly across the fracture site and 0.8 mm screws are placed across the fracture (Fig. 2.7). The finger is splinted for 6 weeks, and then full ROM is instituted. Reporting on 12 patients with >30% of joint involvement and followed for 31 months, Kronlage et al. found that there were no postoperative complications, and the average extensor

lag was 6° with flexion of 70° [83]. Screw head prominence was reported in 30% of the patients. No other complications were reported. A note of caution, even in large intra-articular fractures where there is the temptation to use cannulated interfragmentary 2.0 mm screws, one must be extremely cautious not to comminute the dorsal fragment.

Pull-Out Wires Over a Volar Button

Kang et al. reported on 59 patients who underwent interfragmentary fixation with 4.0 nylon or 24-gauge cerclage wire tied around the fracture, passed through two drill holes in the distal phalanx, and tied over a volar button (Fig. 2.29;

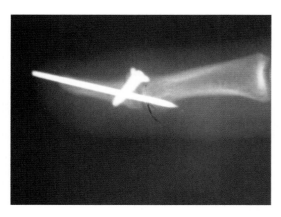

Fig. 2.28 Open interfragmentary screw fixation. Comminution of the dorsal fragment is a real concern in placement of the screws

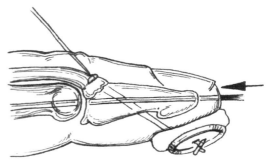

Fig. 2.29 Pull-out wires to a volar button. Care must be taken to pad the button to avoid pressure necrosis of the volar pad. Note the dorsal strand to pull out the wire at 4 weeks (With permission from JR Waterman)

[84]). K-wire of 1.1 mm was used to pin the DIP into extension. After 4 weeks, the pull-out wire was removed at 4 weeks, and the K-wire was removed at 6 weeks. The complication rate was 41%, which included skin breakdown, superficial and deep infection, osteomyelitis, recurrent mallet deformity, radial deviation of the DIP, and nail deformity.

However, Zhang et al. did a variation of the pull-out wire technique in 65 patients, with an average joint involvement of 39% and DIP subluxation [85]. Their technique avoided placement of a button on the volar surface of the finger, such that the pull-out wire was attached to an outrigger composed of a K-wire that runs transarticular through the DIP, and the segment out of the tip is bent volarly at 45° to the long axis of the finger to capture the pull-out wire emerging from the pad. The K-wire is spring-loaded to maintain the pull-out wire in traction. Dorsally, the pullout wire wrapped around the dorsal fragment obliquely to capture it stably (Fig. 2.30). Postoperatively, there was no skin necrosis, breakdown, or any infection. After 27 months, all the fractures had healed uneventfully and without fragmentation. Only one out of 64 patients had noticeable DIP joint pain. The mean extensor lag was 7° and the mean active DIP flexion was 76°. There was comminution of the dorsal fragment, no skin necrosis or infection. The construct was seen to be so stable that no external splinting was needed.

Lu and Jiang et al. described a "pull in suture" technique which requires no volar buttons or knots and was designed to prevent necrosis or dyesthesia of the volar pad of the digit [86]. After opening the dorsum of the distal phalanx, the tendon end (or fracture fragment) are "freshened up." A 1-mm K-wire is placed across the fingertip with the DIP in full extension. It is then bent to receive the 4.0 Prolene sutures that were tied in a "Kessler" stitch pattern at the terminal extensor tendon. If there was a mallet fracture, the suture were then passed through the fragment. Two holes were drilled obliquely with 21-gauge spinal needles through the distal phalanx from volar-distal to proximal-dorsal exiting at the fracture site and the suture is passed through the fracture site and exits the finger through the volar pad. They are then tied over the distal K-wire at its bend. After 6 weeks of immobilization, the K-wire and suture was removed and full active and active assist exercises were begun.

They reported on ten mallet fingers and at 15 months all patients were pain free and final mean active flexion was 60°. However, only two patients were rated as excellent, seven as good, and one graded as fair. There were no complications reported in this study.

"Umbrella Handle" Technique (Fig. 2.31)

Rocchi et al. described a technique in 48 patients followed for 8 years utilizing a single

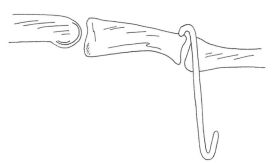

Fig. 2.31 The "umbrella handle" technique. One-millimeter K-wire is passed across the fracture site, out through the distal phalanx and volar skin. After bending the tip of the wire proximally, the wire is pulled from the volar side until the "hook" captures the proximal fragment and holds it in place under a small dorsal skin incision. The volar side of the wire is passed through a small volar thermoplastic cap and bent around the cap to secure the fragment (With permission from Jessica Rose Waterman)

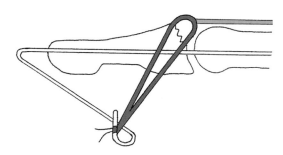

Fig. 2.30 Pull-out wire attached to an extension of the central intramedullary pin set in tension at 45° to the long axis of the distal phalanx. This angle must be maintained to assure that the dorsal fragment does not rotate out of alignment (With permission from Jessica Rose Waterman)

1-mm K-wire passed across the fracture site, out through the distal phalanx and volar skin [87]. After bending the tip of the wire proximally, the wire is pulled from the volar side until the "hook" captures the proximal fragment and holds it in place under a small dorsal skin incision. The volar side of the wire is passed through a small volar thermoplastic cap and bent around the cap to secure the fragment. Patients are allowed immediate active ROM of the DIP without restriction lessening the chance of postoperative DIP joint stiffness as has been reported when the DIP joint is "protected" for 4–6 weeks with a transarticular K-wire in full DIP extension. After the wire was removed at 6 weeks, the authors reported that 35 patients had a mean extension lag of 6° and 11 patients had full pain free DIP flexion and extension. There was one postoperative pin tract infection.

Open Pinning of the Fracture and the DIP

In 2010, Phadnis et al. reported, in 20 patients, their technique of open reduction and pin fixation of mallet fractures, involving greater than 30° of the joint surface with associated subluxation [88]. After opening the fracture site through a dorsal incision, the subluxation is reduced and held with a 1.25 mm K-wire across the DIP to the middle phalanx. Care was taken to drive the wire volar to the fracture site. With converging 0.6 mm K-wires, the fracture is reduced and pinned. The wires are removed at 6 weeks. At 1-year follow-up, 16 patients had good to excellent results, three were fair, and one was poor. There was one superficial wound infection with loss of reduction.

Fritz et al. reported on an open pinning technique in 24 patients where under direct visualization, K-wire was driven antegrade across the fracture site out the tip of the finger [79]. The point of the wire remained at the fracture site. The fracture was then reduced by extending the DIP joint and the wire was driven retrograde across the fragment and into the middle phalanx. The wire was removed at 4 weeks and ROM exercises commenced. At final follow-up, 21/24 had full extension and an average flexion arc of

72°. The remaining three had < 10° extension lag. There were no complications noted.

Reissner, Glenck et al. in 2012 reported on 43 patients, whose fractures involved >30% joint surface [89]. In this technique, the fracture site was exposed through a dorsal "H" or lazy "S" incision. The fracture was reduced closed with a towel clip or 18-gauge needle and pinned with K-wires. A longitudinal transarticular K-wire held the DIP joint in full extension. Follow-up was 28 months. Five patients had superficial wound infections.

Two patients needed early pin removal. Two patients had a nail deformity and two had ulnar deviation of the distal phalanx. The mean extensor lag was 10° but 11 patients had >20° extensor lag. All these had tendon tears by ultrasound. Sixty-three percent of the patients considered their outcome unsatisfactory. The authors recommended abandoning the technique.

Open Reduction Internal Fixation Using a Hook Plate

Teoh and Lee described the use of a "hook plate," which is fashioned from a titanium 1.3-mm plate using one hole, and as the screw is tightened, two hooks grasp the tendon against the bony insertion (Figs. 2.32a, b; [90]). The prongs are used to grip the bony fragment while the intact hole is attached distally with a screw. Immediate active motion is DIP allowed obviating the need for a transarticular K-wire. Patients were issued a thermoplastic splint on postoperative day one and the splint was removed several times daily for controlled active DIP flexion. This protected mobilization went on for 6 weeks after which full use of the finger was permitted. Nine patients were followed at an average follow-up of 17 months, and all the patients had a good or excellent result by Crawford's criteria. There were no implant or skin complications or any infections. However, this technique did necessitate removal of the implant at a later time due to the bulkiness of the implant resulting in tenting of the overlying dorsal skin. There is also concern about the germinal matrix of the nail when placing the distal screw although nail deformity has not been reported yet with this technique.

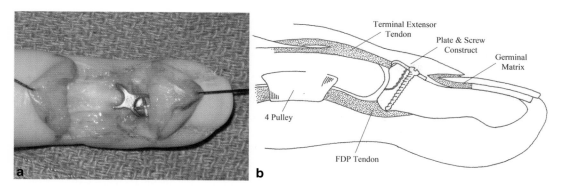

Fig. 2.32 **a** Hook plate securing the terminal extensor and bony fragment. Care must be taken not to put the screw through the germinal matrix of the nail bed. **b** Schematic diagram of the hook plate technique. The screw must be placed proximal to the germinal matrix (By JR Waterman)

Modified Tenodesis Method (Fig. 2.33)

Tung et al. described an open technique where the dorsal fragment was reduced to the distal phalanx and held in place via 4.0 Prolene suture passed through a bone tunnel in the distal phalanx [91]. The finger was immobilized post-op with the DIP joint in full extension for 5 weeks. This was followed by 6 weeks of active and active assist DIP flexion/extension and strengthening exercises. In all, there were 13 mallet fractures and at 5.2-months follow-up, 8/13 were described as excellent by Crawford's criteria and 5/13 were considered good with an extensor lag of 0–10°. DIP flexion ranged between 50–70° with a mean of 67.3°. There were no complications reported.

Lucchina et al. compared three techniques in 58 patients, using interfragmentary K-wires bent dorsally around the fragment and pulled out volarly, extension block K-wire fixation,

and open reduction internal fixation (ORIF) with compression screws [92]. They concluded that screw fixation, while being technically more difficult to perform, allowed earlier return of function. While K-wire fixation is easier to perform, it demands longer periods of immobilization, and one must manage the pin tracts to avoid infection. In the ORIF group, some patients had pulp pain related to the screw lengths, but long-term functional outcome was the same in all three techniques in follow-up mean of 21 months.

A biomechanical cadaveric study by Damron et al. compared three fixation techniques of mallet fractures after creating one utilizing a dorsal oblique osteotomy of the distal phalanx at the tendon insertion under X-ray control so that 45% of the joint surface was involved [93]. There were 40 fresh frozen fingers and the fixation methods included: K-wires, figure-of-eight wires, pull-through wires and pull-through sutures. The fingers were put through numerous cycles of DIP flexion and extension. All of the K-wires lost reduction, 60% of the pull through wires and 50% of the figure-of-eight wires failed. None of the pull through sutures failed [93].

Cheung et al. studied 32 cadaveric fingers looking at four fixation methods for large mallet fractures [94]:

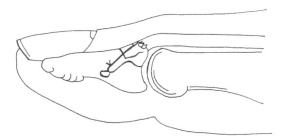

Fig. 2.33 Modified tenodesis method. Sutures are passed through a bone tunnel and tied at the side of the distal phalanx. (By JR Waterman)

1. Transfragmentary K-wire fixation placed diagonally in from the corners.

2. Pull-out wires threaded under the extensor tendon at its insertion and passed volarly through the distal phalanx and tied below.
3. Tension band wiring through a transverse hole in the distal phalanx with the wire threaded under the tendon insertion in a figure-of-eight fashion.
4. Soft anchor fixation 1.4 mm holes into the dorsal fragment and distal phalanx. A suture anchor is placed into the distal phalanx and sutures tied over the dorsal fragment.

All fingers underwent an osteotomy of the articular surface of the distal phalanx so that the dorsal fragment encompassed 50% of the articular surface. The fingers were tested to peak load resistance at 30, 45, and 60°. It was found that tension band wiring was found to be the strongest and the other methods appeared to have similar strength. The conclusion reached in this study can be called into question for several reasons. It is not clear how peak load resistance was measured. There is no possibility of "load to failure" testing here as the specimens were tested multiple times at varying angles and even before the osteotomy. Testing to failure would make impossible to retest a specimen more than once. There is no accounting for testing artifact meaning the viscoelastic effect of previous testing on the terminal extensor tendon. One can however get a general sense of relative strengths of four fixation methods.

Chronic Mallet Fractures

Chronic mallet fractures >3 months after injury must be distinguished from acute injuries because:

• Callous and scar have formed between the dorsal fragment and the distal phalanx making closed reduction impossible.
• There has been remodeling and absorption of the dorsal fragment making anatomic reduction difficult if not impossible.
• There may be a DIP joint flexion contracture.
• If there has been volar subluxation, the collateral ligaments may have contracted thus fixing the deformity.

• There may already be degenerative change in the DIP joint.

Lee et al. reported on 23 patients with a chronic bony mallet fingers with a mean of 53% of the joint surface and >3 months post injury all of whom had unsuccessful splinting regimen [95]. After freeing up the callous and releasing the contractures, they passed a 25-gauge wire carefully through the dorsal fragment avoiding comminution and the distal phalanx exiting volarly and tied over a volar button. The DIP joint was stabilized in extension by a K-wire across the DIP joint. The wires were removed at 6 weeks and full unrestricted activity and active ROM exercises were started. The pre-op mean extensor lag was 36° which was corrected to a mean 4°.

The maximum lag in the series was 7°. Mean DIP flexion was 72°. Two patients had mild pain which resolved after 5 months and four patients had early degenerative changes at the DIP joint. There was one wound infection treated with oral antibiotics. Five patients had transient paresthesias that resolved after 4 months. There was no AVN, wire breakage, flap necrosis, or persistent DIP subluxation. Using Crawford's criteria, 74% had an excellent result, 17% were rated as good, and 9% had a fair result.

DIP Arthrodesis: Final Salvage (Fig. 2.34a, b)

The final common solution for failed reconstruction for mallet fingers and mallet fractures especially those who have gone on to develop degenerative arthritis is DIP arthrodesis. This is commonly done through a transverse dorsal incision. The extensor tendon is incised and the DIP joint is exposed. The distal condyles of the middle phalanx are exposed and rongeured down to cancellous bone removing the flanges of the condyles. The articular surface of the distal phalanx is removed similarly down to cancellous bone. A double pointed guide (0.035, 0.045) wire is drilled from proximal to distal, up the central axis of the distal phalanx and brought out so that only a small point of the wire is in the joint. A hole is made in the distal end of the middle phalanx to allow that point to penetrate the middle phalanx. Under fluoroscopic control, the wire is passed

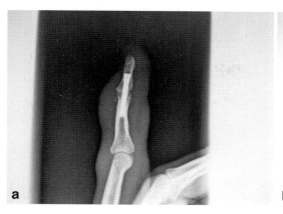
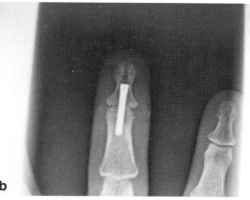

Fig. 2.34 a Lateral view of a DIP fusion. Care must be taken not to pierce either dorsal or volar cortices or damage to the nail bed or volar pad tenderness will result. **b** PA view of a distal interphalangeal fusion. The screw has good purchase in both phalanges and good compression is paramount. The screw should go down the central axis of both phalanges. *DIP* distal interphalangeal joint

into the central axis of the middle phalanx both in the sagittal and coronal planes. It is preferred that the DIP joint is flexed between 10 and 20° prior to full insertion of the wire. At this point, with the DIP compressed into position, either two derotational wires are passed or a central screw can be passed over the K-wire. If the screw is employed, a drill is passed through a stab incision in the fingertip and a window is placed into the distal tuft for screw placement. The screw is passed so that the cortices of the distal phalanx (especially the dorsal cortex) are not disturbed. The screw is driven down under compression until excellent bony purchase is achieved. The dorsal incision is closed in layers. The fingertip is splinted for 3 weeks then wrapped with a self-adhering tape for three more. Full PIP motion is commenced immediately. If K-wires alone are to be used the pins should be cut just proud of the skin and the fingertip should be splinted for about 6–8 weeks when the pins should be removed.

Post-op Management

Complications of Treatment

Complications have been reported for mallet fractures that have been treated operatively or by splinting. Splinting complications have included: dorsal skin maceration, necrosis, ulceration, nail deformities, and persistent flexion deformities.

These have been reported as high as 45 % [24]. Surgical complications include: infection, hardware failure, loss of fixation, persistent deformity, nonunion, nail deformities, and dorsal skin necrosis. In this group, complications have been reported as high as 50 % [95].

Tuft, Shaft, and Pilon Fractures of the Distal Phalanx

Tuft Fractures (Fig. 2.35)

Tuft fractures are generally associated with crush injuries and can exist in open and closed injuries to the nail bed or volar pad. The force of the crush and its duration will determine the extent of the injury. Mild injuries are frequently accompanied by mild swelling and ecchymosis. As the severity of the crush increases, the volar pad can become turgid and a subungual hematoma may develop as the sterile matrix of the nail bed lacerates under a nail plate that is otherwise adherent at the edges (Fig. 2.36). This laceration creates a communication between the tuft fracture and the underside of the nail plate. Eventually, the nail plate avulses and the nail bed lacerates. The bony tuft may or may not rupture through the sterile matrix of the nail bed. The laceration can extend around the nail folds to the volar side. If the crush

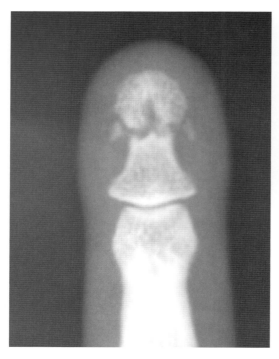

Fig. 2.35 Tuft fracture distal phalanx. Most common mechanism is a crush injury

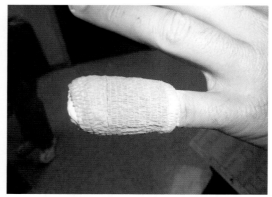

Fig. 2.37 Total contact cast used to splint crush injuries to the fingertip. Three weeks will suffice

is severe enough, the tip will simply amputate with or without the crushed bone.

Generally, if the injury to the soft tissue is mild the tuft requires no open treatment. In these cases, the tuft fracture is nondisplaced and simple immobilization for 2–3 weeks in a total contact plaster cast or splint will suffice (Fig. 2.37). These fractures generally fail to achieve bony union but rather a painless fibrous union results. Immobilization should not include the PIP joint as stiffness there may result. At 3 weeks, the DIP joint should be stretched to achieve maximal ROM.

Subungual hematomas are exquisitely painful and if involving more than 50 % of the sterile matrix will require decompression. Traditionally, a heated paperclip was used to trephine a hole in the nail plate just past the lunula. More recently a battery powered "ophthalmic" cautery provides much higher heat and will painlessly burn a hole in the nail plate. The sense of relief is immediate and intense. The fingertip is immobilized for about 2 weeks and an ROM program is begun.

It must be noted that creating a hole in the nail plate converts the closed tuft fracture into an open one so that there is a risk of developing a subungual abscess that may extend into distal phalanx. The trephination must be done under sterile technique. Recent evidence suggests that prophylactic antibiotics are not necessary unless the nail plate is removed [95].

There has been controversy of late as to whether patients who present with subungual

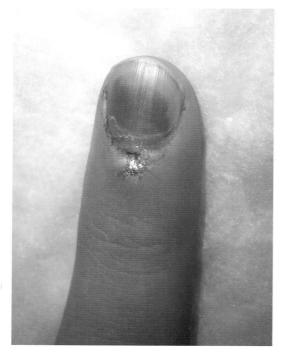

Fig. 2.36 Subungual hematoma from a crush injury. The nail folds are all intact

hematomas can be treated simply with trephination or is complete removal of the nail plate with repair of the nail bed necessary. Roser et al. (1999) compared the two techniques and found no difference in final outcome regardless of the size of the hematoma, or associated fracture [96]. It is now recommended to simply trephine the hematoma if it is greater than 50 % of the nail plate [94]. This assumes that the underlying fracture is undisplaced. If there is displacement, then full open treatment including nail-bed repair and fracture reduction and internal fixation is needed.

Shaft Fractures

There are many types of fractures of the distal phalanx (Fig. 2.38a). Two types of shaft fractures described by Schneider are transverse and longitudinal [5]. Transverse fractures are usually caused by crush injuries accompanied by a bending moment usually in flexion. They can be nondisplaced and stable or displaced and unstable (Fig. 2.38b, c). They can also be entirely closed or the distal fragment while displacing into flex-

ion can herniate through the sterile matrix usually avulsing the proximal nail plate out of the eponychial fold. The extent of the injury can be under appreciated by the ER staff who may simply "tuck" the nail plate back in and stabilize it with a suture. The underlying fracture and sterile matrix laceration is then left untreated with serious consequences for nail growth. The open nail matrix can be a conduit for soft tissue infection and/or osteomyelitis of the distal phalanx. In higher-energy injuries, the nail folds and the volar pulp can be avulsed too. Longitudinal fractures can also be open or closed and are usually a result of a crush injury. They can be extra-articular or may extend into the DIP joint (Fig. 2.39). They can also be widely displaced (Fig. 2.40).

The treatment of these injures vary with the clinical presentation. Nondisplaced closed fractures either transverse or longitudinal are generally treated with a splint or protective covering such as a total contact finger cast from the tip to the proximal end of the middle phalanx for about 2 weeks in order to allow the pain and swelling to subside and to prevent reinjury. Protected ROM exercise to the DIP joint is begun. The tip may

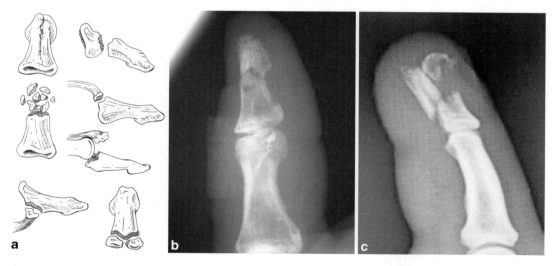

Fig. 2.38 a Distal phalanx fracture patterns. Nondisplaced distal split. Displaced proximal metaphyseal with flexion deformity. Comminuted distal tuft. Avulsion dorsal lip fracture <30 % of articular surface "mallet fracture." Intra-articular fracture >30 % of the joint surface with volar subluxation of the distal phalanx "Mallet fracture." Volar avulsion associated with closed flexor digitorum profundus (FDP) rupture "jersey finger." T-intercondylar basilar fracture (By JR Waterman). **b** Stable distal shaft fracture can be open or closed. If closed can be readily treated with splinting alone. **c** Unstable comminuted fracture of the distal phalanx. Will require an open reduction internal fixation probably with a longitudinal pin

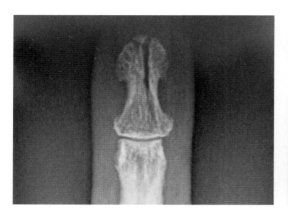

Fig. 2.39 Longitudinal minimally displaced split fracture of the distal phalanx

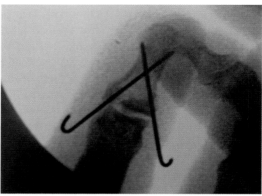

Fig. 2.41 Proximal metaphyseal fracture treated with crossed K-wires sparing the DIP joint. *DIP* distal interphalangeal joint

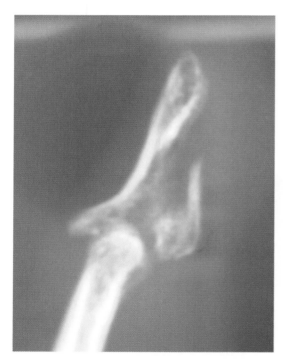

Fig. 2.40 Widely displaced intra-articular fracture of the distal phalanx

This can be accomplished with a longitudinal K-wire or small screw placed distal to proximal. Usually the wire need not extend across the DIP joint into the middle phalanx (Fig. 2.41). If, however, there is insufficient bone in the proximal metaphysis of the distal phalanx the wire can extend to the condyles of the middle phalanx (Fig. 2.42a, b). Wires remain in place for 4–5 weeks. Use of screws must be considered with caution because of the difficulty encountered in their insertion and the ease with which they can cut out of the bone. Frequently, the distal phalanx may be curved compounding the problem.

Nonunion of Distal Phalanx Shaft Fractures

Although most closed distal phalanx shaft or neck fractures are treated with splinting alone until the tip is nontender usually at about 3–4 weeks, there is a subset of patients who have persistent pain and a sense of instability even after 3 months. DaCruz et al. reported that as many as 47 % of shaft fractures of the distal phalanx many develop symptomatic nonunions at 6 months [97]. Many developed numbness, cold sensitivity, hyperesthesia and DIP stiffness, and nail growth abnormalities. Those will require internal fixation. By and large, these fractures are either comminuted, displaced, or have a short oblique

still need protection for an additional 2 weeks with a soft cover such as a Coban wrap.

Displaced closed injuries to the distal phalanx shaft should be reduced anatomically and stabilized in order to prevent subsequent injury to the overlying sterile matrix and late nail deformity.

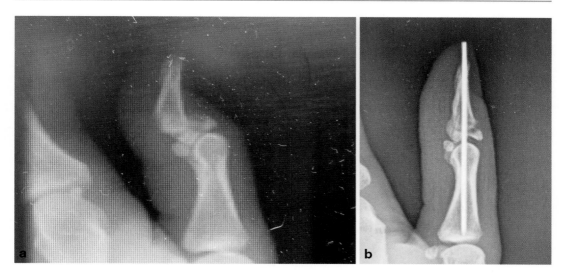

Fig. 2.42 **a** Displaced and angulated proximal metaphyseal fracture of the distal phalanx. **b** Unstable transverse metaphyseal fracture treated with a transarticular longitudinal K-wire

pattern. Open fractures despite soft tissue healing are more prone to the development of a nonunion.

Chim and coworkers utilized cortical miniscrews to internally fix these delayed unions [98]. All but one of their series had an open fracture to begin with but there were no infections. They approached the fracture through the nail bed, debrided the fracture site, and through a separate distal stab incision one or two cortical screws were passed longitudinally through the fracture site with care taken not to breach the DIP joint. Generally, bone graft was not required unless the fracture was comminuted. There were 14 patients in this series. All had painful and unstable pinch at 3 months and no X-ray evidence of fracture union. The fractures healed at an average of 4.2 months but the range was wide (1–10) months with 8/14 still remaining ununited at 3 months. All patients experience some shortening of the distal phalanx with some up to 30%. All but one of the patients had their screws removed after clinical and X-ray evidence of union and despite the surgical approach no patient experienced lasting nail deformity.

Another study, by Ozcelik et al. looked at 11 patients 4 months after injury to the distal phalanx who had developed nonunion [99]. Three had had an infection and four others had resorption at the fracture site. They were grafted with olec-

ranon structural cancellous bone graft through a midlateral approach and fixed with K-wires. At 7 months follow-up, all had bony healing and all were pain and instability free.

Most distal phalangeal nonunions that have been reported in the literature have been atrophic in nature. Meijis reported on two patients who presented with hypertrophic nonunion 1 and 2 years post injury [100]. Both were treated with distally placed 1.5 mm compression screws, placed through a small stab incision, that were removed after 4 months. Both were pain free but needed a second procedure to remove the screw as the screw head protruded from the distal tuft. Others have reported DIP stiffness, sensory loss at the fingertip, degenerative arthritis at the DIP joint and infection necessitating resection of the distal fragment and in one case, fingertip amputation ([101]; Fig. 2.43).

Henry presented a technique in 18 patients where a headless cannulated compression screw was placed across a 4-month-old nonunion site through a distal percutaneous stab incision [102]. The nonunion site was manually compressed under fluoroscopic guidance and stabilized with a guide wire. The screw was advanced across the fracture site so that it countersunk into the distal tuft and remained under the subchondral bone of the DIP joint. All 18 patients went on to painless

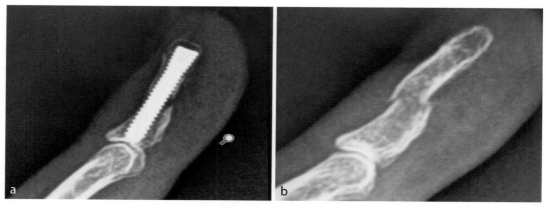

Fig. 2.43 a, b Nonunion distal phalanx fixed with a headless compression screw

bony union at an average of 9 weeks. There were no complications reported.

Profundus Tendon Avulsions

Classification and Diagnosis

FDP terminal avulsions are common injuries that are caused by forced hyperextension of the DIP while the finger is actively flexing. When the eccentric extension load on the FDP exceeds the mechanical strength of its terminal insertion, the flexor tendon either avulses off the bone or pulls off the volar tip of the distal phalanx. The size of the fragment can vary from a fleck of bone to more than 50% of the joint surface. There may also be an associated metaphyseal fracture of the distal phalanx (Figs. 2.44a, b). This injury is known as the "jersey finger," because of the classic mechanism of injury seen in football and rugby players. When a player forcefully grabs the jersey of an opponent to hinder his forward progress, the finger will be wrenched into hyperextension as the opponent advances. The player may hear or feel a sudden pop, usually in the ring finger. On the sidelines, a "jammed finger" is often diagnosed, and the player is sent back out to play. The initial pain and swelling in the finger preclude motion. Therefore, it may take several weeks for the athlete to realize that he is unable to actively flex the DIP joint, and there may be additional difficulty in flexing the PIP joint (Fig. 2.45). Waiting too long to surgically

treat an FDP avulsion can make it impossible to repair the tendon primarily and may necessitate a flexor tendon reconstruction. How long one can delay primary repair depends on how far up the finger the flexor tendon has retracted.

Pertinent Anatomy of FDP Tendon Rupture

The anatomy of the flexor tendon and the mechanism of injury determine what type of injury occurs. Interestingly, the ring finger is the most common digit that sustains an FDP rupture [103]. Several theories have been proposed regarding such ruptures:

1. The ring finger FDP tendon is anatomically most tethered to the other FDP tendons so that hyperextension of that digit will be least accommodated on the flexor side.
2. The insertion of the ring PDP is weaker than the other FDP insertions [104].
3. The lumbrical muscle to the ring FDP is bipennate, further tethering the tendon [105].
4. In full grip, the ring finger juts out 5 mm farther than the other digits making it more vulnerable to injury (longer lever arm).

The extent of retraction of the tendon after rupture is the basis of the classification system of these injuries. Although the presence and size of an accompanying bony avulsion is an important determinant for retraction, the vincular anatomy of the FDP is critical to this process. The FDP possesses and a vinculum longa (VL) at the level

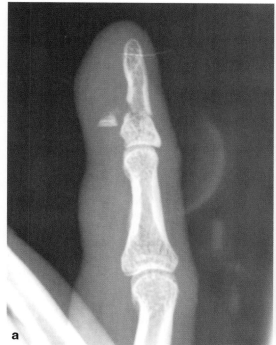
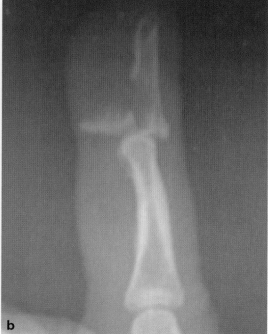

a

b

Fig. 2.44 a Flexor digitorum profundus (FDP) with a "fleck" bony avulsion. The flexor tendon may or may not be attached to the bony fragment. If it is, it is caught at the A-4 pulley. Note the transverse metaphyseal fracture.

b Bony avulsion involving 50% of the joint surface. If the flexor profundus is still attached to the tendon, then it is easily attached with a screw. (Note the dorsal subluxation of the distal phalanx)

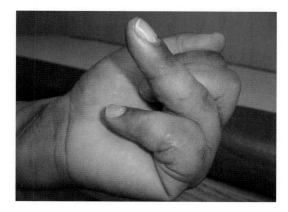

Fig. 2.45 Inability to flex the DIP joint of the ring finger from a closed FDP rupture, the "jersey finger." *DIP* distal interphalangeal joint, *FDP* flexor digitorum profundus tendon

of the PIP joint and a vinculum brevis (VB) just proximal to the DIP joint. When the FDP avulses off its insertion, there will be no retraction with an intact VB. The VB will rupture before the VL and if the VL is intact, the tendon will not retract beyond the PIP. If both vincula are ruptured, assuming there is no attached bone fragment at the tip of the tendon, the tendon will retract into the palm. Rupturing both vinculae has the added significance of detaching critical blood supply to the tendon. It is estimated that one-half of FDP ruptures are bony avulsions.

Leversedge et al. described a "watershed" region near the insertion point of the FDP [106]. There are interosseous vessels at the insertion that arise from the distal phalanx, which feed the terminal tendon at the volar aspect of the tendon. Two millimeters proximal to this, another leash of vessels emanating from the distal phalanx supplies the dorsum of the tendon. Between that complex of vessels and the blood supply coming from the VB, there is an area of hypovascularity measuring about 3.5 mm, which is particularly vulnerable to rupture with eccentric traction. This

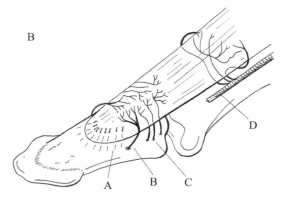

Fig. 2.46 Vascular diagram of the terminal flexor tendon. Note the leash of vessel emanating from the distal phalanx (a, b, c) and the 1-cm hiatus between c and d. That area is a weak zone and prone to rupture. Thus, when the tendon ruptures, there is always a small distal stump still on the distal phalanx (By JR Waterman)

Table 2.3 Modified version of Leddy and Packer classification system of FDP avulsion [107]

Type 1	Full FDP retraction into the palm. Both vincula are torn and there is no bony avulsion
Type 2	FDP retracts to the PIP joint. VB is torn and VL is intact. Small volar avulsion attached to the tendon (Fig. 2.47)
Type 3	FDP retracts to the distal end of the A4 pulley (Fig. 2.44a). VB and VL are intact. Large bony avulsion catches on the end of the pulley preventing further retraction
Type 4	Large volar fragment trapped at the A4 pulley but the FPD detaches from the bone and retracts into the palm. VB and VL are both torn
Type 5	Volar fragment in the presence of either an intra-articular or extra-articular fracture of the distal phalanx (Fig. 2.44b)

Tendon retraction is variable depending on the size of the bony fragment and VB and VL continuity
FDP flexor digitorum profundus tendon, *PIP* proximal interphalangeal joint, *VB* vinculum brevis, *VL* vinculum longa

is also why there is usually a tendon remnant of a few millimeters still left attached to the distal phalanx after an avulsion (Fig. 2.46).

Classification of Injury

Leddy and Packer devised a classification system of FDP avulsion based on the extent of FDP retraction, together with the presence and size of a bone fragment at the end of the tendon [107]. This system has more recently been modified to reflect whether the FDP is still attached to the avulsed bone allowing retraction of FTP to the distal end of the A-2 and A-4 pulleys, as well as whether there was the presence of a separate distal phalanx fracture (see Table 2.3 and Figs. 2.44a, b, 2.47).

Diagnosis

The primary presentation is an inability to actively flex the DIP joint (Fig. 2.45). This is best tested with the hand, palm up on a flat surface and the other joints blocked in extension. At rest, the DIP joint assumes a more extended posture than the other digits. Thus, the "cascade effect" of the digits is disrupted, and the ulnar digits sit in more PIP and DIP flexion than the radial ones.

The clinical examination becomes more unclear if the patient is unwilling or unable to flex the digit because of pain. Additionally, when

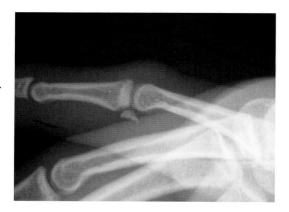

Fig. 2.47 FDP retraction to the PIP joint carrying with it a bony avulsion. *FDP* flexor digitorum profundus tendon, *PIP* proximal interphalangeal joint

there is minimal retraction of the tendon, i.e., type 3, the DIP may appear to flex actively. Injection of a local anesthetic into the finger can assist with the examination but it is important to block (PIP) flexor digitorum sublimis (FDS) flexion when testing for FDP function.

Local palpation along the course of the tendon is important, given that the point of maximal tenderness may be a clue to the location of the

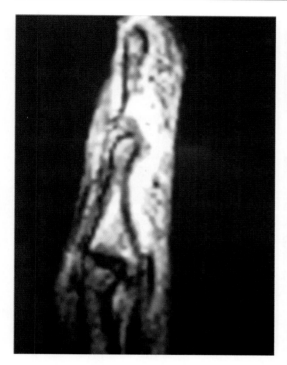

Fig. 2.48 Sagittal view profundus tendon rupture to the PIP joint where it is tethered by the vinculum longa (VL). *PIP* proximal interphalangeal joint

retracted tendon end even in the palm. An X-ray of the finger will locate the location of a bony avulsion but, as we have seen, may not determine the extent of retraction. Although ultrasound has been recommended as a noninvasive method of determining retraction, MRI (sagittal section; Fig. 2.48) is helpful in making the diagnosis and delineating the level of retraction. Locating the source of the retraction obviates the need to make a large exploratory incision [108].

Surgical Indications: Surgical Techniques

Surgical Management

It is wholly unfortunate that so many of these go undetected for 3–4 weeks, considering the simplicity of diagnosing a complete closed FDP rupture. Management decisions hinge on the time interval from injury to treatment, the extent of tendon retraction, and the presence of a bone fragment.

Depending on how far down the actual tendon end has retracted will determine the maximal time that can elapse from the time of the injury until primary repair. If the tendon end has retracted into the palm (type 1), repair should take place within 2 weeks optimally. If the tendon has retracted to the distal end of the A-2 pulley (type 2), the tendon repair can be done within 3 weeks. If the tendon has avulsed with a large volar fragment and the tendon end is still attached to bone, the tendon will not retract beyond the A-4 pulley (type 3). One must be careful to distinguish between a type 3 and type 4 avulsion. X-rays will not be helpful in this case. Ultrasound or MRI will reveal a proximal FDP retraction.

Acute injuries diagnosed within 2 weeks are managed with direct repair, regardless of avulsion type. A variety of techniques have been described. The goal of treatment is secure fixation of the tendon to bone (or bone to bone), so that early postoperative active and passive mobilization can commence.

For pure tendon injuries, the FDP can be secured to the distal phalanx by passing locking sutures (2.0 monofilament/4-strand repair, Bunnell or Kessler) through the tendon end and passing the suture through the distal phalanx, sterile matrix and nail plate distal to the lunula then tying them over a dorsal button. Great care must be exercised to avoid over compressing the nail plate with the button so as to avoid nail necrosis. Also, severe subungual infection and even osteomyelitis has been reported using this technique [109].

When the tendon end is retracted into the palm, it may be difficult to pass the tendon through the intact pulley system or Camper's chiasm. These structures frequently need to be dilated to allow the tendon to go through. The use of a seven-French pediatric feeding tube can aid in passing the tendon through the A-2 pulley. The FDP can be passed either through the chiasm or around it then passed distally under the A-4 pulley. The end of the tendon is secured with a Bunnell or a Kessler stitch pattern using a 3.0-monofilament 2 or 4 strands, and attached to the volar base of the distal phalanx which has been partially decorticated at the attachment site on the volar aspect of the proximal end of the distal phalanx. It is attached to the distal phalanx via suture passed

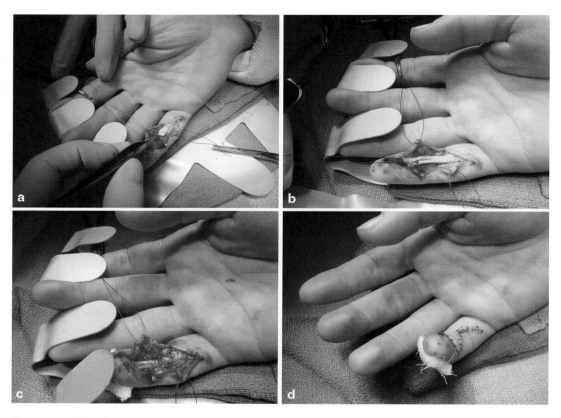

Fig. 2.49 a Closed profundus rupture retracted to the proximal phalanx level. **b** FDP advanced to its insertion checked for tension of the repair. **c** Graft inset and tied over a dorsal button. **d** Repair complete, normal cascade effect reestablished. *FDP* flexor digitorum profundus tendon (Source: [125], Fig. 2.37, [127] Used with permission from The American Society for Surgery of the Hand)

through the distal phalanx with Keith needles and tied over a padded button on the nail plate about 4–5 mm distal to the lunula (Figs. 2.49a–d).

Great care must also be exercised to avoid over-tensioning the repair, since this would lead to the quadriga effect in the other digits where they lose flexion power because of the common muscle belly the FDP tendons share. The distal tendon remnant can then be sutured to the repair using a 3.0 or 4.0 FiberWire. Biomechanical studies by Silva showed that the repair strength exceeded the loads created by early active ROM exercises [110]. The suture and button are removed at 6 weeks. Complications include nail bed injury, skin necrosis under the button, suture rupture at the button, infection, and late tendon rupture. Another problem with the pull-out, dorsal button technique as that the monofilament suture can stretch over time causing the tendon to pull away from the bone and the ensuing gap can lead to rupture of the repair.

Suture anchors can also be used successfully to avoid problems with the nail bed and tendon to bone gapping. Two pilot holes are drilled into the distal phalanx at 45° to the long axis of the finger directed proximally. This increases the pull-out strength and diminishes the probability of gap formation between the tendon and the bone of the construct. Depending on the size of the distal phalanx, two mini or micro sutures are used, each with two strands. If the anchors are metallic, fluoroscopy can be used to ascertain correct placement of the anchors. Biomechanical strength of the construct exceeds the requirements for passive ROM exercise. Failure occurred when the anchors came out of the bone (i.e., in osteoporotic bone) or the suture tore at the attachment site to the anchor.

Contrastively, McCallister et al. in comparing suture anchors and the pull-out button technique, found identical functional outcomes in both groups with regard to ROM and grip strength, active ROM and incidence of contracture [111]. Patients how underwent suture anchor repair returned to work faster than the pull-out group. Ruchelsman et al. have begun to recommend combined use of pull-out wires and bone anchors, resulting in a four-strand repair [112]. This will exhibit greater pull-out strength than anchors alone, especially in osteopenic bone, and less gap formation than pull-out sutures alone.

Lee et al. compared four different anchoring techniques [113]. One was the classic Bunnell pull-out technique with a dorsal button. Two other techniques included suture anchors alone with different suture configurations and a fourth combined both techniques. The combined technique of anchors and pull-out sutures was three-fold stronger than either technique alone. Also, there was no gap formation seen with this technique, something critically important in maintaining the insertional strength of the FDP repair during early active ROM and the long term.

Brustein et al. in a cadaver study compared the pull-out button technique with single mini (1.8 mm) versus dual micro (1.4 mm) anchors and found that both the pull-out button and the single-anchor technique were far inferior in terms of pull-out strength than the dual micro anchors [114]. Also, the failures in the button technique occurred at the knot over the button and the failures of the anchors occurred at the suture anchor junction or by pulling out of the anchor.

Bidwai et al. studied 37 patients treated with the button-over-nail technique in patients who had either closed avulsions or FDP lacerations near its insertion [115]. The final ROM between the groups was not statistically significant at 43° for open lacerations and 35° for closed avulsions. Complications included tendon ruptures, tendon adherence and DIP flexion contracture, wound infection, and one swan-neck deformity. In all 7/37 had complications. There were no cosmetic nail deformities.

When there are bony avulsions, internal fixation techniques using interfragmentary mini-fragment screws, K-wires, and interosseous wires may be used. Assuming that the tendon attachments to the bone are intact, these can be treated with screw fixation (Figs. 2.50a–c).

If the fragment is large enough, a mini-fragment plate can be used in addition.

If patients present more than 2–3 weeks post injury, management decisions are much

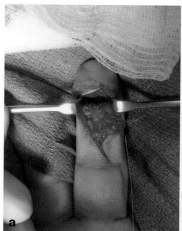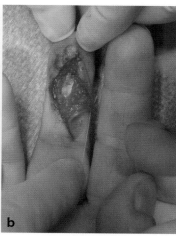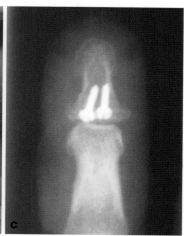

Fig. 2.50 a The Leddy type 3 fracture/FDP avulsion depicted on X-ray in Fig. 2.44. In (a) the tendon bone end is just proximal to the retractors and the dark space above is the recipient bed. **b** The tendon is reattached and secured with cortical screws. **c** X-ray of the volar fragment secured with cortical screws. *FDP* flexor digitorum profundus tendon

less straightforward. In those cases where bony avulsions are large enough to have no retraction or minimal retraction and intact vincular blood supply to the tendon, excellent results can be anticipated, even with delays of 6–8 weeks. However, when retraction has occurred, other considerations must be entertained.

At 3 weeks, it may be impossible to advance the tendon from the palm up to the fingertip. Myostatic contraction and fibrosis of the FDP muscle and collapse of the pulley system are the main obstacles. After the acute rupture, hematoma develops in the flexor sheath, contributing to the fibrosis. If primary advancement is not possible but the pulleys are intact, then a primary tendon graft can be used. Supposing the pulley system has collapsed, then the options include a two-stage tendon reconstruction using Silastic rods, an FDP tenodesis around the DIP joint, or a DIP arthrodesis.

Ruchelsman et al. summarized the evidence-based criteria for the management of terminal FDP avulsions [112]:

- Locking suture configuration are stronger.
- Nonabsorbable braided suture are stronger than monofilament.
- Gapping is a persistent problem with pullout suture.
- Two micro-anchors are stronger than one mini anchor.
- Pull out remains a problem with suture anchors.
- A technique combining suture anchors and pull-out buttons is much stronger than either technique separately.

Post-op Management

Rehabilitation

Initially, a dorsal-blocking splint is worn with the wrist in neutral flexion, MPs at 90° flexion, and the PIPs in extension. At 7–10 days, passive ROM exercises and active finger motion with wrist tenodesis can be started. At 4 weeks, one can begin place-and-hold and joint blocking exercises with the PIP and DIP in flexion. This will help to isolate motion at a given joint by stabilizing adjacent joints. The dorsal clocking splint can be removed at 6 weeks. Resistive grip is started at 10–12 weeks. No heavy lifting is allowed for 6 months.

Outcomes and Complications of Treatment

Although several studies have reported long-term loss of extension of 10–15° at the DIP, others have had no loss of motion at all [116]. Moiemen et al. showed in their study that nearly 70 % of their patients lost more than half their normal DIP motion at final follow-up [117]. Variables include type of repair, interval from injury to treatment, type of injury, and quality of the rehabilitation regimen. To date, there has been no level 1 or level 2 evidence to recommend a course of treatment.

Patients who present late for treatment cannot be treated by primary repair. The timing of primary repair has already been discussed and it depends on the type of rupture. There are patients who remain asymptomatic despite the loss of DIP flexion. Those can be left alone. If the DIP becomes unstable or hyperextends when a patient tries to grip an object, a DIP tenodesis or arthrodesis should be considered. In young patients or high-performance athletes or musicians, secondary one- or two-stage tendon reconstructions should be considered understanding that the tendon graft will have to be placed through or around an intact FDS tendon.

DIP Joint Dislocations

Introduction

Dislocations of the DIP joint are quite unusual owing to the short lever arm of applied stresses to the tip of the finger but when they occur these forces can hyperflex, hyperextend, shear, or cause lateral stress to the fingertip tearing the collateral ligaments. These dislocations can be open or closed. Many of these dislocations are irreducible by closed means due to soft tissue interposition. Early intervention is key to restoration of a functional pain free joint. These dislocations can be open as well with the head of the middle phalanx herniating through the volar DIP crease.

Classification and Diagnosis

Stability of the DIP joint relies on its primary and secondary stabilizers. The ligamentous apparatus, the collateral ligaments, and the volar plate, which are intimate with the joint, provide a checkrein to hyperextension and lateral stress. The arrangement of the ligaments is similar to the PIP joint. Secondary restraint is provided by the insertions of the terminal flexor and extensor tendons. Curiously, the volar plate in the DIP joint, which is confluent with the terminal extent of the FDS insertion, has no formal checkrein ligaments, and is relatively weaker than the volar plate in the PIP joint. This explains the proximal avulsion of the volar plate from the middle phalanx during dorsal DIP dislocation (Fig. 2.51a).

Nonoperative Treatment

The mechanism of injury is hyperextension, hyperflexion, and shear or lateral deviation. These are generally closed, but sometimes the head of the middle phalanx can herniate volarly through the skin. If the injuries are indeed closed, they can be reduced under digital block anesthesia. Reduction of the dislocation is accomplished by longitudinal traction, volarly directed pressure on the dorsal rim of the proximal distal phalanx, and then downward pressure to flex the DIP joint. The reduction should be "crisp" and allow full active ROM. Any "soft" or "rubbery" feel signals that the reduction is incomplete and in all likelihood a result of soft tissue interposition either tendon or ligament.

Hyperextension of the DIP joint should be avoided, given that it can irreducibly alter the dislocation, secondary to volar plate interposition. A post reduction X-ray is necessary to confirm a stable, congruent reduction. If the reduction is unstable but congruent, the joint can be stabilized with a longitudinal K-wire for 3 weeks. If the reduction is stable, treatment is closed, and the DIP joint is placed into an extension block splint for about 3 weeks, at about 20° of flexion, using a dorsal-blocking splint. Full flexion is allowed at 1 week. After 3 weeks, full ROM exercises can begin. If the dislocation is open, a meticulous incision and drainage (I&D) prior to reduction must be done or the reduction will force the outside contamination into the wound predisposing to infection.

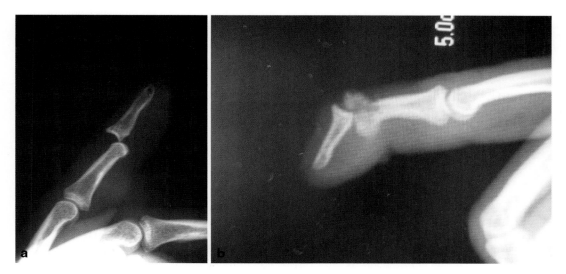

Fig. 2.51 a Dorsal dislocation of the distal interphalangeal joint. These can be usually reduced closed. **b** Irreducible DIP dislocation with soft tissue interposition. *DIP* distal interphalangeal joint

Surgical Indications: Surgical Techniques

One should be suspicious of any residual increased joint space. Soft tissue interposition will render the dislocation irreducible (Fig. 2.51b), for which there may be several causes.

For instance, the volar plate may avulse off the middle phalanx and interpose into the site. Additionally, the FDP terminus may be entrapped, either pushing the head of the middle phalanx to the ulnar side or having the head herniate through the FDP itself, which may or may not rupture the tendon [118]. Sesamoid bones have been found interposed in the DIP joint. Abouzahr et al. found 12 irreducible dorsal dislocations of the DIP in the literature, the majority of which were sports injuries (e.g., attempting to catch a ball) [14, 119]. The ring and long fingers were most affected. Nine of the 12 were open injuries. The mechanism of irreducibility was due to volar plate avulsion and interposition and FDP entrapment. In this case, longitudinal traction will only tighten the FDP, making it even more entrapped. Also, there may be fracture fragments or even sesamoid bones interposed ([120]; Fig. 2.52).

Though most dislocations are dorsal, volar dislocations have been described. These usually coincide with terminal extensor disruption leading to the view that they are nothing more than mallet fingers. Irreducible volar dislocation with extensor tendon interposition in the joint has also been reported [121]. If the closed reduction is congruent but unstable, stabilize with a K-wire for 4 weeks then start ROM.

Irreducible and open dislocations must be treated open. All joint structures must be addressed, and if the FDP is ruptured, it must be repaired.

Simultaneous Dislocations of the DIP and PIP Joints (Fig. 2.53)

These are usually high-energy, dorsal dislocations resulting from sports injuries. These are more common in males than females, affect the dominant hand, and primarily involve the fifth finger but has even been described in the thumb [122]. The mechanism of injury is a hyperextension force applied to the fingertip tearing the volar plate, dislocating the DIP. If the force is still not dissipated, the energy will be transmitted to the PIP, which will result in further dislocation. This is generally treated with gentle longitudinal traction on the finger under a digital block. The PIP is reduced, first easing the tension on the ORL then the DIP is addressed [123].

Single and double dislocations involving the DIP joint must be addressed promptly. Any delay will make closed reduction difficult, if not impossible [116]. Even if the joint is reduced, it is

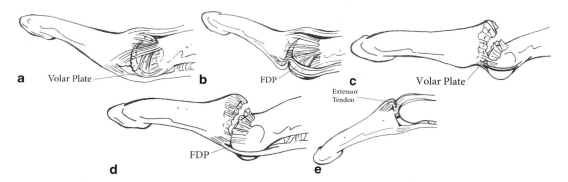

Fig. 2.52 Mechanism of soft tissue entrapment into DIP joint rendering the dislocation irreducible. *DIP* distal interphalangeal joint. **a** Volar plate entrapment. **b** Flexor tendon interposition, the condyle can push the tendon radially too. **c** Herniation of the condyle through the volar plate. **d** Herniation of the condyle through the flexor tendon. **e** Extensor tendon interposition (With Permission from JR Waterman)

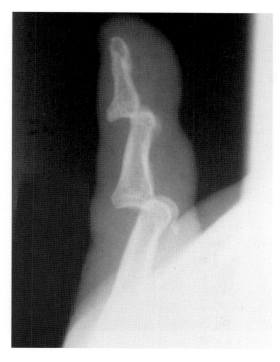

Fig. 2.53 Simultaneous double dislocation of the PIP joint and DIP joint. *PIP* proximal interphalangeal joint, *DIP* distal interphalangeal joint

difficult to maintain, since the joint capsule contracts and disruption in the joint space will significantly derange the metabolism of the hyaline cartilage and synovium in the joint. Following this, degenerative change in the joint surfaces is very rapid.

If a patient presents more than 1–2 weeks after injury with a DIP dislocation, closed reduction of any kind will be impossible because of scar formation. These will always require open reduction internal fixation. In these cases, degenerative joint disease is likely and arthrodesis of the DIP joint is the likely outcome [123].

Pilon Fracture Dislocations of the DIP joint

Dorsal fracture dislocations of the DIP joint can result in impaction of the volar base of the distal phalanx on the dorsal head of the middle phalanx. There is usually significant comminution at the base. Similar to the PIP joint, there may be a large volar lip fracture of the distal phalanx with or

without FDP rupture. This fragment may be large enough to render the joint unstable, even after closed reduction. The goal is to establish enough congruent surface to allow a functional ROM of the DIP joint and to prevent dorsal subluxation of the distal phalanx. Closed reduction is often unsuccessful There have been several methods proposed in the literature for dealing with distal phalangeal volar lip deficits in the face of dorsal dislocations. These have included:

1. *Closed Reduction and Extension Block Splinting.* This involves a closed reduction under X-ray control and dorsal splinting at 45° for about 3 weeks. Then the DIP joint is released at about 10° a week afterward. While stability was achieved, DIP motion remained extremely limited [124].
2. *Open Reduction Internal Fixation.* Through a lateral approach, the DIP is reduced and stabilized with a K-wire for 4–6 weeks and the bony step off is back filled with bone graft. The ROM loss at follow-up was up to 45° flexion [116]. All too frequently the fragments may be too small to fix (Fig. 2.54a, b).
3. *Extension Block Pinning.* Allows early active and passive ROM of the DIP joint [125]. Through a mid-lateral approach, the DIP joint is reduced by traction and slight flexion. A 0.045 K-wire is inserted into the terminus of the extensor tendon into the middle phalanx just beyond the rim of the distal phalanx with the DIP joint flexed 5°. The wire is driven distal to proximal, dorsal to volar at an angle of 30° to the long axis of the finger. The finger is taken through a full ROM under fluoroscopy to ensure that the joint stays reduced through the entire range. Immediate full active and PIP joint blocking passive motion was started and the pins were removed at 5 weeks. In this case, the final ROM was 74°. Interestingly, at final follow-up, the volar articular step-off filled in with calcified fibrocartilage recreating the volar lip restoring stability.
4. *Volar Plate Arthroplasty.* In the event that less than 40% of the joint surface remains intact the DIP becomes unstable, volar plate arthroplasty similar to which has been described

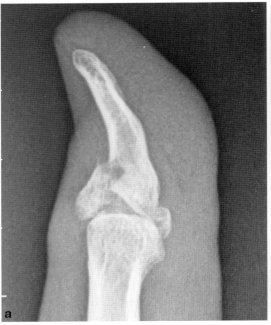

Fig. 2.54 a Pilon fracture of the distal phalanx of the thumb. There is significant disruption of the joint surface despite the absence of dislocation. **b** After open reduc-

tion longitudinal pinning in traction through a lateral approach, restoration of the joint surface and back grafting the resultant bony defect in the metaphysis

in the PIP joint has been tried and met with success. Rettig et al. treated ten patients with chronic fracture dislocations of the DIP joint with significant volar articular surface involvement [126]. At follow-up, his patients had a 12° flexion contracture and an average of 42°. Volar plate arthroplasty, however, is very technically difficult at the DIP joint because of the FDP insertion there.

5. *Primary Arthrodesis.* Primary arthrodesis of the DIP can be considered and affords the patient just one operation to salvage an otherwise irreparable injury.

References

1. Peterson JJ, Bancroft LW. Injuries of the fingers and thumb in the athlete. Clin Sports Medicine. 2006;25(3):527–42.
2. Handoll HHG, Vaghela M. Interventions for treating mallet finger injuries. The Cochrane Database of Systematic Reviews 2004;1.
3. Maitra A, Dorani B. The conservative treatment of mallet finger with a simple splint: a case report. Arch Emerg Med. 1993;10:244–8.
4. Grundberg AB, Reagan DS. Central slip tenotomy for chronic mallet deformity. J Hand Surg Am. 1987;12(4):545–7.
5. Schneider LH. Fractures of the distal phalanx. Hand Clin. 1988;4:537–47.
6. Clayton RA, Court-Brown CM. The epidemiology of musculoskeletal tendinous and ligamentous injuries. Injury. 2008;39:1338–44.
7. Wehbe MA, Schneider LH. Mallet fractures. J Bone Joint Surg. 1984;66A:658–69.
8. Simpson D, McQueen MM, Kumar P. Mallet deformity in Sport. J Hand Surg Br. 2001;26(1):32–3.
9. Costello J, Howes M. Best evidence topic report. Prophylactic antibiotics for subungual hematoma. Emerg Med J. 2004;21:503.
10. Schweitzer TP, Rayan GM. The terminal tendon of the digital extensor mechanism: part 2, Kinematic Study. J Hand Surg. 2004;29A:903–8.
11. Doyle JR. Extensor tendons: acute injuries. In: Green DP, Hotchkiss RN, Peterson WC, editors. Greens operative hand surgery. 4th ed. New York: Churchill Livingston; 1999. p. 195–8.
12. Abouna JM, Brown H. The treatment of mallet finger, the results in a series of 148 consecutive cases and review of the literature. Br J Surg. 1968;55:653–67.
13. Evans RB. Therapeutic management of extensor tendon injuries. Hand Clin. 1984;2(1):157–69.
14. Bunnell SB. Surgery of the hand. 1st ed. Philadelphia: Lippincott. 1944. p 490–3.

15. Katzman BM, Klein DM, Mesa J, Caligiuri DA. Immobilisation of the mallet finger. Effects on the extensor tendon. J Hand Surg Br. 1999;24(1):80–4.

16. Evans D, Weightman B. The Pipflex splint for treatment of mallet finger. J Hand Surg. 1988;13(2):156–8.

17. Mason ML. Ruptures of tendons in the hand: with a study of the tendon insertions in the fingers. Surg Gynecol Obstet. 1930;50:611–24.

18. Smillie IS. Mallet finger. BR J Surg. 1937;24:439–45.

19. Hallberg D, Lindholm A. Subcutaneous rupture of the extensor tendon of the distal phalanx of the finger: "Mallet finger". Brief review of the literature and report on 127 cases treated conservatively. Acta Chir Scand. 1960;119:260–7.

20. Stack G. Mallet finger. Lancet. 1968;2:1303.

21. Pulvertaft RG. Mallet finger. Proceedings of the Second Hand Club. British Society for Surgery of the Hand, 1975; 156.

22. Auchincloss JM. Mallet-finger injuries: a prospective, controlled trial of internal and external splintage. Hand. 1982;14:168–72.

23. Evans RB. Early active short arc motion for the repaired central slip. J Hand Surg. 1994;19A:991–7.

24. Patel MR, Desai SS, Bassini-Lipson L. Conservative management of chronic mallet finger. J Hand Surg Am. 1986;11:570.

25. Okafor B, Mbubaegbu C, Munshi I, Williams DJ. Mallet deformity of the finger. Five year follow-up of conservative treatment. J Bone Joint Surg. 1997;79B:544–7.

26. Garberman SF, Diao E, Peimer CA. Mallet finger: results of early vs. delayed closed treatment. J Hand Surg. 1994;19(5):850–2.

27. Kinninmouth AW, Holbourn FA. A comparative controlled trial of a new perforated splint and a traditional splint in the treatment of mallet finger. J Hand Surg Br. 1986;11(2):261–2.

28. Tocco, Silvio et al. (2013) Effectiveness of cast immobilization in comparison to the gold-standard self-removal orthotic intervention for closed mallet fingers: A randomized clinical trial. J Hand Ther, Volume 26(3):191–201.

29. Villeco JP, Mackin EJ, Hunter JM. Edema: therapists management. In: Hunter JM, Mackin EJ Callahan AD, editors. Rehabilitation of the hand: surgery and therapy. 5th ed. St. Louis: Mosby; 2002. p. 183–93.

30. Colditz JC. Plaster of Paris: the forgotten hand splinting material. J Hand Ther. 2002;15(2):144–57.

31. Warren RA, Norris SH, Ferguson DG. Mallet finger: a trial of two splints. J Hand Surg. 1988;13B:151–3.

32. Pike J, Mulpuri K, Metzger M, Ng G, Wells N, Goertz T. Blinded, prospective, randomized clinical trial comparing volar, dorsal, and custom thermoplastic splinting in treatment of acute mallet finger. J Hand Surg. 2010;35A:580–8.

33. O'Brien L, Bailey M. Single blind, prospective, randomized, controlled trial comparing dorsal aluminum and custom thermoplastic splints to stack splint for acute mallet finger. Arch Phys Med Rehabil. 2011;92:191–8.

34. Flint MH. Some observations on the vascular supply of the nail bed and terminal segments of the finger. Br J Plast Surg. 1955;8:186–95.

35. Rayan GM, Mullins PT. Skin necrosis complicating mallet finger splinting and vascularity of the distal interphalangeal joint overlying skin. J Hand Surg. 1987;12A:548–52.

36. Groth GN, Wilder DM, Young VL. The impact of compliance on the rehabilitation of patients with mallet finger injuries. J Hand Ther. 1994;7(1):21–4.

37. Jablecki J, Syrko M. Zone 1 extensor tendon lesions: current treatment methods and a review of the literature. Orthop Traumatol Rehab. 2007;9(1):52–62.

38. Eliott RA. Injuries to the extensor mechanism of the hand. Orthop Clin North Am. 1970;1:282–5.

39. Fowler SB. Extensor apparatus of the digits. J Bone Jt Surg Br. 1949;31:477.

40. Maklouf V, Al Deek N. Surgical treatment of chronic mallet finger. Ann Plast Surg. 2011;66:670–2.

41. Bowers HW, Hurst LC. Chronic mallet finger: the use of fowler's central slip release. J Hand Surg. 1978;3:373–6.

42. Chao JD, Sarwahi V, Da Silva YS, Rosenwasser MP, Strauch RJ. Central slip tenotomy for the treatment of chronic mallet finger: an anatomic study. J Hand Surg. 2004;29A:216–9.

43. Hiwatari R, Kuniyoshi K, Aoki M, Hashimoto K, Suzuki T, Takahashi K. Fractional Fowler central slip tenotomy for chronic mallet finger: a cadaveric biomechanical study. J Hansd Surg. 2012;37A:2263–8.

44. Rozmaryn LM. Central slip tenotomy with distal repair in the treatment of severe chronic mallet fingers. J Hand Surg Am. 2014;39(4):773–8.

45. Albertoni WM. The Brooks and Graner procedure for correction of mallet finger. In: Tubiana R, editor. The hand. Vol 3. Philadelphia: WB Saunders; 1988. p. 97–100.

46. Boeck HD, Jaeken R. Treatment of chronic mallet deformity in children by tenodermodesis. J Ped Orthop. 1992;12:351–4.

47. Kardestucer T, Bae DS, Waters PM. The restults of tendermodesis for severe chronic mallet finger deformity in children. J Ped Ortho. 2008;28(1):81–5.

48. Iselin F, Levame J, Godoy J. Simplified technique for treating mallet finger: tenodermodesis. J Hand Surg. 1977;2(2):118–21.

49. Kon M, Bloem JJ. Treatment of mallet fingers by tenodermodesis. Hand. 1982;14(2):174–6.

50. Sorene E, Goodwin D. Tenodermodesis for established mallet finger deformity. Scad J Plast Surg Hand Surg. 2004;38:43–5.

51. Kaleli T, Ozturk C, Ersozlu S. External fixation for surgical treatment of a mallet finger. J Hand Surg. 2003;28B(3):228–30.

52. Lind J, Hansen B. A new operation for chronic mallet finger. J Hand Surg. 1989;14:347–9.

53. Ulker E, Cengiz A, Ozge E. Repair of chronic mallet finger using Mitek micro arc bone anchor. Ann Plastic Surg. 2005;5:393–6.

54. Thompson JS, Littler JW, Upton J. The spiral oblique retinacular ligament reconstruction (SORL). J Hand Surg Am. 1978;3(5):482–7.

55. Kleinman WB, Petersen DP. Oblique retinacular ligament reconstruction for chronic mallet finger deformity. J Hand Surg. 1984;9A:399–404.

56. Kayana K, Wada T, Yamashita T. The Thomson procedure for chronic mallet deformity. J Hand Surg Am. 2013;38(7):1295–300.

57. Gu YP, Zhu SM. A new technique for repair of acute or chronic extensor tendon injuries in Zone I. J Bone Joint Surg Br. 2012;94(5):668–70.

58. Wang L, Zhang X, Liu Z, Huang X, Zhu H, Yu Y. Tendon-bone graft for tendinoous mallet fingers following failed splinting. J Hand Surg Am. 2013;38(12):2353–9.

59. Robb WAT. The results of treatment of mallet finger. J Bone Joint Surg. 1959;41B:546–9.

60. Tabbai GN, Bastidas N, Sharma S. Closed mallet thumb injury: a review of the literature and case study of the use of MRI in deciding treatment. Plast Recon Surg. 2009;124:222–6.

61. Miura T. Extension block pinning using a small external fixator for mallet finger fractures. J Hand Surg Am. 2013;38(12):2348–52.

62. Din KM, Meggit BF. Mallet thumb. J Bone Joint Surg. 1983;65B:606–7.

63. Verdan DE. In: Flynn JE, editor. Hand surgery. 2nd ed. Baltimore: Williams & Wilkins; 1975. p. 152.

64. Nishumura R, Metsuava S, Miyauki T, Uchida M. Bony mallet thumb. Hand Surg. 2013;18(1):107–9.

65. Zancolli E. Structural and dynamic bases of hand surgery. 2nd ed. Philadelphia: JB Lippincott; 1979.

66. Husain SN, Dietz JF, Kalainov DM, Lautenschlager EP. A biomechanical study of distal interphalangeal subluxation after mallet fracture injury. J Hand Surg. 2008;33A:26–30.

67. Kalainov, David M. et al. . Nonsurgical Treatment of Closed Mallet Finger Fractures. J Hand Surg Am. 2005; 30(3):580–6.

68. Geyman JP, Fink K, Sullivan SD. Conservative versus surgical treatment of mallet finger: a pooled quantitative literature evaluation. J Am Board Fam Prac. 1998;11(5):382–90.

69. Weber P, Segmüeller H. Non-surgical treatment of mallet fractures involving more than one third of the joint surface: 10 cases. Handchir Mikrochir Plast Chir. 2008;40:145–8.

70. Stern PJ, Kastrup JJ. Complications and prognosis of treatment of mallet finger. J Hand Surg. 1988;13A:329–34.

71. Lubahn JD. Mallet finger fractures: a comparison of open and closed technique. J Hand Surg. 1989;14A:394–6.

72. Niechayev IA. Conservative and operative treatment of mallet fingers. Plastic and Reconstr Surg. 1985;76(4):580–5.

73. Hofmeister EP, Mazurek MT, Shin AY, Bishop AT. Extension block pinning for large mallet fractures. J Hand Surg. 2003;28A:453–9.

74. Pegoli L, Toh S, Arai K, Fukuda A, Nishikawa S, Vallejo IG. The Ishiguro extension block technique for the treatment of mallet finger fracture: indications and clinical results. J Hand Surg Br. 2003;28:15–7.

75. Lee SK, Kim KJ, Yang DS, Moon KH, Choy WS. Modified extension–block fixation technique for the treatment of bony mallet finger. Orthopedics. 2010;33(10):728.

76. Chung DW, Lee JH. Anatomic reduction of mallet fractures using extension block and additional intrafocal pinning techniques. Clin Orthop Surg. 2012;4:72–6.

77. Jupiter JB, Sheppard JE. Tension wire fixation of avulsion fractures in the hand. clinical Orthop and Relat Res. 1987; (214):113–20.

78. Bischoff R, Buechler U, De Roche R, Jupiter J. Clinical results of tension band fixation of avulsion fractures of the hand. J Hand Surg. 1994;19A:1019–26.

79. Fritz D, Lutz M, Arora R. Delayed single Kirschner wire compression technique for mallet fracture. J Hand Surg. 2005;30B:180–4.

80. Badia A. Riano F. A simple fixation method for unstable bony mallet finger. J Hand Surg Am. 2004;29:1051–5.

81. Kang HJ, Lee SK. Open accurate reduction for irreducible mallet fractures through a new pulp traction technique with primary tendon repair. J Plast Surg Hand Surg. 2012;46:438–43.

82. Yamanaka K, Sasaki T. Treatment of mallet fractures using compression fixation pins. J Hand Surg. 1999;24B:358–60.

83. Kronlage SC, Faust D. Open reduction and screw fixation of mallet fractures. J Hand Surg Br. 2004;29(2):135–8.

84. Kang HJ, Shin SJ, Kang ES. Complications of operative treatment for mallet fractures of the distal phalanx. J Hand Surg. 2001;26B:28–31.

85. Zhang X, Meng H, Shao X, Wen S, Zhu H, Mi X. Pull-out wirefixation for acute mallet finger fractures with k-wire stabilizationof the distal interphalangeal joint. J Hand Surg. 2010;35A:1864–9.

86. Lu J, Jiang J, Xu L, Xu W, Xu J. Modification of the pull in suture technique for mallet finger. Ann Plast Surg. 2013;70:30–3.

87. Rocchi L, Genitiempo M, Fanfani F. Percutaneous fixation of mallet fractures by the "umbrella handle" technique. J Hand Surg. 2006;31B:407–12.

88. Phadnis J, Yousaf S, Little N, Chidambaram R, Mok D. Open reduction internal fixation of the unstable mallet fracture. Tech Hand Up Ext Surg. 2010;14:155–9.

89. Reissner L, Gienck M, Weishaupt D, Platz A, Kilgus M. Clinical and radiological results after operative treatment of mallet fracture using Kirschner wire technique. Handchir Mikrochir Plast Chir. 2012;44(1):6–11.

90. Teoh LC, Lee JYL. Mallet fractures: a novel approach to internal fixation using a hook plate. J Hand Surg. 2007;32B:24–30.

91. Tung KY, Tsai MF, Chang SH, Huang WC, Hsiao HT. Modified tenodesis method for treatment of mallet fractures. Ann Plast Surg. 2012;69:622–6.

92. Lucchina S, Badia A, Nistor A, Fusetti C. Surgical treatment options for unstable mallet fractures. Plast Recon Surg. 2011;2:599–600.

93. Damron TA, Engber WD, Lange RH, McCabe R, Damron LA, Ulm M. Biomechanical analysis of mallet finger fracture fixation techniques. J Hand Surg Am. 1993;18(4):600–7.

94. Cheung PYC, Fung B, Ip WY. Review on mallet finger treatment. Hand Surg. 2012;3(17):439–47.

95. Lee SK, Kim HJ, Lee KW, Kim KJ, Choy WS. Modified pull out wire suture technique for the treatment of chronic bony mallet finger. Ann Plast Surg. 2010;65:466–70.

96. Roser SE, Gellman H. Comparison of nail bed repair versus trephination for subungual hematomas in children. J Hand Surg. 1999;24A:1166–70.

97. DaCruz DJ, Slade RJ, Malone W. Fractures of the distal phalanges. J Hand Surg. 1988;13B:350–2.

98. Chim H, Teoh LC, Yong FC. Open reduction and interfragmentary screw fixation for symptomatic nonunion of distal phalangeal fractures. J Hand Surg. 2008;33(1):71–6.

99. Ozcelik B, Kabakas F, Mersa B, Purisa H, Sezer I, Erturer F. Treatment of nonunions of the distal phalanx with olecranon bone graft. J Hand Surg. 2009;34E:638–42.

100. Meijis CM, Verhofstad MH. Symptomatic nonunion of a distal Phalanx fracture: treatment with a percutaneous compression screw. J Hand Surg. 2009;34A:1127–9.

101. Voche P, Merle M. Pillot D. Pseudoarthrosis et. retards de consolidation de la phlanage distale des doigts longs. A propose de 13 cas. Rev Chir Orthop Repatriace Appar Mot. 1995;81:485–90.

102. Henry M. Variable pitch headless compression screw treatment of distal phalangeal nonunions. Tech Hand Surg. 2010;14:230–3.

103. Kovacic J, Bergfeld J. Return to play issues in upper extremity injuries. Clin Surg J Sports Med. 2005;15:448.

104. Manske PR, Lesker PA. Avulsion of the ring finger flexor digitorum profundus rendon: an experimental study. Hand. 1978;10:52.

105. LunnPG LDW. "Rugby finger" avulsion of the profundus ring finger. J Hand Surg Br. 1984;9:69.

106. Leversedge FJ, Ditsios JH, Goldfarb CA, Silva MJ, Gelberman RH, Boyer MI. Vascular anatomy of the human flexor digitorum profundus tendon insertion. J Hand Surg. 2002;5A:806–12.

107. Leddy JP, Packer JW. Avulsion of the profundus tendon insertion in athletes. J Hand Surg. 1977;1A:66–9.

108. Boyer M. Flexor tendon injury In: Green DP, editor. Operative hand surgery. Philadelphia: Elsevier Churchill Livingstone; 2005. p. 218.

109. Kang N, Marsh D, Dewar DJ. The morbidity of the button over nail technique for zone I flexor repairs. Should we still be using this technique? J Hand Surg Eur. 2008;33:566–7.

110. Silva MJ, Hollstein SB, Fayazi AH, Adler P, Gelberman RH, Boyer MI. The effects of multiple-strand suture techniques on the tensile properties of repair of the flexor digitorum profundus tendon to bone. J Bone Joint Surg. 1998;10A:1507–14.

111. McCallister WV, Ambrose HC, Katolik LI, Trumble TE. Comparison of pullout button versus suture anchor for zone I flexor tendon repair. J Hand Surg. 2006;2A:246–51.

112. Ruchelsman DE, Christoforou D, Wasserman B, Lee S, Rettig ME. Avulsion injuries of the flexor digitorum profundus tendon. J Am Acad Orthop Surg. 2011;19:152–62.

113. Lee SK, Fajardo M, Kardashian G, Klein J, Tsai P, Christoforo D. Repair of flexor digoitorum profundus to distal phalanx: a biomechanical evaluation of four techniques. J Hand Surg. 2011;36A:1604–9.

114. Brustein M, Pellegrini J, Choueka J, Heminger H, Mass D. Bone suture anchors versus the pullout button for repair of distal profundus tendon injuries: a comparison of strength in human cadaveric hands. J Hand Surg Am. 2001;26(3):489–96.

115. Bidwai ASC, Feldberg L. The button-over-nail technique for zone I flexor tendon injuries. Hand Surg. 2012;17(3):365–9.

116. Horiuchi Y, Itoh Y, Sasaki T. Dorsal dislocation of the DIP joint with fracture of the volar base of the distal phalanx. J Hand Surg. 1989;14B:177–82.

117. Moiemen NS, Elliot D. Primary flexor tendon repair in zone 1. J Hand Surg Br. 2000;25(1):78–84.

118. Rayan GM, Elias LS. Irreducible dislocation of the distal interphalangeal joint caused by long flexor tendon entrapment. Orthopedics. 1981; 4:35–7.

119. Abouzahr MK, Poalete JV. Irreducible dorsal dislocation of the distal interphalangeal joint: case report and literature review. J Trauma. 1947;42(4):743–5.

120. Sabapathy SR, Bose VC, Rex C. Irreducible dislocation of the interphalangeal.

121. Inoue G, Maeda N. Irreducible palmar dislocation of the distal interphalangeal joint of the finger. J Hand Surg. 1987;12A:1077–9.

122. Hutchinson JD, Hooper G, Robb JE. Double dislocation of the digits. J Hand Surg Br. 1991;16:114–5.

123. Kim YS, Song HS, Kim HM, Chung E, Park IJ. Simultaneous double dislocation of the interphalangeal joint in a finger. Arch Orthop Trauma Surg. 2009;129:1387–90.

124. Hamer DW, Quinton DN. Dorsal fracture subluxation of the distal interphalangeal joint of the finger and the interphalangeal joint of the thumb treated by dorsal block splintage. J Hand Surg. 1992;17B:591–4.

125. Xiong G, Zheng W, Wang S. Extension block pinning for the treatment of a dorsal fracture dislocation of the distal interphalangeal joint: case report. J Hand Surg. 2008;33A:869–72.

126. Rettig ME, Dassa G, Raskin KB. Volar plate arthroplasty of the distal interphalangeal joint. J Hand Surg. 2001;26A:940–4.

127. Rozmaryn LM. Distal phalangeal and fingertip injuries. In: Seitz WH, editor. Fractures and dislocations of the hand and fingers. Chicago: American Society for Surgery of the Hand; 2013.

Injuries to the Nail Apparatus

3

Nicole Z. Sommer, M. Colin Rymer and Ryan W. Schmucker

Anatomy

The nail apparatus or perionychium consists of the eponychium, paronychium, hyponychium, nail bed, and nail fold (Fig. 3.1). The nail bed is the soft tissue beneath the nail plate and can be divided into the sterile matrix distally and the germinal matrix proximally. The germinal matrix produces about 90 % of the nail [1] and the sterile matrix keeps the nail adherent to the nail bed by producing a thin layer of cells added to the nail undersurface. [2–4] The nail fold consists of a ventral floor and dorsal roof. The ventral floor is the location of the germinal matrix and the dorsal roof produces the shine on the nail. The hyponychium is the soft tissue distal to the nail bed and the paronychium is the soft tissue on each side of the nail. The soft tissue that covers the nail proximally is referred to as the eponychium. The cuticle extends from the eponychium onto the proximal nail surface, underneath this is the white lunula which marks the distal extent of the germinal matrix.

The radial and ulnar digital nerves trifurcate at the level of the *distal interphalangeal* (DIP) joint with the dorsal branches supplying sensation to the nail. [5] The blood supply to the nail apparatus is provided by terminal branches of the volar digital arteries and the capillary loops they form. [6] Venous drainage is concentrated toward the proximal nail bed and nail fold and then continues along the dorsum of the finger. [7, 8] The lymphatics drain parallel to the venous system. The hyponychium is extremely dense with lymphatics to protect from frequent exposures. [9, 10]

Epidemology

The nail apparatus is the most commonly injured structure in the hand. Injuries occur most often in older children or young adults. The long finger is the most frequently injured digit and distal injuries to the nail apparatus are the most common. Doors are the most encountered method of traumatic injuries to the nail apparatus. [11] Injuries can be subdivided into subungual hematoma, simple laceration, stellate laceration, crush injury or nail avulsion. [12, 13] Crush injuries are the most frequent. There is a 50 % chance of bone involvement with nail bed injuries so X-ray examination is always recommended.

N. Z. Sommer (✉) · M. C. Rymer · R. W. Schmucker
Southern Illinois University School of Medicine,
Institute for Plastic Surgery, 747 N. Rutledge St, 62702
Springfield, IL, USA
e-mail: nsommer@siumed.edu

M. C. Rymer
e-mail: mrymer@siumed.edu

R. W. Schmucker
e-mail: rschmucker@siumed.edu

L. M. Rozmaryn (ed.), *Fingertip Injuries*, DOI 10.1007/978-3-319-13227-3_3,
© Springer International Publishing Switzerland 2015

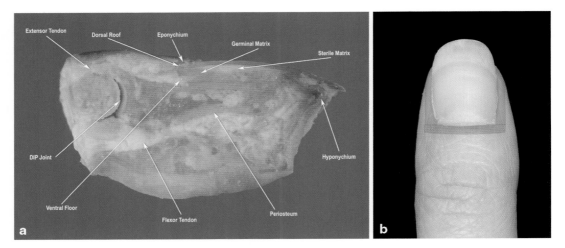

Fig. 3.1 a Nail bed anatomy shown in sagittal section. **b** Surface anatomy of the perionychium consists of the paronychium, hyponychium, eponychium, and nail bed.

Injuries

Subungual Hematoma

Compression injuries to the nail often result in nail bed lacerations with bleeding beneath the nail leading to a subungual hematoma (Fig. 3.2). This fluid collection beneath the nail can lead to severe throbbing pain which is an indication for hematoma drainage. The decision to drain the hematoma versus nail plate removal with exploration has evolved over time. Currently, the recommendation is to remove the nail plate with exploration and repair of the nail bed laceration if the nail edges are disrupted. If the nail edges are intact then hematoma drainage without nail plate removal and exploration is preferred. The percentage of hematoma is no longer an indication for exploration. This is supported by a prospective 2-year study of 48 patients with subungual hematomas that demonstrated no complications of nail deformity with conservative treatment of drainage only, regardless of the hematoma size. [14] More recently, a systematic review of the literature by Dean et al. showed there was no difference in aesthetic outcome when comparing nail bed repair and simple decompression (drainage) [15].

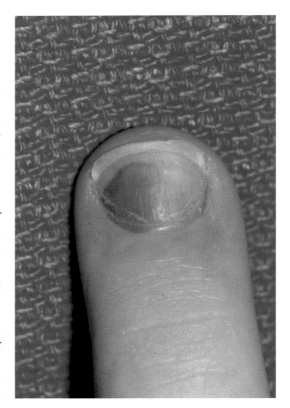

Fig. 3.2 Subungual hematoma.

Subungual hematoma drainage should begin with surgical preparation of the finger or entire hand. This decreases the chance of bacterial inoculation during drainage. We prefer povidone–iodine (betadine) scrub followed by trephination over the hematoma with a battery powered microcautery unit (Fig. 3.3). Once the heated tip is passed through the nail it is cooled by the hematoma which decreases iatrogenic injury to the nail bed. The trephination hole must be large enough to allow continued drainage of the hematoma.

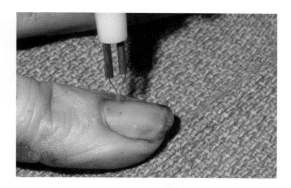

Fig. 3.3 The author's preferred method of subungual hematoma drainage with a battery operated electrocautery unit. Published with kind permission of © Nicole Z. Sommer, MD [2014]. All rights reserved

Nail Bed Injury and Repair

Nail bed lacerations can occur from a sharp injury or crush. The resultant injuries can be subcategorized into simple lacerations, stellate lacerations, or severe crush (Fig. 3.4). Stellate lacerations and crush injuries often involve fragmentation of the nail plate. Great care is taken during nail plate removal to prevent iatrogenic injury to the nail bed. Repair of stellate lacerations can have good outcomes with meticulous approximation of the nail bed segments. The prognosis for crush injuries is poorer because of the nail bed contusion in addition to laceration. A study by Gellman demonstrated that simple nail plate trephination of crush injuries in children produced equal to, or superior results, when compared to nail removal and formal nail bed reconstruction. [16]

Nail bed repair is performed under sterile technique and repair can be successfully performed up to 7 days after injury although early repair is recommended (Fig. 3.5). A digital block is performed with 1 % lidocaine with epinephrine and the finger or entire hand is prepped and draped. The digit is exsanguinated and a tourniquet is placed around the proximal phalanx region of the finger . The nail plate is removed atraumatically with iris scissors or a Kutz elevator. Care is taken to avoid inadvertent injury to the nail bed

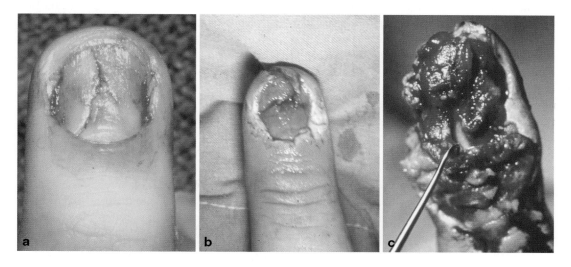

Fig. 3.4 Nail bed laceration classification. **a** Simple nail bed laceration. **b** Stellate nail bed laceration. **c** Crush injury. Published with kind permission of © Nicole Z. Sommer, MD [2014]. All rights reserved

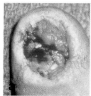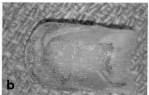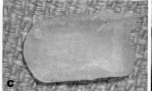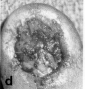

Fig. 3.5 Nail bed repair. **a** Nail bed stellate laceration. **b** Removal of the nail plate. **c** Debridement of the nail plate undersurface. **d** Nail bed following repair with 7–0 chromic sutures. **e** Replacement of the nail plate with drainage hole. Published with kind permission of © Nicole Z. Sommer, MD [2014]. All rights reserved

during nail plate removal with iris scissors. The tips of the scissors should be pointed toward the nail plate and careful spreading in the plane of the nail should be performed distal to proximal. Once removed, the undersurface of the nail is cleaned of any fibrinous debris and the nail plate is soaked in povidone–iodine solution for reapplication if the nail plate is salvageable. Loupe magnification is utilized to inspect the nail bed surface. Conservative debridement is performed along with copious wound irrigation. Repair is performed with simple sutures of 7–0 chromic on a spatulated needle. An alternate method, is the utilization of 2-octylcyanoacrylate (dermabond) for repair. Strauss et al. described this technique and cited equivalent aesthetic and functional results when compared to suture repair. [17]

Postoperatively the nail bed repair must be protected. If the native nail plate is intact, it can be replaced and held either proximally with a horizontal mattress suture through the nail fold or distally with an interrupted suture through the hyponychium. If the eponychial fold is badly damaged, Bristol and Verchere described a figure of eight suture to secure the nail plate that is placed laterally through the paronychial folds [18]. If the nail plate is too badly injured we recommend the use of silicone sheeting or, as a secondary option, non-adherent gauze or suture packet material. Every effort should be made to preserve the native nail, because the use of silicone sheeting is associated with an increased rate of nail deformities, with split nail being the most common. [19] Replacement of the nail, or protection with a secondary material, allows the nail bed repair to be anatomically molded and can splint any associated distal phalanx fracture. [20]

Non-adherent dressings are then applied and an aluminum splint is placed. The patient is seen 5–7 days after the repair and dressings are removed at that time. Continued splinting may be required for pain management and distal phalanx fracture management for an additional 2–3 weeks.

Nail Bed Avulsion

A nail bed avulsion injury presents with the nail bed attached to the undersurface of the nail plate (Fig. 3.6). Often the nail bed laceration is located beneath the eponychial fold and the nail plate remains attached to the distal aspect of the nail bed. A common avulsion injury seen in children is associated with Salter–Harris type I fracture. The distal aspect of the fracture remains attached to the nail plate and the nail plate is displaced above the proximal nail fold. Radiographic evaluation is essential in this type of injury. Adequate reduction of the fracture is accomplished with replacement of the nail plate beneath the nail fold and repair of the nail bed.

The avulsion nail bed injury is managed with removal of the avulsed nail bed from the undersurface of the nail plate and replacement of the nail bed as a free graft. The nail bed survives in a similar fashion to skin grafts by serum imbibition, inosculation, and revascularization. Suture of the free nail bed graft often requires mobilization of the nail fold due to the proximal location of the injury. Two incisions can be placed laterally and perpendicular to the nail fold. This allows elevation of the eponychial fold and visualization of the proximal extent of the injury (Fig. 3.7). After repair of the nail bed avulsion, the nail fold

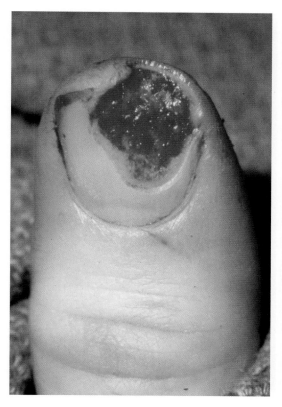

Fig. 3.6 Nail bed avulsion injury. Published with kind permission of © Nicole Z. Sommer, MD [2014].

incisions are approximated. If multiple small pieces of nail bed are avulsed they are all placed as free grafts. The nail bed can be placed directly onto distal phalanx cortex and survive. Rarely, a situation arises where there are multiple small nail bed pieces and removal from the fragmented nail plate could result in further injury. In this case, the nail plate is replaced without an attempt to separate the fragments from the undersurface of the nail plate.

Nail Bed Defect

Assessment of nail bed defects begins with the recognition of involvement of the sterile matrix or germinal matrix and identification of the depth of injury. Partial-thickness injuries to the sterile

or germinal matrix will heal without intervention. Non-repaired full-thickness injuries often result in scarring and nail deformity. For central full-thickness defects, Johnson [21] described releasing incisions at the lateral paronychial fold with nail bed advancement. This technique works for a defect that is less than one third the nail bed width, usually 3–5 mm in size, and good condition of the remaining nail bed [22].

Full-thickness nail bed defects of the sterile matrix can be reconstructed with split-thickness nail bed grafts (Fig. 3.8) [23, 24]. Split-thickness grafts can be obtained from the remaining uninjured nail bed if the defect is less than 50% in size. For defects greater than 50%, a graft must be obtained from an adjacent finger or toe (Fig. 3.9). Harvesting the graft from the toe is more favorable because of the lower risk of nail deformity resulting from grafts harvested too deeply.

Nail bed defects of the germinal matrix require full-thickness germinal matrix grafts, because the deep cells of the germinal matrix are necessary for a new nail to grow. The biggest disadvantage of a full-thickness germinal matrix graft is the loss of nail growth at the donor site.

To harvest a nail bed graft the finger or toe to be used as a donor is anesthetized with a digital block of 1% lidocaine with epinephrine. After prepping and draping the finger or toe, a tourniquet is placed at the base of the proximal phalanx. The nail plate is removed atraumatically with scissors or a Kutz elevator and preserved for reapplication at the end of the procedure. For split-thickness grafts, it is helpful to outline the donor graft size with a surgical marker. A No. 15 blade scalpel is then used to tangentially raise the split-thickness graft. The blade should be visualized through the graft during the harvest to prevent full-thickness injuries. It is better to harvest a graft that is too thin than to create a full-thickness nail bed injury. For larger graft harvests small forceps can be used to provide counter traction because the curve of the nail bed makes harvest with the scalpel alone difficult. The graft is then sutured to the defect with 7–0 chromic suture, and the nail plate replaced for bolstering of the graft.

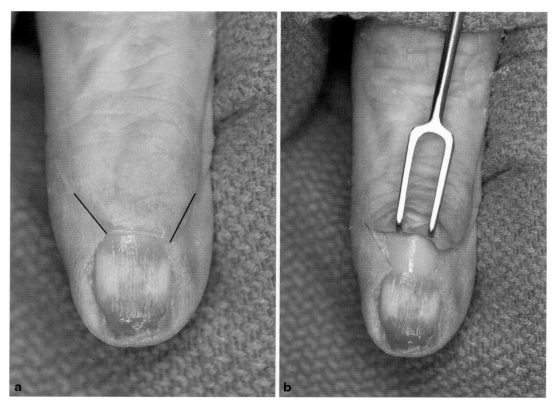

Fig. 3.7 Elevation of the eponychial fold. **a** Incisions are placed at 90°angles to the eponychial fold for proximal nail bed exposure. **b** Elevation of the eponychial fold ex-poses the proximal germinal matrix.

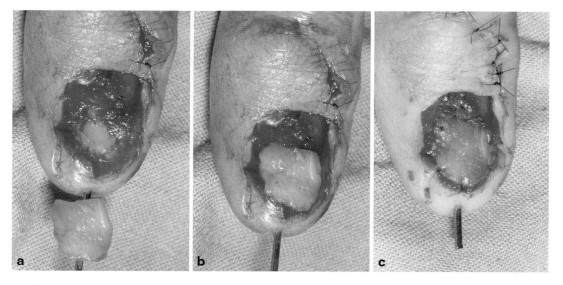

Fig. 3.8 Nail bed grafting. **a** Nail bed with full-thick-ness defect of the sterile matrix and split-thickness graft. **b** Placement of graft. **c** Graft sutured to defect.

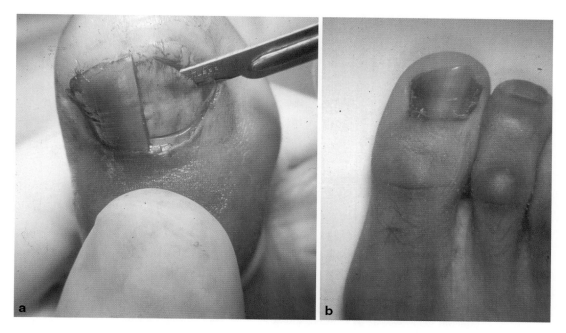

Fig. 3.9 Graft harvest. **a** Harvest of split-thickness sterile matrix graft from toe. **b** Postoperative donor site. Published with kind permission of © Nicole Z. Sommer, MD [2014].

Distal Phalanx Fracture

Fifty percent of nail bed injuries have an associated distal phalanx fracture. [13] Radiographic evaluation is a key component of fingertip injury evaluation. Distal tuft fractures and non-displaced distal phalanx fractures can be treated with nail bed repair and replacement of the nail plate which will act as a splint for the fracture. If the nail plate is missing or badly damaged additional pin fixation may be needed for fracture stability. Displaced fractures and fractures proximal to the nail fold are best treated with operative fixation utilizing 0.028-inch Kirschner wires (Fig. 3.10). Two longitudinally oriented or crossed K-wires should be placed to prevent rotation, the wires should not pass through the DIP joint, if possible, to avoid long-term DIP joint stiffness. Pins are removed at 3–4 weeks in the office.

Comminuted fractures often have small pieces of bone which are adherent to the nail bed. Repair of the nail bed injury allows approximation of the bony fragments. Replacement of the nail or, if unavailable, placement of a piece of silicone acts as a splint for fracture healing. The goal is bony union with an anatomic dorsal cortex for the nail bed to rest on. Although comminuted tuft fractures often result in fibrous nonunion, they are mostly asymptomatic.

Seymour fracture is a unique injury that occurs in children. This is a Salter–Harris type I fracture through the physis if the distal phalanx base, which often is associated with an avulsion nail bed injury. Reduction of the distal segment beneath the proximal nail fold often results in anatomic reduction. Splinting is usually satisfactory but there are some circumstances in which supplemental fixation is required for unstable fractures. Kirchner wires can be used for fracture stability but the DIP joint should be left free if possible (Fig. 3.11). [25].

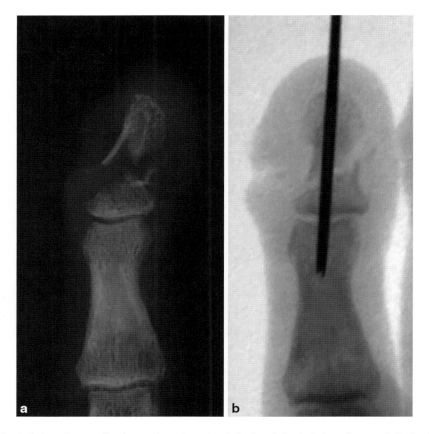

Fig. 3.10 Distal phalanx fracture fixation. **a** Comminuted and displaced distal phalanx fracture. **b** Reduction and percutaneous pinning. Published with kind permission of © Nicole Z. Sommer, MD [2014]. All rights reserved

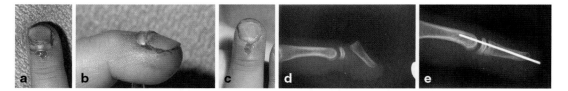

Fig. 3.11 Seymour fracture repair. **a** and **b** Seymour fracture with avulsion nail bed injury. **c** Following reduction of the fracture and replacement of the nail beneath the nail fold. **d** Radiographic imaging of a Seymour fracture. **e** Following reduction and percutaneous pinning. Published with kind permission of © Nicole Z. Sommer, MD [2014]. All rights reserved

Amputation

Injuries to the nail apparatus occur with distal amputations. Management depends on the level of injury and the integrity of the remaining structures. Reconstructive management entails a variety of procedures including revision amputation, skin and nail bed graft placement, local flap reconstruction and replantation. The reconstructive methods that affect the nail apparatus will be discussed in this section.

If the injury involves exposure of the distal phalanx, there are several methods of management for bony coverage. Revision amputation with bone shortening and suturing the remaining skin over the distal phalanx is one option. Local flap advancement is another option [26]. With either of these choices it is essential that the suturing of the skin to the nail bed edge is done in a tension-free manner. If there is any tension at this junction the nail bed will grow in a volar direction and the nail plate will follow creating a hook nail deformity. Similarly, if the nail bed is left longer than the distal phalanx, the nail bed will collapse volarly and a hook nail will develop. The distal phalanx length is crucial in supporting the overlying nail bed. Therefore, when shortening an amputation, the nail bed should be cut to the same length as the distal phalanx.

Volar VY advancement flaps are often used to replace lost hyponychium in a distal amputation injury. [27] Distal nail bed injuries can be reconstructed with the addition of a nail bed split-thickness or full-thickness graft to the distal de-epithelialized portion of the VY flap [28]. The entire nail bed can be reconstructed with this method. Another option is the reverse homodigital artery flap that has been recently described for coverage of a partially amputated distal phalanx with exposed bone. [29] This technique can be used with or without the addition of a nail bed graft.

Replantation of the fingertip can be attempted if the injury is at or proximal to the eponychial fold. Revision amputation is usually preferred for amputation distal to the level of the nail fold. Management of the nail depends on the percent of nail remaining. If greater than 25 % of the nail is still present distal to the nail fold, the nail should be preserved. If less than 25 % of the nail remains then a nail bed ablation should be performed. Ablation requires removal of the dorsal roof and the ventral floor of the nail fold. The eponychial fold skin is preserved and used for additional soft tissue coverage.

Amputation in children can present with fingertip avulsions with the nail bed present on the avulsed digit. In this unique circumstance, the fingertip and nail bed are sutured back into place with minimal or no debridement. Often the avulsed segment will survive from serum imbibition and inosculation in a similar manner to a skin graft. Composite graft take is most successful in children younger than 3 years old. In older children, tip amputations can be defatted and replaced as a "cap" graft [30] for better success than composite grafting.

Postoperative Management

Patients with nail apparatus injuries are often seen in follow up 5–7 days from the injury. At this visit the bandages are soaked off and the repair is inspected. Any sutures securing the nail plate are removed to prevent a sinus tract from forming. Often chromic sutures are used for re-approximation of skin but occasionally nylon sutures are present and can be removed at 10–14 days from the operation.

If the nail was reapplied, the patient should be informed that the nail will slowly be pushed off by the advancing nail in approximately 1–3 months. Silicone or suture material falls off earlier. The nail grows at a rate of 0.1 mm/day and the patient can expect a delay of 3–4 weeks prior to nail growth resumption. [31] Two to three millimeters of total nail growth occurs per month and the nail has a bulge at its leading edge during growth (Fig. 3.12). It takes 6–9 months for a new nail to completely grow. Toenails grow more slowly than fingernails with their linear growth being 30–50 % that of finger nails. [32, 33]

Distal phalanx fractures are protected with splinting for 3–4 weeks. Often a "cap splint" is provided for all patients to protect the fingertip

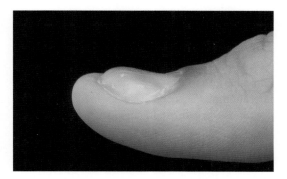

Fig. 3.12 The nail grows at a rate of 0.1 mm/day and has a bulge at its leading edge during growth. Published with kind permission of © Nicole Z. Sommer, MD [2014]. All rights reserved

which will remain sensitive for several months after the injury. Sensitivity is reduced if the nail plate was reapplied. Nail bed repair increases the chance for normal nail growth but all patients should be counseled on the complications that can occur from nail bed injuries and the potential for scarring and a permanent abnormal nail.

Complications

Postoperative complications can be functional, aesthetic, or a combination of the two. These complications can be divided into problems of nail growth and nail support. Problems with nail growth can originate from injuries to the germinal matrix, the sterile matrix, or the nail fold itself. Scar or disruption of the germinal matrix can lead to complete absence of nail growth. Injuries to the sterile matrix, which normally facilitates adherence of the nail plate to the nail bed, can bring about various deformities in the nail including elevation, notching, splitting, and nonadherence. Cicatricial adherence of the dorsal roof to the ventral floor of the nail fold can cause splitting or absence of the nail. This is why we recommend the placement of a temporary spacer under the eponychial fold after repair of the nail bed as a crucial step to prevent future nail deformities. The primary support of the nail bed is the distal phalanx, and when injured in conjunction with the nail bed can cause nail irregularities. An uneven dorsal cortex, loss of bony support due to intentional shortening or unintentional overdebridement, nonunion of a tuft fracture, or osteomyelitis can all cause inadequate or irregular bony support, which can lead to nail abnormalities.

The importance of an anatomical primary repair is emphasized when examining outcomes of late attempts to reconstruct the nail bed. These operations are difficult and often yield results that are not satisfactory for the patient or the surgeon. Reconstruction of the nail apparatus is possible; however it requires a comprehensive understanding of the anatomy and physiology of the perionychium along with an individualized approach to the patient and their problem.

Nail Ridges

Nail growth follows the shape of the nail bed. Any uneven surface will cause irregularity of the nail bed and ridging of the nail plate. Anatomically, the reason ridges occur is most commonly scarring of the nail bed itself or an uneven dorsal cortex of the distal phalanx. Longitudinal ridges are common post injury and represent a mostly cosmetic problem. Transverse nail ridges are also classified as an aesthetic problem unless they cause nonadherence, as can sometimes occur with a ridge that raises the nail plate off of the nail bed and prevents re-adherence distally. This can turn into a functional problem if the separated nail begins to catch on objects and become painful.

Minor nail ridging can also be caused by hypoxic injury to the cells of the germinal matrix, such as occurs with extended tourniquet time during a procedure or general hypoxic illness. These ridges will often resolve with time. Ridging that occurs because of the anatomic abnormalities discussed above is unlikely to resolve with time. Correction of these ridges often necessitates removal of the nail plate and direct examination of the nail bed. Excision of a scarred bed with primary repair or grafting, or leveling of an uneven dorsal cortex can accomplish creation of a flat nail bed.

Split Nail

The split nail deformity occurs when there is a longitudinal split of the nail, dividing it into distinct radial and ulnar sections. This can originate proximally in the germinal matrix causing a split of the entire nail, or can occur distally with only a partial split resulting. Because the scarred area does not produce nail cells, there is a blank area between the surrounding regions of normal nail production. Split nails are cosmetically unappealing but can also cause functional problems, including pain with sharp edges compressing the nail bed, catching on clothing, or serving as a nidus for fungal infection.

Repair should focus first on identifying the etiology of the split. This should be done by thorough preoperative examination and then subsequently by visualizing the entire nail bed at the time of surgery (Fig. 3.13a, b and c). This is done by removal of the entire nail plate. Elevation of the eponychium using radial relaxing incisions will be necessary if the germinal matrix is involved. Once the entire nail bed is visualized under loupe magnification, the scar can then be identified and excised.

The size of the gap in the germinal or sterile matrix is then examined. Some authors recommend wide undermining above the level of the periosteum and primary closure of most defects. [34] However in our experience the bed is often scarred down to the distal phalanx in a way that prevents adequate undermining and tension-free closure. [4] Primary closure of large gaps can also result in significant narrowing of the nail bed. For these reasons, we recommend nail bed grafting for any gaps 2 mm (Fig. 3.13d, e, f, i and

j). The patient must be willing to accept not having a nail at the donor site.

Grafts that involve the germinal matrix are required to be full thickness, as no nail growth will result from a split-thickness germinal matrix graft. A full-thickness germinal matrix graft should be harvested from a toe, and be similar in size and shape to the resected scar. In our experience the second toe is often the most ideal donor site, as deformities of the great toe are less acceptable to patients and the third through fifth toes often do not have an adequate amount of matrix to be harvested [35].

Full-thickness grafts are not required in the replacement of defects of the sterile matrix. Split-thickness sterile matrix grafts harvested for replacement of excised sterile matrix scar can be taken from the remaining normal nail bed of the injured finger, if there is adequate area to harvest a graft, or from adjacent fingers or toes [36]. There should be no donor-site morbidity from these types of grafts. [37, 38]

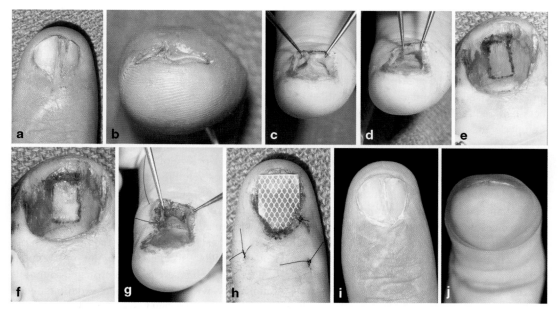

Fig. 3.13 (**a** and **b**) Pterygium causing split nail deformity. **c** Posttraumatic nail bed deformity viewed after nail plate removal and radial relaxing incisions. **d** Nail bed after excision of scarred area. (**e** and **f**) Marking and subsequent harvest of a toe split-thickness nail bed graft (**g**) Placement of split-thickness nail bed graft on dorsal roof to prevent adherence. **h** Placement of silicone sheet for stabilization of the repair and stenting of the eponychial fold. **i** and **j** Postoperative views showing improved adherence and contour. Residual split nail deformity will improve over time. Published with kind permission of © Nicole Z. Sommer, MD [2014]. All rights reserved

Nonadherence

As previously discussed, the sterile matrix produces the cells on the undersurface of the nail that result in adherence of the nail plate to the nail bed. Any scar or disruption of the sterile matrix can cause loosening of this attachment and subsequent elevation of the nail off of the bed distal to the scar. Repair is similar to a split nail, where the scar is resected and the defect repaired, likely with a split-thickness sterile matrix graft from the same finger, a toe or adjacent finger.

Chronic nonadherence can occur at the distal nail bed with repetitive trauma, such as when the nail is used to repeatedly pry open objects. In these cases, the nails are trimmed short and the patient is advised to avoid the activity causing the trauma. If nonadherence persists despite patient compliance, excision, and placement of a graft is the next step.

Absence

Absence of the nail may be congenital or the result of a post-traumatic deformity. Partial absence of the nail distal to the germinal matrix is treated in a similar fashion to the nail deformities discussed above. The area of scar or nonadherence is excised and replaced with a split-thickness nail bed graft from a toe or adjacent finger. Lemperle and associates [39] have reported success with serial crescentic excisions of 4-mm wide full-thickness segments of nail bed. The area of excision is left unrepaired and allowed to heal in secondarily, resulting in distal migration of the nail bed by wound contraction. Lemperle reported aesthetically pleasing results is obtained without the morbidity of a donor site for the graft. However, this technique does require patient cooperation and willingness to undergo multiple procedures.

Complete absence of the nail remains a challenging reconstructive problem. Reconstruction of the germinal matrix, support, and the nail fold itself must be considered as an individualized treatment plan is designed. Simple treatments such as the application of a full-thickness or split-thickness skin graft used to mimic the appearance of the nail are suboptimal and produce aesthetically unappealing results. [40] The application of nail prosthetics secured with glue has been largely unsuccessful. [41] In an attempt to overcome problems associated with artificial nail adherence, Buncke and Gonzalez [42] advocated for reconstruction of a nail-fold pouch. Over time, though this reconstructed pouch attenuates and is unable to contain the edge of the prosthetic. [41] Baruchin and colleagues published on the use of an osseointegrated titanium implant that anchored to the distal phalanx and functioned to attach the prosthetic nail. [43] Their series showed favorable results, however the insertion of a foreign body allows for the possibilities of infection, extrusion, and loosening over time.

The second toenail can be the source of a composite graft for treatment of the absent nail, with the graft containing germinal matrix, sterile matrix, and the dorsal roof of the nail complex. The second toenail most closely approximates the width of a fingernail, however for reconstruction of a thumb nail the great toe is the most likely donor site. Since a toenail is often shorter than a fingernail, a split-thickness sterile matrix graft is placed distally to the composite graft to allow for adequate nail length in the finger. Transfer of these composite grafts yields variable results, and patients should be informed beforehand regarding the unpredictability of the results and the certainty of the donor-site deformity. In our experience, outcomes do not seem to be related to patient age or size of the graft used. [44]

The most reliable treatment to produce a growing nail is also the most technically demanding: Free microvascular transfer of the dorsal tip of the toe including the nail bed. [45–49] These procedures can be lengthy and require meticulous microvascular surgical technique to complete successfully. There can be significant donor-site morbidity with this technique. Additionally as with any microsurgical procedure, there is a risk of total flap loss. Modifications of this technique seek to decrease donor-site morbidity by transferring smaller dorsal flaps with shorter pedicles, limiting the proximal dissection on both the toe and the finger. Nakayama [50] successfully transferred a venous only flap, while Iwasawa and associates [51] anastomosed a venous flap to a digital artery and vein. These procedures do decrease donor- and recipient-site morbidity, but require expert microsurgical skill due to the small vessel size encountered distally. [52–55]

Nail Spikes, Cysts, and Cornified Nail Bed

When completing a revision amputation of a fingertip, the entire germinal matrix and sterile matrix must be removed. Failure to complete this essential step can result in nail cysts, spikes, and cornified nail beds. A nail cyst forms when a stump is closed over a functional germinal matrix that continues to produce a nail while encased within the skin. Nail cysts present as painful enlarging masses at the site of the previous nail fold. Treatment consists of complete resection of the cyst wall with obliteration of any remaining germinal matrix.

Nail spikes occur similarly after incomplete removal of the germinal matrix. These often result from the removal of one side of the nail bed, such as in the case of an ingrown toenail. If incomplete, a nail will still be produced in the area, resulting in an accessory nail structure on the lateral fold of the paronychia. These are also painful and require removal of the spike and residual germinal matrix.

A cornified nail bed results in cases where the germinal matrix was completely excised but all or part of the sterile matrix was left intact. The sterile matrix continues to produce kertanizing material, which would normally provide for adherence of the nail plate. Treatment involves resection of the remaining sterile matrix and application of a split-thickness skin graft.

Eponychial Deformities

The eponychium overlies and protects the proximal portion of the nail and the germinal matrix. Loss of the eponychial fold from trauma can be a functional or aesthetic problem. The dorsal roof is responsible for producing nail shine, and loss of the eponychial fold will cause loss of this shine, which is primarily an aesthetic concern. Notching of the eponychium can occur secondary to improper repair of a laceration or tissue loss in that area. This is usually of little consequence to patients except in the rare instance where the free edge of eponychium catches on objects during regular activities. Revision of these edges can be considered if this is a significant disturbance.

Pterygium is a term used to describe scarring and adherence of the nail fold to the nail bed. These can be small, causing splitting of the nail, or larger encompassing the entire fold and causing total absence of the nail. The most common cause of a pterygium is trauma, although there are reports of associations with ischemia and collagen vascular diseases. Whether the etiology is trauma or another cause, we recommend operative treatment for a persistent pterygium. This is done by freeing up the dorsal roof in the area that is scarred down and placing a spacer, such as a silicone sheet, that is sutured into place to allow for sufficient time for the dorsal roof to epithelialize. This is usually successful, but in cases where the pterygium recurs it may be necessary to place a small split-thickness sterile matrix graft on the undersurface of the eponychium to prevent adherence. At this point the nail bed should again be examined to ensure that absent nail growth is not secondary to a damaged germinal matrix.

Defects in the eponychium can be reconstructed by a composite toe eponychial graft [44], helical rim graft [56], or local rotational flaps [57]. We recommend the use of an eponychial composite graft from an appropriately matched toe to replace the missing eponychium. With these grafts there is only a small raw surface proximally through which revascularization of the graft occurs. For this reason, we harvest the eponychial graft with a large dorsal skin paddle and place it on a corresponding de-epithelialized area of the recipient finger proximal to the defect (which allows for better revascularization of the composite graft). The donor defect is left to heal secondarily.

Hyponychial Deformities

Pterygia of the hyponychium can occur secondary to trauma and cause significant pain and a functional defect. We recommend removal of the distal 5 mm of nail, and subsequent excision of the distal nail bed and hyponychium with placement of a split-thickness skin graft. This results in resolution of pain and also causes nonadherence, which is helpful if there is a concomitant hook nail deformity.

Hooking of the nail occurs with tight closure of the nail bed over an amputation stump (Fig. 3.14). When the nail bed is pulled over the tip of the amputated distal phalanx, the nail follows the matrix into a hook nail formation. Hook nail can also occur when distal hyponychium and nail bed are preserved but loss of support of the

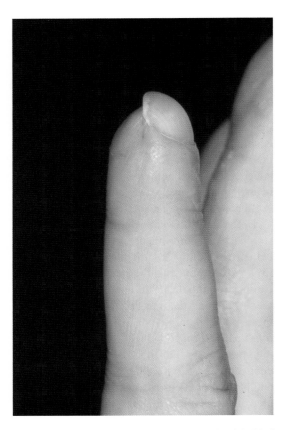

Fig. 3.14 Hook nail deformity. Published with kind permission of © Nicole Z. Sommer, MD [2014]. All rights reserved

tuft of the distal phalanx has occurred. Without support, the nail curves volarly. For this reason, it is never advisable to pull the distal nail bed over the distal phalanx for closure. Instead the better option is to shorten the distal phalanx and corresponding nail bed to avoid abnormal closure patterns.

Once a hook nail has occurred the decision regarding reconstruction must be made. Patients are often dissatisfied with the appearance of the nail, and it may cause functional problems depending on their occupation. Some patients opt for revision amputation with shortening of part of the nail complex and preservation of the base of the distal phalanx where the flexor digitorum profundus (FDP) and terminal extensor tendon insert. This is the least time intensive option and provides the quickest return to function for manual laborers. Other options for reconstruction of the soft tissue of the hyponychium include VY advancement flaps, cross-finger flaps, or full-thickness skin grafts with subsequent trimming back of the distal nail bed [58]. Complete correction is often elusive although improvement in the deformity can be achieved. If the idea of a shortened nail is unsatisfactory to the patient, attempts can be made to maintain length by bone grafting the distal phalanx for additional support. As with most bone grafts that do not have apposition on both ends, significant resorption tends to occur over time, and initial improvements will often dissipate. Free vascularized transfer of the second toe tip has been described, and although this is by far the most complex procedure it does achieve good results [59].

Hyponychial nonadherence occurs when the hyponychial barrier is lost secondary to the chronic exposure of the fingertips to acids, alkali, or other caustic liquids. Without this barrier in place the subungual space is exposed to bacteria, fungus, and all manner of other contamination that can occur on a daily basis and cause nonadherence. Removal of the causative agent should be the first step in treatment. If this is not successful, there is likely keratinous material embedded in the hyponychium that is preventing readherence of the nail. The nail should be removed proximal to this point and the keratin material scraped from the nail bed to allow for adherence of the plate as the nail grows back out to its full length.

Dull Nail

Dull nail is considered a minor complication that can occur with nail bed injury that is only aesthetic in nature. As mentioned previously, the dorsal roof is responsible for producing nail shine, and scar in that area can cause streaks of dullness on the nail. No treatment is necessary as this causes no functional problems.

References

1. Lewis BL. Microscopic studies of fetal and mature nail and surrounding soft tissue. AMA Arch Dermatol. 1954;70:732–47.
2. Barron JN. The structure and function of the skin of the hand. Hand. 1970;2:93–6.
3. DeBerker D, Mawhinney B, Sviland L. Quantification of regional matrix nail production. Br J Dermatol. 1996;134:1083–6.
4. Johnson M, Shuster S. Continuous formation of nail along the bed. Br J Dermatol. 1993;128:277–80.
5. Yates YJ, Concannon MJ. Fungal infections of the perionychium. Hand Clin. 2002;18:631–42.
6. Hasegawa K, Pereira BP, Pho R. The microvasculature of the nail bed, nail matrix, and nail fold of a normal human fingertip. J Hand Surg [Am]. 2001;26:283–90.
7. Moss SH, Schwartz KS, von Drasek-Ascher G, Ogden LL 2nd, Wheeler CS, Lister GD. Digital venous anatomy. J Hand Surg [Am]. 1985;10:473–82.
8. Zook EG. Discussion of "nail fungal infections and treatment." Hand Clin. 2002;18:629.
9. Smith DO, Oura C, Kimura C, Toshimori K. The distal venous anatomy of the finger. J Hand Surg [Am]. 1991;16:303–7.
10. Zook EG. Fingernail injuries. In: Strickland JW, Steichen JB, editors. Difficult problems in hand surgery. St. Louis: CV Mosby; 1982.
11. Wolfe SW, Hotchkiss RN, Pederson WC, Kozin SH. Green's operative H and surgery. 6th ed. Philadelphia: Elsevier Churchill and Livingstone; 2011. (Chapter 10, The Perionychium;). p. 333–45.
12. Guy RJ. The etiologies and mechanisms of the nail bed injuries. Hand Clin. 1990;6:9–21.
13. Zook EG. Reconstruction of a functional and aesthetic nail. Hand Clin. 2002;18:577–94.
14. Seaberg DC, Angelos WJ, Paris PM. Treatment of subungual hematomas with nail trephination: a prospective study. Am J Emerg Med. 1991;9:209–10.
15. Dean B, Becker G, Little C. The management of the acute traumatic subungual haematoma: a systematic review. Hand Surg. 2012;17:151–4.
16. Gellman H: Fingertip-nail bed injuries in children: current concepts and controversies of treatment. J Craniofac Surg. 2009;20:1033–5.
17. Strauss EJ, Weil WM, Jordan C, Paksima N. A prospective, randomized, controlled trial of 2-Octylcyanoacrylate versus suture repair for nail bed injuries. J Hand Surg Am. 2008;33(2):250–3.
18. Bristol SG, Verchere CG. The transverse figure-of-eight suture for securing the nail. J Hand Surg Am. 2007;32(1):124–5.
19. Weinand C, Demir E, Lefering R, Juon B, Voegelin E. A comparison of complications in 400 patients after native nail versus silicone nail splints for fingernail splinting after injuries. World J Surg. 2014;38(10):2574–9..
20. Schiller C. Nail replacement in fingertip injuries. Plast Reconstr Surg. 1957;19:521–30.
21. Johnson RK. Nailplasty. Plast Reconstr Surg. 1971;47:275.
22. Antony AK, Anagnos DP. Matrix-periosteal flaps for reconstruction of nail deformity. Plast Reconstr Surg. 2002;109:1663–6.
23. Saito H, Suzuki Y, Fujino K, Tajima T. Free nail bed graft for treatment of nail bed injuries of the hand. J Hand Surg [Am]. 1983;8:171–8.
24. Shepard GH. Nail grafts for reconstruction. Hand Clin. 1990;6:79–102.
25. Krusch-Mandl I, Kottstorfer J, Thalhammer G, Aldrian S, Erhart J, Platzer P. Seymour fractures: retrospective analysis and therapeutic considerations. J Hand Surg [Am]. 2013;38:258–64.
26. Brown RE, Zook EG, Russell RC. Reconstruction of fingertips with combination of local flaps and nail bed grafts. J Hand Surg [Am]. 1999;24:345–51.
27. Brown RE. Acute nail bed injuries. Hand Clin. 2002;18:561–75.
28. Hwang E, Park B, Song S, Jung H, Kim C. Fingertip reconstruction with simultaneous flaps and nail bed grafts following amputation. J Hand Surg [Am]. 2013;38:1307–14.
29. Alagoz M, Uysal C, Kerem M, Sensoz O. Reverse homodigital artery flap coverage for bone and nailbed grafts in fingertip amputations. Ann Plast Surg. 2006;56:279–83.
30. Rose EH, Norris MS, Kowalski TA, Lucas A, Fleegler EJ. The "cap" technique: non-microsurgical reattachment of fingertip amputations. J Hand Surg [Am]. 1989;14:513–8.
31. Baden HP. Regeneration of the nail. Arch Dermatol. 1965;91:619–20.
32. Krull E, Zook E, Baran R, Haneke E. Nail surgery: a text and atlas. New York: Lippincott Williams & Wilkins; 2001. p. 12. (Chapter 1).

33. Pardo-Castello V. Disease of the nail. 3rd ed. Springfield: Charles C Thomas; 1960.

34. Desciak EB, Eliezri YD. Split nail deformities: a surgical approach. Dermatol Surg. 2001;27:252–6.

35. Clark WE, Buxton LHD. Studies in nail growth. Br J Dermatol. 1938;50:221–35.

36. Rai A, Jha M, Makhija L, Bhattacharya S, Sethi N, Baranwal S. An algorithmic approach to post-traumatic nail deformities based on anatomical classification. J Plast Reconstr Aesthet Surg. 2014;67:540–7.

37. Pessa JE, Tsai TM, Li Y, Kleinert HE. The repair of nail deformities with the nonvascularized nail bed graft: indications and results. J Hand Surg [Am]. 1990;15:466–70.

38. Shepard GH. Perionychial grafts in trauma and reconstruction. Hand Clin. 2002;18:595–614.

39. Lemperle G, Schwarz M, Lemperle SM. Nail regeneration by elongation of the partially destroyed nail bed. Plast Reconstr Surg. 2003;111:167–72.

40. Hanraham EM. The split-thickness skin graft as a covering following removal of a fingernail. Surgery. 1946;20:398–400.

41. Beasley RW, deBeze GM. Prosthetic substitution for fingernails. Hand Clin. 1990;6:105–11.

42. Buncke HJ Jr, Gonzalez RI. Fingernail reconstruction. Plast Reconstr Surg. 1962;30:452–61.

43. Baruchin AM, Nahlieli O, Vizethum F, Sela M. Harnessing the osseointegration principle for anchorage of fingernail prostheses. Hand Clin. 2002;18(4):647–54.

44. Lille S, Brown RE, Zook EE, Russell RC. Free nonvascularized composite nail grafts: an institutional experience. Plast Reconstr Surg. 2000;105:2412–5.

45. Endo T, Nakayama Y, Soeda S. Nail transfer: evolution of the reconstructive procedure. Plast Reconstr Surg. 1997;100:907–13.

46. Morrison WA: Microvascular nail transfer. Hand Clin 6:69–76, 1990.

47. Morrison WA, O'Brien BM, McLeod AM. Thumb reconstruction with a free neurovascular wrap-around flap from the big toe. J Hand Surg [Am]. 1980;5:575–83.

48. Shibata M, Seki T, Yoshizu T, Saito H, Tajima T. Microsurgical toenail transfer to the hand. Plast Reconstr Surg. 1991;88:102–9.

49. Wilgis EF, Maxwell GP. Distal digital nerve graft: clinical and anatomical studies. J Hand Surg [Am]. 1979;4:439–43.

50. Nakayama Y. Vascularized free nail grafts nourished by arterial inflow from the venous system. Plast Reconstr Surg. 1990;85:239–45.

51. Iwasawa M, Furuta S, Noguchi M, Hirose T. Reconstruction of fingertip deformities of the thumb using a venous flap. Ann Plast Surg. 1992;28:187–9.

52. Dautel G, Corcella D, Merle M. Reconstruction of fingertip amputations by partial composite toe transfer with short vascular pedicle. J Hand Surg [Br]. 1998;4:457–64.

53. Endo T, Nakayama Y. Short pedicle vascularized nail flap. Plast Reconstr Surg. 1996;97:656–61.

54. Endo T, Nakayama Y. Microtransfers for nail and finger tip replacement. Hand Clin. 2002;18:615–22.

55. Koshima I, Soeda S, Takase T, Yamasaki M. Free vascularized nail grafts. J Hand Surg [Am]. 1988;13:29–32.

56. Rose EH. Nailplasty utilizing a free composite graft from the helical rim of the ear. Plast Reconstr Surg. 1980;66:23–9.

57. Achauer BM, Welk RA. One stage reconstruction of the postburn nailfold contracture. Plast Reconstr Surg. 1990;85:937–40.

58. Kumar VP, Satku K. Treatment and prevention of "hook nail" deformity with anatomic correlation. J Hand Surg [Am]. 1993;18:617–20.

59. Koshima I, Moriguchi T, Umeda N, Yamada A. Trimmed second toetip transfer for reconstruction of claw nail deformity of the fingers. Br J Plast Surg. 1992;45:591–4.

High-Pressure Injection Injuries

4

David H. Wei and Robert J. Strauch

Introduction

High-pressure injection injuries were described nearly 80 years ago in the English literature by Rees, who reported a mechanic who sustained a 4000 psi injection injury of fuel oil [1]. The patient was testing the jet from a diesel engine about 1 in. from the tip of his right middle finger when he accidentally tripped the valve. Despite an initial benign appearance with minimal bleeding at the distal tip, the finger became intensely swollen and painful within 24 h. Subsequently, the affected tissues underwent necrosis, developed a superimposed infection, and ultimately required amputation at the level of the mid-metacarpal bone.

High-pressure injection injuries to the hand and upper extremity often appear innocuous with only minor punctate wounds in laborers using pressurized tools (Fig. 4.1). These patients frequently present with minimal pain, resulting in under appreciation of the severity of the soft tissue injury that was sustained from the dissection of the foreign substance.

D. H. Wei (✉) · R. J. Strauch
Department of Orthopaedic Surgery,
Columbia University Medical Center,
622 West 168th Street, New York, NY 10032, USA
e-mail: davidwei.md@gmail.com

R. J. Strauch
e-mail: robertjstrauch@hotmail.com

The Evidence

Epidemiology

The incidence of reported high-pressure injection injuries in the medical literature coincides with the development of more complex machinery in the last half of the twentieth century, when increasingly higher-pressure guns were used to inject paint, grease, concrete, plastic, and fuel [2]. Some authors noted that paint gun injuries usually occurred in painters who were accustomed to low-pressure guns and switched to high-pressure airless guns [3]. On average, 1 of 600 hand traumas are due to high-pressure injection injuries, and 1–4 cases present to large surgical hand centers annually [4]. The patient is most commonly a young male laborer involved in industrial cleaning, painting, lubricating, or fueling, and injuries are sustained when the operator attempts to clean the nozzle with a finger or a cloth. The nondominant hand is most commonly injured with more than 50 % of these injuries sustained in the index finger [5, 6]. The thumb is the second most commonly injured digit, followed by the palm, but high-pressure injection injuries may occur anywhere along the upper extremity [7].

Pathophysiology

The injury process from high-pressure injections may be divided into four main components: (1)

L. M. Rozmaryn (ed.), *Fingertip Injuries*, DOI 10.1007/978-3-319-13227-3_4,
© Springer International Publishing Switzerland 2015

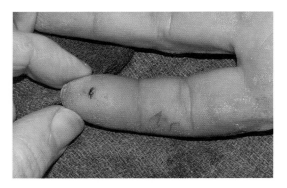

Fig. 4.1 Preoperative photograph of a pinpoint wound on the volar aspect of the distal phalanx of the index finger on the nondominant hand secondary to high-pressure injection of paint (From: Rosenwasser and Wei [41], with permission from Wolters Kluwer Health. Courtesy Robert Strauch, MD, New York, NY)

initial injury, (2) chemical irritation, (3) inflammation, and (4) secondary infection.

Initial Injury

High-pressure injection injury begins with the initial force delivered to the tissues. A pressure of 100 psi (7 bar) is sufficient for skin penetration, while high-injection pressures can range from 3000 to 12,000 psi depending on the specific application of the apparatus with velocities up to 400 mph [7–9]. Examples of systems that operate around 3000 psi include airless high-pressure spray guns first developed in the 1950s that use hydraulic pumps to deliver paint, as well as reinforced hydraulic pipes used in many industries such as coal mining, agriculture, and construction, that contain pressurized oils [10]. The higher end of pressurized systems includes diesel engines that compress fuel up to 12,000 psi before releasing its contents through a nozzle to the combustion chamber. In the event of nozzle malfunction or blockage, these pressures may even be higher [11]. The kinetic injury of a grease gun injury to the finger is calculated to be equivalent to a 1000-kg (2205-lb) weight falling from a height of 25 cm (9.8 in.) [12]. Injuries are less severe when a small distance separates the injection source from the skin. Nevertheless, high-pressure jets can penetrate and infiltrate the subcutaneous tissues even without direct bodily contact [13, 14].

The force of the injection dissects along planes of least resistance that tend to follow neurovascular bundles in the digits. When the fibrous sheaths of the stouter annular pulleys are encountered, the force of the injected substance usually deflects and passes around the tendon sheath and underlying bone [15]. However, if the force penetrates the tendon sheath over the thinner, membranous cruciate pulleys that overlie the joints of the hand, the injected material may distend and disrupt the tendon sheath itself. Mid-palmar injections are usually limited to material superficial to the palmar aponeurosis, with occasional deposition in the deep palmar space injuring bones, muscles, and vessels, and through and through penetration entering the dorsum of the hand [11].

Following the forceful entry of the injected substance, compression, decreased perfusion pressure, venous hypertension, and capillary leaking initiate a cycle of swelling, edema, and further compression much like a typical compartment syndrome. Caustic chemical reaction, secondary to the injected material, initiates a second hit with a violent inflammatory response magnifying the injury. This then cycles back as increased tissue pressures further compromise blood flow, triggering vasospasm, thrombosis, and ultimately ischemia.

Local Chemical Irritation

Paint, grease, hydraulic fluid, diesel fuel fluid, paint thinner, mud, toluene, molding plastic, paraffin, and cement are the most commonly injected substances. Many of these chemicals are intrinsically cytotoxic, causing necrosis and inciting inflammatory responses. In particular, paint and turpentine have been shown to be particularly harmful agents, and the severe toxicity of paint has led some authors to recommend primary amputation as the initial treatment [16].

The chemical composition of paint can consist of up to 40 raw materials, but they may be divided into three main parts: a solvent that evaporates shortly after it is applied, a pigment that provides color, and a transport vehicle or binder that acts as an adherent [10]. Each of these constituents can damage tissue directly. The vehicle or binder may be an unsaturated or drying oil, or it may be a synthetic polymer such as an alkyd resin.

Water-based latex paints were introduced in the late 1940s, and they differ in solvent and vehicle compared with oil-based paints, with substantially lower rates of amputation following latex paint injection than following oil paint injection (6 and 58%, respectively) [10]. This difference is thought to be due to the reduced inflammatory potential of acrylic latex vehicles compared with the alkyd resins of oil-based paints. Turpentine and other paint thinners are a mixture of alkylated aromatic hydrocarbons designed to dissolve fats, and they cause lipid dissolution without a high-pressure etiology [17, 18]. The powerful detrimental nature of turpentine is demonstrated through its effects even when not injected into the body. The fumes can cause irritation of exposed mucous membranes and bronchial inflammation, predisposing individuals with chronic exposure to pneumonia, chronic nephritis, and dermatitis [14].

In contrast, the chemical contents of grease are less inflammatory than both paint and paint solvents. Grease contains 88% mineral oil, along with graphite and detergent, and produces chronic granulomas rather than direct chemical irritation [19]. Water, air, and small quantities of veterinary vaccine have been reported to produce minimal damage and good outcomes even with nonsurgical management, further emphasizing the impact of direct chemical irritation on treatment and outcomes [7, 20, 21].

Systemic Inflammatory Response

Experimental injection of oils, waxes, diesel oil, and turpentine into human and animal tissues have been shown to cause acute and chronic inflammation with granulomatous changes [11, 14, 22]. Soya alkyd, a polymeric resin vehicle for paint, produces greater inflammatory responses and is more caustic than mineral spirits, turpentine, xylol, and acrylic latex [10]. Postinjection sectioning of resected tissue shows substitution of normal connective tissue and fat, with whorls of proliferative granulation tissue and fibroblasts. Macrophages containing vacuoles of the injected material, as well as polymorphonuclear leukocytes, lymphocytes, and plasma cells are present [17].

Secondary Infection

The ischemic conditions and tissue necrosis that occur following the initial injury creates an environment for bacteria to thrive [10, 23]. However, some authors have found wound infection to be rare, due to the injected material being an organic chemical that does not support bacterial growth [8]. Although wound cultures have not been consistently obtained for injection injuries, infection rates have ranged widely from 1.6 to 60% [6, 11, 24, 25]. In the literature review performed by Hogan and Ruland, wound cultures were reported for 126 out of 435 patients, of which 53 were positive (42%) [20]. Most of the infections were polymicrobial. Infection is fostered by necrotic tissue and the reluctance to aggressively debride these injection injuries early may allow infection to take hold.

Clinical Presentation and Indications

Initially, small punctate lesions may be the only visible sign of injury on the skin, with minimal or no pain. Some patients have seen as many as seven doctors before the significance of their injury was recognized. Such innocuous presentation of a painless wound often delays patients from seeking medical evaluation. The average time to physician evaluation averages nearly 9 h. However, as swelling develops, pain and paresthesias occur with loss of perfusion, and the urgency of the clinical presentation becomes obvious as the finger becomes bloated, edematous, tense, pale, and cold [7].

Appropriate initial management of this injury mandates a high index of suspicion by the physician who first encounters the patient. In the presence of radiopaque materials, radiographs can be effective and helpful in determining the spread of injected material; however, some material may be radiolucent, or lucent areas may represent air [26, 27] (Fig. 4.2a, b). If laboratory evaluation occurs within a few hours after injury, it may reveal an elevated white blood cell count and be accompanied by lymphadenitis and lymphangitis [16].

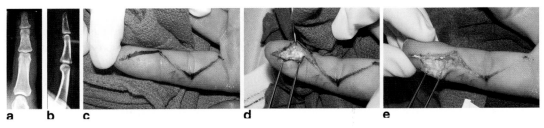

Fig. 4.2 The injected material is radiolucent and therefore cannot be seen on the preoperative AP (**a**) and lateral (**b**), radiographs of the index finger. **c** Intraoperative photograph of the markings for a planned Bruner incision for debridement. **d** Photograph of the incision of the volar aspect of the finger showing the appearance of the injected material in the subcutaneous space. **e** Post-debridement photograph following the removal of foreign injected material with careful preservation of neurovascular structures (From: Rosenwasser and Wei [41], with permission from Wolters Kluwer Health. Courtesy Robert Strauch, MD, New York, NY)

Initial management should include elevation of the limb, tetanus prophylaxis, systemic prophylactic antibiotics, and analgesia. Digital blocks should be avoided because they may add to swelling and vasospasm in a digit that is already at risk. Wounds should be left open, with no attempt to obtain primary closure in the emergency department setting, and ice is discouraged due to the need to optimize perfusion of the injected hand [4].

Nonsurgical treatment is reserved only for injections of air, water, or chicken vaccine; these injuries may be managed with close observation, unless signs of compartment syndrome are present, in which case surgical decompression is indicated [28–30].

Management

Surgical Debridement

The benefits of early and aggressive surgical debridement have been known since the initial reports of injection injuries [1]. Ensuring the entire zone of injury is debrided, decompressing compartments, exploring and incising tendon sheaths, removing injected material, and using ample saline irrigation are all critical steps in the management of high-pressure injection injuries to the hand (Figs. 4.2c–e and 4.3a–k). Surgical removal of foreign material to avoid ischemic gangrene and to reduce fibrosis and scarring are also im-

portant steps [16]. Delayed surgery has been associated with increased morbidity and higher amputation rates [2, 16, 27].

Some authors have recommended amputation as the primary treatment for high-pressure injection injuries to the hand [31]. However, Pinto et al. reported an 84 % salvage rate with open wound packing, repeat debridement, and delayed closure with only four amputations in 25 patients [6]. They utilized a wide exposure with Bruner palmar digital incisions and thoroughly debrided all devitalized tissue in the zone of injury, while removing injected material and preserving the neurovascular structures. Repeat debridement was performed at 24–72 h later as necessary. Alternative incisions may be used such as a midaxial incision to achieve full exposure and in some cases may be preferred over palmar flaps that might be compromised from the injury itself (Fig. 4.4). Following debridement and excision of injected material, irrigation with normal saline or lactated Ringer injection may be used, whereas organic solvents should be avoided, as they lead to further inflammation and tissue damage.

Steroids and Anti-Inflammatory Agents

Treatment of high-pressure injection injuries with systemic steroids was reported as early as 1962, when Bottoms advocated the use of dexamethasone, reporting the effectiveness of its anti-inflammatory properties [32]. However, more

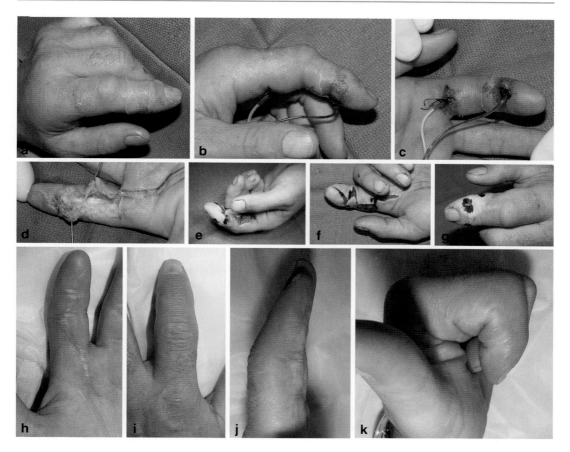

Fig. 4.3 **a** through **c**: Photographs of the left index finger of a patient who was transferred from another institution after having had only catheter irrigation of a paint injection injury without formal debridement. **d** Intraoperative photograph during thorough surgical debridement. **e** through **g**: Photographs showing that the wounds were left open to heal by secondary intention. **h** through **k**: Follow-up clinical photographs of the healed wound. The patient had excellent motion (From: Rosenwasser and Wei [41], with permission from Wolters Kluwer Health. Courtesy Robert Strauch, MD, New York, NY)

recent evidence challenges the utility of steroid use in the setting of high-pressure injection injuries. Some authors advocate the routine use of steroids in all patients, while others voice concerns that steroid suppression of the leukocyte response will increase the risk of superinfections [14, 33, 34].

Gillespie et al. studied the effects of dexamethasone on albino rabbits injected with subdermal paint, and found less inflammation but no difference in bacterial count [10]. Waters et al. injected saline, toluene, and turpentine into guinea pigs, and on histologic sectioning noted an intense acute inflammatory reaction with vascular congestion and marked infiltration of polymorphonuclear leukocytes [14]. In the same article, the authors include a clinical case report of steroid use that may have led to an infection and did not prevent tissue necrosis. In contrast, Kaufman reported a small benefit from the nonsteroidal anti-inflammatory drug, oxyphenbutazone, but the drug has been removed from the formulary because of other toxicities [31].

Schoo et al. reviewed 127 case reports and found variable regimens of steroid use, but found their anti-inflammatory effects of steroids to be impressive [11]. Their own regimen consisted of routine use of hydrocortisone sodium succinate

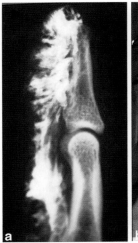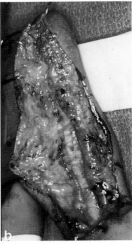

Fig. 4.4 A lateral radiograph (**a**) and clinical photograph (**b**) of an index finger demonstrating the appearance of radiopaque paint in a patient who sustained a high-pressure injection injury. An extensile midaxial incision was used to ensure adequate exposure of the zone of injury (From: Rosenwasser and Wei [41], with permission from Wolters Kluwer Health. Courtesy Robert Strauch, MD, New York, NY)

100 mg intravenously every 6 h until swelling and erythema improved, followed by oral prednisone 25 mg twice daily, with further intravenous doses as necessary and a tapered protocol thereafter.

Empiric Antibiotics

The role of prophylactic empiric antibiotics in high-pressure injection injuries was examined by Mirzayan et al., who found wound cultures to be positive at initial debridement in 15 of 35 patients, with 58% of isolates being gram-negative bacteria [35]. On this basis, they recommended the routine use of prophylactic antibiotics to cover both gram-positive and gram-negative organisms.

Despite the potential intrinsic antibacterial properties of injected substances, animal studies by Gillespie et al. demonstrated that the ability of the host to fight infection was still compromised after injection injury [10]. Thus, they recommended antibiotic prophylaxis for all patients. Similarly, Hogan and Ruland recommended pro-

phylactic broad-spectrum intravenous antibiotics to minimize the deleterious effects of bacterial contamination of the wound, despite finding no correlation between infection and the rate of amputation [20].

Postoperative Care

Postoperative care varies from early and intensive physical therapy with active range of motion to immobilization with splinting of the fingers in a resting position on a volar slab with the metacarpophalangeal joints flexed to 90° and the interphalangeal joints fully extended [11]. Twice-daily hand soaks in povidone-iodine or sterile water whirlpools are also used to promote a clean environment for healing, and wounds may be left open for healing by secondary intention.

Prognostic Factors

Several factors are correlated with the patient's ultimate outcome; these include location of the injury, the type and volume of injected material, as well as the time interval between injury and debridement [6, 16, 25]. Higher injection pressures, the presence of secondary infection, and more distal site of infection have also been correlated with poorer prognosis [2].

Location of Injury and Volume

Injuries to the fingers are significantly more likely to require amputation than are injuries to the thumb and palm, with some studies reporting sixfold greater likelihood of amputation of the finger [20]. One possible anatomic explanation for this difference is the larger potential volume of the palm and thumb, resulting in higher tolerance of swelling and limited detrimental effects of high pressure. However, this difference may also simply reflect surgeon selection bias, due to the greater morbidity associated with loss of opposition without a thumb as well as the fact that the thumb may still be quite useful even with stiff metacarpophalangeal and interphalangeal joints.

In contrast, a stiff proximal interphalangeal joint in a palmar digit may significantly limit or interfere with functional grasp.

Higher volumes of injected material, involvement of the tendon sheath, and proximal spread of the injected substance have been associated with worse outcomes [8, 25]. In a cadaver study, the final location of injected material was found to be dependent on the angle of entry, depth of penetration, and resistance of the anatomic structures encountered [15]. Injuries over the thinner parts of the flexor sheaths that overlie the joints of the digit allow entry into the tendon sheaths, further dispersing both the injected material and the force of injury over a greater zone. In the thumb and small finger, where the tendon sheaths are in continuity with the radial and ulnar bursae, injected material may travel into the forearm, sometimes as far proximal as the mediastinum. Temple et al. reported the frightful case of a laborer who suffered a high-pressure injection injury to the hypothenar region from an air pressure hose, resulting in pneumomediastinum [36]. During the injury, the patient felt an immediate sensation from his hand to his face and then trunk. The path of the air followed the ulnar artery up to the brachiocephalic artery, along the neck to the common carotid, then back down the thorax along the aortic arch to the posterior mediastinum. In contrast, injected material in the index, long, and ring fingers may be trapped in the tendon sheath, leading to increased pressures in a confined space.

Injected Material

In a meta-analysis of 127 cases of high-pressure injection injuries of the hand, the most important factor in determining outcome was the material injected [11]. This study reported an overall amputation rate of 48%, with an amputation rate of 80% for turpentine injections, 58% for paint injections, and 20% for grease injuries. A review of the literature by Hogan and Ruland also demonstrated that the material injected is a significant factor in determining the risk of amputation [20]. Amputation was required in >40% of cases involving organic solvents including paint thinner, paint, diesel fuel, gasoline, jet fuel, and oil.

Mirzayan et al. retrospectively reviewed the records of 35 patients and correlated amputation rate with type of paint [35]. The rate of amputation was significantly higher following injuries involving oil-based paints than following injuries involving water-based paints (100 and 0%, respectively).

In comparison, high-pressure injection of water and air is likely much less toxic than injection of other materials [37]. Veterinary vaccine injection injuries are sometimes classified as high-pressure injection injuries, but many authors believe that they should be a separate category because the amount injected is limited, the pressure and velocity are low, and nonsurgical treatment is usually adequate [28].

Time to Debridement

Delay to surgical debridement and irrigation has often been deemed a critical factor in the morbidity of high-pressure injection injury. However, the exact timing from injury to treatment in the operating room is difficult to estimate. In a recent meta-analysis of 166 high-pressure injection injuries with adequate reporting of the interval between injury and surgery, the authors found no significant difference in amputation rate overall. However, the subgroup of patients injected with the most inflammatory organic solvents demonstrated a significantly higher rate of amputation when surgery was delayed >6 h than in those treated within 6 h (58 and 38%, respectively) [18]. In 1967, Stark et al. found the interval from injury to treatment to be correlated with amputation rate, with delays of >10 h leading to higher rates of amputation [16].

Pressure

It is unclear whether the intensity of the pressure during the time of injury may reliably correlate with morbidity or prognostic markers such as amputation rate. While higher pressures are important in the wider distribution of material, it has not been a consistent independent prognostic factor for amputation [38]. In one series with a small patient cohort, pressures of >7000 psi were associated with a 100% amputation rate [11]. In contrast, in a meta-analysis of 435 cases, two patients with documented pressures of >7000 psi both did not require amputation [20]. Their study revealed a greater risk of amputation for injuries greater than 1000 psi, although they stated there is no pressure threshold above which amputation is inevitable.

Clinical Outcomes and Complications

The clinical outcomes of high-pressure injection injuries are heterogeneous in the published literature with amputation rates ranging from 16 to 80% [4, 11, 24, 39]. Pinto et al. reported an amputation rate of 16% (4 of 25 patients) and attributed their relatively better results to consistent and extensive surgical debridement [6]. In their series, 64% of patients had "essentially normal" hand function at last follow-up, with final flexion lag of <2.5 cm in 16 patients.

A few studies have reported subjective or objective functional outcomes on high-pressure injection injuries, such as patient-reported outcome measures, range of motion, or strength. Christodoulou et al. followed up 15 patients and found a nearly 20% decrease in grip, a 23% reduction in lateral pinch, and a 25% reduction in three-point pinch strength compared with the contralateral uninjured side [21]. Four patients were unable to return to their occupation, and all but one patient had abnormal peripheral nerve function with decreased two-point discrimination. Wieder et al. followed 23 patients for a mean of 1 year and reported significant loss of grip and pinch strength compared with the contralateral side (12 and 35%, respectively) [7]. They also noted significant loss of range of motion compared with the contralateral side, with 30% loss of distal interphalangeal joint motion, 24% of proximal interphalangeal joint motion, and 8% of metacarpophalangeal motion. Patients also reported cold intolerance, hypersensitivity, paresthesias, constant pain, and impairment of activities of daily living. Long-term peripheral neurologic dysfunction and infection may also occur after high-pressure injection injuries due to injection of water and air. Thus, despite the lack of urgency for surgical intervention, these injuries still warrant close observation and management [36, 40].

Summary

High-pressure injection injuries to the hand can have devastating sequelae, leading to eventual amputation and poor functional outcomes. Strong clinical suspicion and prompt wide surgical debridement as needed are critical to the long-term preservation and restoration of function. Empiric broad-spectrum antibiotic coverage is also reasonable to prevent infection. Although the use of steroids cannot be fully recommended based on current evidence, our understanding of the pathophysiology of this injury has provided some insight into the potential determinants of prognosis with steroid use.

References

1. Rees CE. Penetration of tissue by fuel oil under high pressure from diesel engine. J Am Med Assoc. 1937;109(11):866.
2. Neal NC, Burke FD. High-pressure injection injuries. Injury. 1991;22(6):467–70.
3. Blue A, Dirstine M. Grease gun damage: subcutaneous injection of paint, grease, and other materials by pressure guns. Northwest Med. 1965;64:342–4.
4. Verhoeven N, Hierner R. High-pressure injection injury of the hand: an often underestimated trauma: case report with study of the literature. Strategies Trauma Limb Reconstr (Online). 2008;3(1):27–33.
5. Sirio CA, Smith JS, Graham WP. High-pressure injection injuries of the hand. A review. Am Surg. 1989;55(12):714–8.
6. Pinto MR, Turkula-Pinto LD, Cooney WP, Wood MB, Dobyns JH. High-pressure injection injuries of the hand: review of 25 patients managed by open wound technique. J Hand Surg Am. 1993;18(1):125–30.
7. Wieder A, Lapid O, Plakht Y, Sagi A. Long-term follow-up of high-pressure injection injuries to the hand. Plast Reconstr Surg. 2006;117(1):186–9.
8. Lewis HG, Clarke P, Kneafsey B, Brennen MD. A 10-year review of high-pressure injection injuries to the hand. J Hand Surg Br. 1998;23(4):479–81.
9. McClinton MA, Wright S. High-pressure tool injection injuries. Md Med J (Baltimore, Md: 1985). 1985;34(3):289–91.

10. Gillespie C a, Rodeheaver GT, Smith S, Edgerton MT, Edlich RF. Airless paint gun injuries: definition and management. Am J surg. 1974;128(3):383–91.

11. Schoo MJ, Scott FA, Boswick JA. High-pressure injection injuries of the hand. J Trauma. 1980;20(3):229–38.

12. Kaufman HD. High pressure injection injuries, the problems, pathogenesis and management. Hand. 1970;2(1):63–73.

13. Scott AR. Occupational high-pressure injection injuries: pathogenesis and prevention. J Soc Occup Med. 1983;33(2):56–9.

14. Waters WR, Penn I, Ross HM. Airless paint gun injuries of the hand: a clinical and experimental study. Plast Reconstr surg. 1967;39(6):613–8.

15. Kaufman HD. The anatomy of experimentally produced high-pressure injection injuries of the hand. Br J surg. 1968;55(5):340–4.

16. Stark HH, Ashworth CR, Boyes JH. Paint-gun injuries of the hand. J Bone Joint Surg Am. 1967;49(4):637–47.

17. Dickson RA. High pressure injection injuries of the hand. A clinical, chemical and histological study. Hand. 1976;8(2):189–93.

18. Rimmer MG, King JB, Franklin A. Accidental injection of white spirit into the hand in golfers. J Hand Surg Br. 1993;18(5):654–5.

19. Green SM. Injection injuries of the hand. Bull Hosp Jt Dis Orthop Inst. 1981;41:48–58.

20. Hogan CJ, Ruland RT. High-pressure injection injuries to the upper extremity: a review of the literature. J Orthop Trauma. 2006;20(7):503–11.

21. Christodoulou L, Melikyan EY, Woodbridge S, Burke FD. Functional outcome of high-pressure injection injuries of the hand. J Trauma. 2001;50(4):717–20.

22. Dial DE. H and injuries due to injection of oil at high pressures. JAMA. 1938;110(21):1747.

23. Valentino M, Rapisarda V, Fenga C. Hand injuries due to high-pressure injection devices for painting in shipyards: circumstances, management, and outcome in twelve patients. Am J Ind Med. 2003;43(5):539–42.

24. Schnall SB, Mirzayan R. High-pressure injection injuries to the hand. Hand Clin. 1999;15(2):245–8, viii.

25. Gelberman RH, Posch JL, Jurist JM. High-pressure injection injuries of the hand. J Bone Joint Surg Am. 1975;57(7):935–7.

26. Crabb DJ. The value of plain radiographs in treating grease-gun injuries. Hand. 1981;13(1):39–42.

27. Pai CH, Wei DC, Hou SP. High-pressure injection injuries of the hand. J Trauma. 1991;31(1):110–2.

28. Couzens G, Burke FD. Veterinary high pressure injection injuries with inoculations for larger animals. J Hand Surg Br. 1995;20(4):497–9.

29. Weltmer JB, Pack LL. High-pressure water-gun injection injuries to the extremities. A report of six cases. J Bone Joint Surg Am. 1988;70(8):1221–3.

30. Curka PA, Chisholm CD. High-pressure water injection injury to the hand. Am J Emerg Med. 1989;7(2):165–7.

31. Kaufman HD. The clinicopathological correlation of high-pressure injection injuries. Br J Surg. 1968;55(3):214–8.

32. Bottoms RW. A case of high pressure hydraulic tool injury to the hand, its treatment aided by dexamethasone and a plea for further trial of this substance. Med J Aust. 1962;49(2):591–2.

33. Gutowski KA, Chu J, Choi M, Friedman DW. High-pressure hand injection injuries caused by dry cleaning solvents: case reports, review of the literature, and treatment guidelines. Plast Reconstr Surg. 2003;111(1):174–7.

34. Wong TC, Ip FK, Wu WC. High-pressure injection injuries of the hand in a Chinese population. J Hand Surg Br. 2005;30(6):588–92.

35. Mirzayan R, Schnall SB, Chon JH, Holtom PD, Patzakis MJ, Stevanovic MV. Culture results and amputation rates in high-pressure paint gun injuries of the hand. Orthopedics. 2001;24(6):587–9.

36. Temple C, Richards R, Dawson W. Pneumomediastinum after injection injury to the hand. Ann Plast Surg. 2000;45(1):64–6.

37. Subramaniam RM, Clearwater GM. High-pressure water injection injury: emergency presentation and management. Emerg Med (Fremantle, WA). 2002;14(3):324–7.

38. Ramos H, Posch JL, Lie KK. High-pressure injection injuries of the hand. Plast Reconstr Surg. 1970;45(3):221–6.

39. Lewis RC. High-compression injection injuries to the hand. Emerg Med Clin North Am. 1985;3(2):373–81.

40. Markal N, Celebioğlu S. Compression neuropathy of the hand after high-pressure air injection. Ann Plast Surg. 2000;44(6):680–1.

41. Rosenwasser MP, Wei DH. High-pressure injection injuries to the hand. J Am Acad Orthop Surg. 2014;22(1):38–45. doi:10.5435/JAAOS-22-01-38 (with permission from Wolters Kluwer Health. Copyright Robert Strauch, MD, New York, NY).

Fingertip Amputations: Supermicrosurgery and Replantation

Alexander B. Dagum

Introduction

The possibility of reattaching a completely severed part has been the dream of reconstructive surgeons for centuries [1, 2]. It was not until 1965 that Komatsu and Tamai replanted a digit, in this case, a completely amputated thumb [3]. The subsequent establishment of replantation centers throughout the world has led to viability rates of 80–90 %. Many early pioneers of microsurgery advised against reattaching single digits, as it was felt that the digit would get in the way and be bypassed by the patient [4, 5]. By the mid-80s and early 90s, reports started to appear that single digit replantation distal to the flexor digitorum superficialis (FDS) provided better function than a revision amputation [6–10]. However, replantation of fingertips has been late to gain acceptance in hand surgery, in particular when it is an isolated injury. Many hand surgeons perceive that these technically challenging, lengthy procedures provide little functional gains over a revision amputation. Fingertip replantation allows for the restoration of length, function, and esthetics while avoiding a painful stump neuroma. The intricate function of the fingertip and nail cannot otherwise be restored as well [11].

Classification

Fingertip amputations are classified by the mechanism of injury and the anatomic level.

There are three types of amputations: guillotine, crush, and avulsion. A guillotine amputation refers to a clean-cut amputation such as those seen with a knife and has a narrow zone of injury. A crush amputation is usually caused by a compressive force and has a larger zone of injury. An avulsion amputation has the largest zone of injury and is caused by tearing and degloving as seen after rotating machine or rope injuries [1, 2]. Guillotine amputations have the best survival and functional outcomes, while avulsions have the worst [1, 2].

There are various anatomic classifications for fingertip amputations. These include those of Allen, Foucher, Tamai, Ishikawa, Hirase, and others [6, 12–16]. The one most often used probably because of its simplicity and preferred at our institution is that of Tamai. He classified fingertip amputations into two zones by level: zone I, distal to the base of the nail, and zone II, from the base of the nail to the distal interphalangeal joint (DIPJ). Ishikawa et al. expanded on Tamai's classification into four subzones. Subzone I distal to the midpoint of the nail, subzone II from the nail base to the midpoint, subzone III from midway of the nail base and DIPJ to the nail base, and subzone IV from the DIPJ to the midway point (Fig. 5.1).

A. B. Dagum (✉)
Department of Surgery, Stony Brook Medicine,
HSC T-19 Rm 60, Stony Brook, NY 11791-8191, USA
e-mail: alexander.dagum@stonybrook.edu

L. M. Rozmaryn (ed.), *Fingertip Injuries,* DOI 10.1007/978-3-319-13227-3_5,
© Springer International Publishing Switzerland 2015

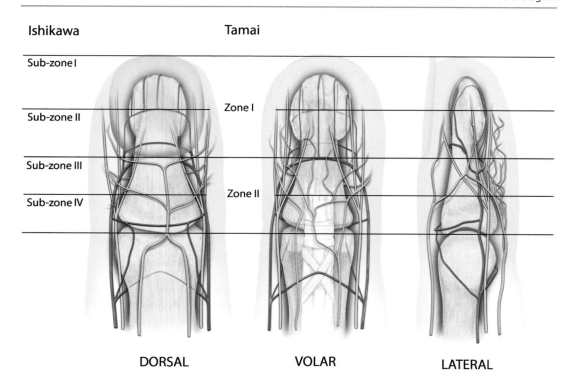

Ishikawa   Tamai

Sub-zone I

Sub-zone II   Zone I

Sub-zone III

Sub-zone IV   Zone II

DORSAL   VOLAR   LATERAL

Fig. 5.1 **a**, **b**, **c** Fingertip arterial, venous, and nerve anatomy by Tamai and Ishikawa zones (with permission by Alexander B. Dagum)

Surgical Anatomy

A thorough knowledge of the vascular anatomy of the fingertip is necessary for successful fingertip replantation. The arterial anatomy is relatively constant and has been well described in the classic paper by Strauch and de Moura and others [17–19]. The ulnar digital artery is dominant in the thumb, index, and long fingers and the radial digital artery is dominant in the ring and small fingers. The ulnar and radial arteries are connected by three transverse palmar arches in the finger: two Gothic-like (pointed) arches at the level of the C1 and C3 cruciate pulleys and a rounded (Romanesque) arch just distal to the insertion of the flexor digitorum profundus (FDP) tendon. At the level of the distal transverse palmar arch (DTPA), the digital arteries measure 0.85 ± 0.1 mm in diameter. There are approximately three or more arteries that takeoff from the distal arch measuring 0.58 ± 0.1 mm with

the center one being dominant and known as the terminal central artery (Fig. 5.1). These terminal arteries are in close proximity to the periosteum, travel longitudinally before turning dorsally, and communicate with the distal matrix arch. There is some tortuosity to these distal pulp arteries which allows for some extra length to be gained with dissection [19, 20].

The venous anatomy is more variable and consists of a dorsal and palmar system [21, 22] (Fig. 5.1). The dorsal system is dominant and commences in the paronychial area as one or two venules on each side of the nail fold measuring approximately 0.2 mm distally and 0.4 mm proximally. They unite at the level of the nail bed in the middle forming a central vein known as the dorsal terminal vein measuring (0.5–0.8 mm). This dorsal vein increases slightly in size before dividing into two or three veins at the level of the DIPJ.

The palmar venous network commences at the tip and forms multiple anastomosing veins in the subcutaneous tissue with no consistent pattern.

They converge at the level of the base of the distal phalanx into one to three veins, with the central vein measuring 0.4–0.6 mm in diameter and lateral veins 0.3–0.5 mm in diameter. The palmar and dorsal systems are connected by the lateral commissural veins which measure 0.5–0.8 mm at the level of the DIPJ.

The digital nerve trifurcates 60 % of the time just distal to the DIPJ crease in 78 % of digit [23]. There may be anywhere from two to five branches in the digits and as many as seven in the thumb [23]. In the thumb, they consist of the proximal dorsal, distal medial, and lateral ungal branches [24]. There is an extensive crossover distal to this of the territory supplied by each nerve branch.

Indications and Contraindications

The decision to replant a part should be made at a replantation center. A careful evaluation of the patient and the part needs to be made. The patient needs to be aware of the limitations of replantation surgery. In patients with serious life-threatening conditions or illnesses, replantation is contraindicated [1, 2]. In fingertip amputations, the part needs to be evaluated with the operating microscope as surgical loop magnification is usually insufficient to assess the vessels.

In general, fingertip replantation is indicated in all children because of their great regenerative potential, in musicians or patients in whom digital length is very important for their employment or hobbies, or where esthetic concerns are paramount. Replantation is contraindicated in crush avulsion injuries where there has been significant soft tissue injury or contamination or injury at multiple levels. Nevertheless, the part should be scrutinized for their salvage potential and the spare part's concept used. A nonmicrovascular replantable distal fingertip amputation can sometimes be reattached as a composite graft after appropriate debridement, yielding a reasonable result (Fig. 5.2). The results of composite fingertip grafts, Tamai zone I for adults, are in the order of 20 versus 50 % for children and depend on various factors [25–27]. Several techniques have been proposed to improve survival of composite grafts including hyperbaric oxygen, cooling, and the pocket principle.

In the pocket method, the part is de-epithelialized, reattached, and then buried into a subcutaneous pocket in the abdomen, axilla, chest, and more recently the palm. This increases the surface area contact and thus blood supply. At 2–3 weeks, the part is detached from the pocket and allows to re-epithelialize over a 3-week period or a thin split thickness skin graft applied. The pocket principle has not gained widespread acceptance despite being first described by Brent in 1979, and subsequently modified by several authors with reported success rates from 14 to 90 %. It would appear to be best suited for non-replantable fingertip amputations distal to the lunula [28–31].

Care of the Amputation Part and Patient

Appropriate care of the amputated part is extremely important. Cooling of the part to 4 °C lowers the metabolic rate and doubles the allowable ischemia time. The part should be gently cleaned with saline, then wrapped in saline-soaked gauze and placed in a bag and into a container consisting of ice slurry, which will be at approximately 4 °C. The part can also be placed in a container of saline, which is then placed in an ice bucket. The part must not rest on pure ice because this can lead to a frostbite injury making the part no longer replantable. Although there have been isolated reports of longer ischemia times with successful outcomes, in general, digits will tolerate 12 h of warm ischemia and up to 24 h of cold ischemia time [1, 2, 32].

The overall management of the patient takes precedence. This mandates a thorough history and physical examination. The tetanus status should be checked and given as per protocol if needed. Antibiotics are given. This usually consists of cefazolin except in farm injuries for which Gram-negative coverage with gentamicin is usually added. The appropriate laboratory workup is performed and radiographs of the part and amputation stump are obtained. An axillary block is used to provide for pain relief and vasodilation.

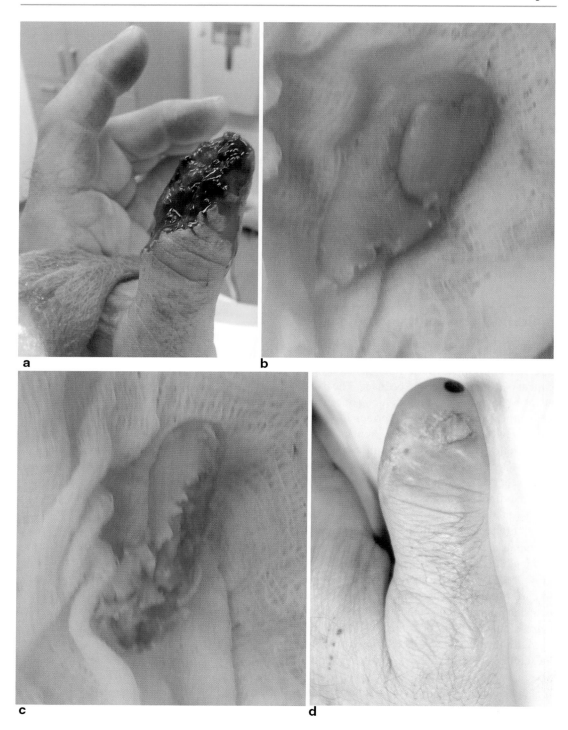

Fig. 5.2 Fifty-one-year-old male with a Tamai zone II fingertip amputation. **a** The part consisted of skin, pulp germinal matrix, and sterile matrix and contained a small amount of tuft distally. No suitable vessels were available for arterial anastomosis as it was superficial to the digital artery and terminal arteries. **b**, **c** The part was carefully debrided and the small piece of tuft removed and then the remaining part was reattached as a composite graft. **d** Three months post injury, showing a healed composite graft with a new nail growing in

The part is carefully assessed for the type and extent of injury, presence of a second level of injury, and contamination. Red streaks or bruising along the skin in the course of the digital arteries, the so-called Chinese red lines, represent the tearing of the small side branches of the digital arteries and signify extensive digital vessel injury. If the digital artery is elongated, twisted, and curled up like a pigtail (the ribbon sign), this signifies extensive intimal damage to the vessel. Both of these signs usually preclude successful replantation unless the zone of injury can be bypassed with a vein graft.

Technique

The use of two teams is optimal when multiple fingertips/digits have been amputated. One team works on the amputated part and the other on the amputation stumps. In isolated fingertip amputations, one team suffices, as in general the part can be assessed and prepared in under an hour. This in general is less than the time it takes to prepare the patient and bring him from the emergency room to the operating room. At our institution, we have performed fingertip replantations under local anesthesia with IV sedation, regional anesthesia, and general anesthesia.

The part is carefully assessed for its replant potential. In fingertip amputations, a significant crush or avulsion component will usually preclude successful replantation, as once one is out of the zone injury, very little fingertip will be left to work with. A clean-cut injury with at most a limited crush component will yield best results.

Ishikawa subzone I amputations, i.e., distal to the midpoint of the nail, are extremely challenging, but good reconstructive options are available for fingernail preservation such as composite graft, V–Y advancement flaps, etc. Subzone II amputations from the nail base to midpoint of the nail are very challenging as well, but reconstructive options diminish as the injury proceeds proximally (Fig. 5.3). A similar approach is used in Ishikawa subzones I and II or Tamai zone I injuries. The part is examined for its replant potential under the microscope. The part can be stabilized by suturing the nail plate to a suture package; the suture package can then be held by an assistant [33]. We have modified this technique and held the suture package with a lead hand, thus freeing up the assistant. A search for the terminal central artery which runs close to the midline just superficial to the periosteum is carried out in both the part and the stump by gently dissecting and elevating the soft tissue. The stump is assessed for any area of pulsation which, if seen,

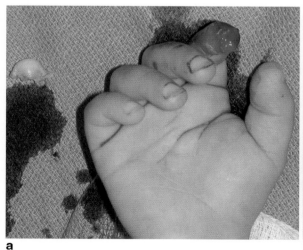
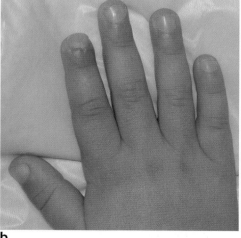

a **b**

Fig. 5.3 **a** A child sustained a Tamai zone I, Ishikawa subzone II fingertip amputation. **b** Three months post replantation, showing some mild pulp atrophy, but otherwise a good result

will indicate the location of the proximal artery. Matching the part to the stump can then facilitate locating the terminal artery if one is having difficulties. Although, in general, the distal artery is very consistent in its location and not difficult to find, the central artery has a certain amount of tortuosity which provides for added length when dissected distally [19, 20]. Occasionally, at subzone II, a palmar vein of suitable quality or lateral commissural vein will be found. Pressure on the pulp will sometimes lead to a small venous ooze facilitating the location of the vein. In the author's experience, a suitable vein is often not found at these levels and the strategies delineated below will need to be applied for venous drainage. The vascular structures are tagged with 10–0 nylon. A 028 K-wire or just sutures are used to secure the part. A dorsal-to-volar sequence of repair is used. Care is taken to repair the sterile matrix with 6–0 chromic gut. It is not always feasible or necessary to apply a microvascular clamp. The repair starts with the back wall first as one may not be able to easily flip the vessel. A small nylon suture can be used to stent the vessel and facilitate repair [34]. The anastomoses are performed with four to five 11–0 nylon sutures around the vessel wall; care is taken during the anastomosis as the vessel walls are thin and can easily tear. No nerve anastomosis is performed at this level, as the branches will have arborized with no suitable size branch available for repair. Nevertheless, good sensory recovery occurs at this level probably through spontaneous neurotization from the multiple branches [12].

Tamai zone II or Ishikawa subzones III and IV are amputations between the DIPJ and nail base (Figs. 5.4, 5.5 and 5.6). At these levels, no good option exists for fingertip and nail reconstruction, but the vessels are larger and replantation easier. Adequate debridement is performed with appropriate bone shortening (Fig. 5.4). If the repair is through the germinal matrix, meticulous repair is essential to avoid late fingernail deformities. Injuries through the DIPJ level or in very close proximity are arthrodesed (Figs. 5.5 and 5.6). One or two K-wires are used for bony osteosynthesis, occasionally a circlage wire with one K-wire is used for more proximal injuries. The FDP tendon,

if lacerated, is repaired if adequate distal tendon is available for repair. At the level of the DIPJ, curvilinear midlateral incisions both in the part and in the stump are adequate to expose the distal digital vessels, digital nerve branches, and dorsal veins. Distal to the DIPJ, a thin oblique flap is preferred for exposure of the vessels as described by Tsai et al. [35]. The oblique flap is made very thin to avoid injuring the palmar veins in case these are necessary for venous anastomosis. It is important to keep in mind that in the fingers the DTPA was found on average at 13.7 mm from tip or at the level of germinal matrix [19]. In a distal subzone III amputation, the repair will be at the level of the distal digital artery as it is forming the arch. Attention is then turned to isolating the terminal dorsal vein which is found along the dorsal midline from the DIPJ to the level of the germinal matrix [21]. Usually, one large vein, a few millimeters proximal to the nail fold, greater than 5 mm distally and more often 8 mm proximally will be found. We also look laterally and search for a lateral commissural vein and palmar for palmar veins. All structures are tagged with 10–0 nylon. In proximal subzone III and subzone IV, we look laterally to isolate a nerve branch for repair. Usually, one nerve branch is found without too much effort radially and ulnarly and tagged. At these more proximal levels, repair of one branch will lead to good sensory recovery and is better than no repair in the author's experience.

An opposing curvilinear or oblique incision, depending on the zone, is performed on the part to identify the proximal neurovascular structures. Prior to elevating the tourniquet, the distal stump is observed for pulsation which helps in identifying the distal digital arteries. If pulsations are observed, this bodes well for the success of the replantation [2]. Matching the stump to part and vice versa can help in isolating structures. The bony osteosynthesis is then performed, followed by repair of the flexor and extensor tendons if necessary in more proximal injuries, and germinal matrix in more distal injuries. The tourniquet is deflated and the proximal artery assessed for good pulsatile flow, i.e., a good squirt test if this was not assessed on the stump prior to elevation of the tourniquet. Both in the part and in the

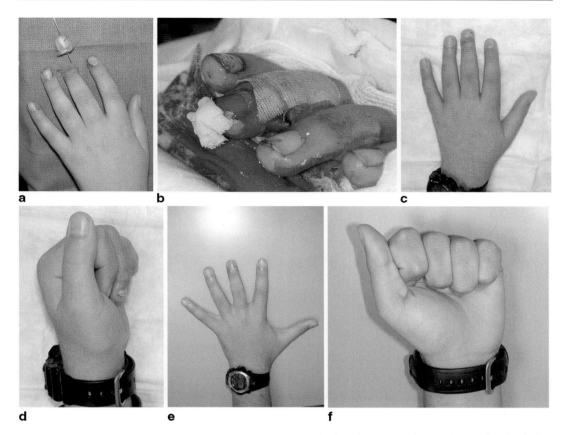

Fig. 5.4 a, b Fourteen-year-old boy with a clean-cut Ishikawa Sub-zone III fingertip amputation through the growth plate from a zip line. **c, d** Three months later and **e, f** 5 years post operation, the digit was slightly shorter than the contralateral side from premature closure of the growth plate; he recovered normal two-point discrimination and 30° of DIPJ motion. (From: [2]. Used with permission from Alexander B. Dagum and The American Society for Surgery of the Hand). DIPJ distal interphalangeal joint

stump, it is important to dissect the vessels out of the zone of injury back to healthy-appearing vessels. There should be no clots in the vessels, petechiae, or other evidence of vascular injury. If it is apparent that vein grafts are going to be necessary, it is best to perform the vein graft to the distal artery prior to bony osteosynthesis. Vein grafts are harvested from the volar aspect of the thenar eminence or distal wrist [2, 36]. Because vein grafts have valves, they need to be reversed and should be marked with a small Ligaclip on the proximal end, which will signify the distal end when placed as a graft.

Once the preparation is complete, the tourniquet is deflated and the arteries assessed for pulsatile bleeding. If there is no pulsatile bleeding and the vessels appear of good quality, there may be an element of vasospasm. Before sectioning proximally, one must check with the anesthesiologist that the patient is not cold, dry, hypotensive, or on vasoconstrictors to maintain his or her blood pressure. If so, these factors need to be reversed. The amputation stump should be warmed with saline and topical papaverine or lidocaine applied to help vasodilate the vessel. If these methods are not successful in restoring pulsatile flow, the vessel should be dissected and sectioned more proximally and vein grafts used [1, 2].

The tourniquet is reinflated and the arterial and nerve repairs performed. It is our preference to repair both digital arteries and two veins

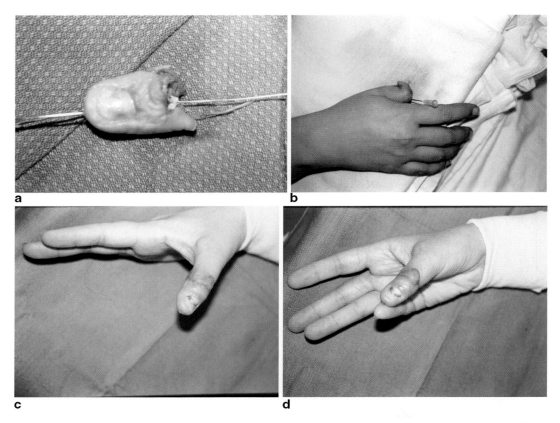

a   b   c   d

Fig. 5.5 a, b A watch jeweler sustained a thumb avulsion injury at the IPJ level Tamai zone II from a rein on a horse that was spooked. **c, d** Replantation was successful in restoring good hand function and 12 mm of two-point discrimination. However, the sensation was not good enough for her to return to her prior occupation. (From: [2]. Used with permission from Alexander B. Dagum and The American Society for Surgery of the Hand). *IPJ* interphalangeal joint

if possible. If a large terminal central vein was isolated, this is repaired next prior to letting the tourniquet down. The patient is given a loading dose of 5000 units of heparin before digital artery repair and then started on a heparin drip at 1000 units/h, adjusted to an activated partial thromboplastin time (aPTT) of 1.5 times the control. The tourniquet is deflated, the arterial anastomosis is assessed for flow, and the fingertip evaluated for perfusion. Deflating the tourniquet facilitates isolating adequate distal veins for anastomosis. These veins are tagged and the tourniquet usually reinflated to facilitate venous repair. As long as the patient has been heparinized, the author has not encountered problems with thrombosis of the digital arterial anastomosis with reinflation of the tourniquet.

An arterial-only repair has an approximately 40% chance of survival depending on the level; therefore, it is imperative to find some form of venous outflow to improve survival of the replanted part [37]. Various techniques are available to achieve venous outflow. The classic methods involve heparinization and external bleeding by the use of medicinal leeches, or rubbing heparin pledgets on a pulp stab wound or nail bed until normal venous connections are reestablished between the amputation part and the stump. If medicinal leeches (*Hirudo medicinalis*) are used, the patient should be started on gentamicin, ciprofloxacin, trimethoprim-sulfamethoxazole, tetracycline, or third-generation cephalosporin to prevent an infection from *Aeromonas hydrophilia*, from the leech which can lead to not

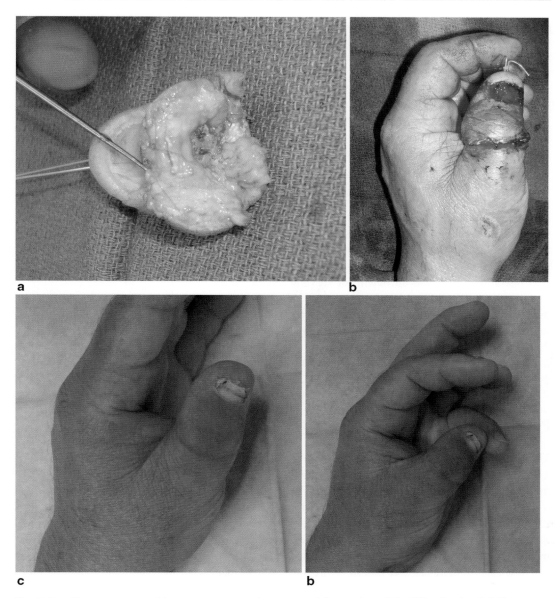

Fig. 5.6 a Forty-seven-year-old carpenter, two-pack a day smoker, sustained a Tamai zone II complete amputation of his thumb. The part was debrided, the structures tagged for repair, and the IPJ arthrodesed. **b** Status post replantation. **c, d** Seven months later, showing a solid fusion with good function

only loss of the part but also sepsis. *A. hydrophilia* is not sensitive to cefazolin. A leech is applied four to five times a day for 5–7 days. Placement of a Styrofoam cup with a hole to isolate the congested digit will prevent the leech from attaching to an inappropriate digit. It will feed for 15–30 min before detaching. It injects a very powerful anticoagulant known as

Hirudin that allows the puncture wound to bleed for 8–12 h, thus preventing congestion. The alternative is to rub the sterile matrix or a puncture wound on the fingertip with heparin-soaked pledgets every half an hour for 5–7 days. Leech or the pledgets are continued until the fingertip has normal capillary refill with no evidence of congestion and pinprick of the tip yields slow red oxygenated bleeding. These techniques will increase the survival of the arterial-only fingertip replantations to 80% [12, 38–41]. Because there will be continuous oozing, the majority (77%) of patients will require a blood transfusion [40, 41].

The alternatives consist of use of an arteriovenous fistula with anastomosis of a distal artery to a proximal vein or creation of a venocutaneous fistula [42, 43]. A venocutaneous fistula involves suturing a vein graft distally to a surgically created punch wound on the replanted parts of the pulp and running the vein graft proximally to a dorsal vein on the digit. The vein graft is covered with a film dressing or split thickness skin graft to prevent desiccation. In one study, the vein graft was found to stay patent 4 or more days post operation which was sufficient for survival of the replanted part [43]. Another option that has been advocated is that of waiting 24 h to perform the venous repair [44]. This allows for the distal draining veins to become engorged and easier to isolate but has the disadvantage of a second surgery.

Postoperative Care

The patient is transferred from the recovery room to a microsurgical step-down unit for postoperative monitoring. The patient is kept on nil per os (NPO, meaning nothing by mouth) status for 12–24 h in case a take-back to the operating room is necessary. It is important to keep the patient well hydrated, warm, and on a caffeine-free diet, with complete smoke cessation to prevent vasospasm. A warming blanket is placed over the dressing and the patient is given lactated Ringer's solution at 150 mL/h for 48 h to keep him or her vasodilated and well perfused and to prevent vasospasm. The patient is kept anticoagulated with heparin to aPTT of 1.5 times control for 5–7 days and on aspirin at 81 mg/day for 6 weeks. The patient is kept on strict bed rest for 3 days, then progresses with ambulation as tolerated. The dressing is not changed until day 7 to prevent any disruption in the vascular anastomosis. The patient is usually discharged on day 7 [1, 2].

The replanted part is monitored hourly for 48 h and then every 4 h thereafter. This involves assessing the capillary refill, temperature, turgor, and color (CTTC). The author no longer uses continuous monitors for digital replantation and relies solely on good clinical observation. If the digit is pale with no capillary refill and diminished turgor (prune like) and cold, an arterial thrombosis is suspected. If the digit is blue, engorged with rapid capillary refill, and cool, a venous thrombosis is suspected. If there is cause for concern, the digit is pricked with a 21-gauge needle for bleeding; slow, bright red (oxygenated) bleeding signifies a well-perfused digit; rapid, dark blue bleeding signifies a venous problem; and poor or no bleeding, an arterial problem[1, 2].

Complications

Early complications in fingertip replantation are primarily vascular and lead to loss of the replant. At the first evidence of vascular insufficiency, the dressing should be loosened to make sure there is no constriction on the digit or part. This is followed by release of a few sutures, as there may be compression of the vessel from postoperative edema or a small hematoma. If this fails to restore perfusion, the patient should be immediately taken back to the operating room for re-exploration, and the vessel in question is assessed. This means redoing the anastomosis with vein grafts if needed. If this restores adequate perfusion, there is no need to assess the other vessel. For example, if it is an arterial problem and repairing the artery restores normal perfusion, the vein repair need not be explored and vice versa. Although the need for re-exploration is uncommon, if done early, it is associated with a 50–60% salvage rate. At our institution, we will re-explore Tamai zone II and more proximal replantation if warranted; however, in Tamai zone I injuries, we do not re-explore. If venous re-exploration fails to provide adequate venous drainage, medicinal leeches should be used or the nail plate should be removed with application of heparin-soaked pledgets as outlined previously. Infection is uncommon in digital replantations.

Bleeding can be a major postoperative complication even in a fingertip. It may be caused by excessive anticoagulation, inadequate hemostasis, an arterial or venous anastomotic leak, or a thrombosed vein. If reversal of the anticoagulation does not reverse the bleeding, the patient should be taken back and assessed in the operating room where adequate lighting and equipment allow for appropriate hemostasis.

Bony nonunion is related to inadequate fixation and shortening. This can be a problem in proximal, Tamai zone II amputations. It has been reported to occur up to rates of 21 % with cross K-wires, 8 % with a single K-wire and interosseous wire, and 0 % with perpendicular interosseous wires. Nevertheless, with prolonged splinting, one third of early nonunions will go on to bony union [45].

The most common late complications include cold intolerance, numbness, and nail deformity and pulp atrophy, in particular, in Tamai zone I and distal zone II amputations.

Outcomes

In a recent systematic review by Sebastin and Chung, of 30 studies representing 2273 distal replantation, the overall survival rate was 86 % with no difference in the survival rate between Tamai zone I and zone II amputations [11]. Clean-cut amputations had a better survival at 92 % versus crush at 80 %, and avulsion at 75 %. Zone 1 amputations with vein repair had a 92 % survival and without an 83 % survival rate. Zone 2 amputations had an 88 % survival with vein repair versus 78 % without. The average two-point discrimination was reported to be 7 mm despite that in 50 % of patients, no digital nerve was repaired, 24 % one nerve, and 26 % both digital nerves. In zone 1 injuries, there is most likely significant neurotization with very short regeneration distances and extensive branching that account for the high success of reinnervation. In the author's experience, Tamai zone I injuries do well, but proximal zone II injuries

without nerve repair and a crush component do not recover such good sensation and cold intolerance can be a significant problem particularly in northern climates. Ninety-eight percent of patients returned to work.

Nail abnormalities were in the order of 24 %. These are primarily related to the level of injury, sterile matrix versus germinal matrix, and the type of injury—clean cut versus crush—as well as the return of adequate perfusion. Pulp atrophy was reported to occur 14 % of the time and is again likely related to the type and extent of injury and the postoperative circulation status. Hahn and Jung in a large study of 450 zone 1 injuries felt that this was primarily a vascular issue and that repairing as many veins as possible decreased the chances of developing these complications [46].

In a level 3 study, Hattori et al. compared the functional outcome of distal replantation versus revision amputation. In their study of 46 patients of which half underwent replantation and half revision amputation, they found that the successful replantation group had a greater range of motion at the PIPJ, had less pain, better disabilities of the arm, shoulder and hand (DASH) score, and all were highly or fairly satisfied compared to 54 % of the revision amputation group [11]. There was no difference in grip strength, paresthesia, and cold intolerance. The time spent off work, in hospital, was longer and the cost five times as much for the replantation group versus the revision amputation.

Conclusions

Fingertip replantation can be challenging, but in the right patient, has a better functional and esthetic outcome than a revision amputation by providing increased length and preservation of nail function while avoiding a painful neuroma. Appropriate patient selection, firm knowledge of the vascular anatomy, and good microsurgical skills will often lead to a successful and rewarding outcome.

References

1. Dagum AB, Mirza MA. Replantation surgery in the upper extremity. In: Dee R, Hurst LC, Gruber MA, Kottmeier SA, editors. Principles of orthopedic practice. 2nd ed. New York: McGraw-Hill, 1997. pp. 1187–92 (Chap. 64).
2. Dagum AB. Replantation: indications and rationale. In: Seitz WH, editor. Fractures and dislocations of the hand and fingers. Chicago: American Society for Surgery of the Hand, 2013. pp. 260–76 (Chap. 17).
3. Komatsu S, Tamai S. Successful replantation of a completely cut-off thumb. Plast Reconstr Surg. 1968;42:374–7.
4. Morrison WA, O'Brien BM, MacLeod AM. Evaluation of digital replantation: a review of 100 cases. Orthop Clin North Am. 1977;8:295–308.
5. Weiland AJ, Villarreal-Rios A, Kleinert HE, Kutz J, Atasoy E, Lister G. Replantation of digits and hands: analysis of surgical techniques and functional results in 71 patients with 86 replantations. J Hand Surg. 1977;2A:1–12.
6. Foucher G, Henderson HR, Maneaud M, Merle M, Braun FM. Distal digital replantation: one of the best indications for microsurgery. Int J Microsurg. 1981;3:263–70.
7. Yamano Y. Replantation of the amputated distal part of the fingers. J Hand Surg. 1985;10A:211–8.
8. Urbaniak JR, Roth JH, Nunley JA, Goldner RD, Koman LA. The results of replantation after amputation of a single finger. J Bone Joint Surg. 1985;67A:611–9.
9. Goldner RD, Stevanovic MV, Nunley JA, Urbaniak JR. Digital replantation at the level of the distal interphalangeal joint and the distal phalanx. J Hand Surg. 1989;14A:214–20.
10. Foucher G, Norris RW. Distal and very distal digital replantations. Br J Plast Surg. 1992;45:199–203.
11. Hattori Y, Doi K, Ikeda K, Estrella EP. A retrospective study of functional outcomes after successful replantation versus amputation closure for single fingertip amputations. J Hand Surg. 2006;31A:811–8.
12. Sebastin SJ, Chung KC. A systematic review of the outcomes of replantation of distal digital amputation. Plast Reconstr Surg. 2011;128:723–37.
13. Allen MJ. Conservative management of fingertip injuries in adults. Hand. 1980;12:257–65 [PubMed: 7002744].
14. Tamai S. Twenty years' experience of limb replantation review of 293 upper extremity replants. J Hand Surg. 1982;7A:549–56 [PubMed: 7175124].
15. Ishikawa K, Ogawa Y, Soeda H, Yoshida Y. A new classification of the amputation level for the distal part of the fingers. J Jpn Soc Microsurg. 1990;3:54–62.
16. Hirase Y. Salvage of fingertip amputated at nail level: new surgical principles and treatments. Ann Plast Surg. 1997;38:151–7 [PubMed: 9043584].
17. Strauch B, de Moura W. Arterial system of the fingers. J Hand Surg. 1990;15A:148–54.
18. Chaudakshetrin P, Kumar VP, Satku K, Pho RWH. Digital artery diameters: an anatomic and clinical study. J Hand Surg. 1987;6B:740–3.
19. Smith DO, Oura C, Kimura C, Toshimori K. Artery anatomy and tortuosity in the distal finger. J Hand Surg. 1991;16A:297–302.
20. Smith DO, Tajima N, Oura C, Toshimori K. Digital artery tortuosity and elasticity: a biomechanical study. J Reconstr Microsurg. 1991;7:105–8.
21. Smith DO, Oura C, Kimura C, Toshimori K. The distal venous anatomy of the finger. J Hand Surg. 1991;16A:303–7.
22. Lucas GL. The pattern of venous drainage of the digits. J Hand Surg. 1984;9A:448–50.
23. Zenn MR, Hoffman L, Latrenta G, Hotchkiss R. Variations in digital nerve anatomy. J Hand Surg. 1992;17A:1033–6.
24. Johnson RK, Shrewsbury MM. Neural pattern in the human pollical distal phalanx. Clin Anat. 2005;18:428–33.
25. Elsahy NI. When to replant a fingertip after its complete amputation. Plast Reconstr Surg. 1977;60(1):14–21.
26. Moiemen NS, Elliot D. Composite graft replacement of digital tips. 2. A study in children. J Hand Surg. 1997;22B(3):346–52.
27. Imaizumi A, Ishida K, Arashiro K, Nishizeki O. Validity of exploration for suitable vessels for replantation in the distal fingertip amputation in early childhood: replantation or composite graft. J Plast Surg Hand Surg. 2013;47(4):258–62.
28. Brent B. Replantation of amputated distal phalangeal parts of fingers without vascular anastomoses, using subcutaneous pockets. Plast Reconstr Surg. 1979;63:1–8.
29. Arata J, Ishikawa K, Soeda H, Sawabe K, Kokoroishi R, Togo T. The palmar pocket method: an adjunct to the management of zone I and II fingertip amputations. J Hand Surg. 2001;26A:945–50.
30. Yabe T, Tsuda T, Hirose S, Ozawa T. Treatment of fingertip amputation: comparison of results between microsurgical replantation and pocket principle. J Reconstr Microsurg. 2012;28(4):221–6.
31. Muneuchi G, Kurokawa M, Igawa K, Hamamoto Y, Igawa HH. Nonmicrosurgical replantation using a subcutaneous pocket for salvage of the amputated fingertip. J Hand Surg. 2005;30A(3):562–5.
32. Wei FC, Chang YL, Chen HC, Chuang CC. Three successful digital replantations in a patient after 84, 86, and 94 hours of cold ischemia time. Plast Reconstr Surg. 1988;82:346–50.
33. Venkatramani H, Sabapathy SR. A simple technique for securing the amputated part in fingertip replantation. Br J Plast Surg. 2004;57:592–3.
34. Narushima M, Mihara M, Koshima I, et al. Intravascular stenting (IVaS) method for fingertip replantation. Ann Plast Surg. 2009;62:38–41.

35. Tsai TM, McCabe SJ, Maki Y. A technique for replantation of the finger tip. Microsurgery. 1989;10:1–4.

36. Hattori Y, Doi K, Ejiri S, Baliarsing AS. Replantation of very distal thumb amputations with pre-osteosynthesis interpositional vein graft. J Hand Surg. 2001;26B:105–7.

37. Susuki K, Matsuda M. Digital replantation distal to the distal interphalangeal joint. J Reconstr Microsurg. 1987;3:291.

38. Gordon L, Leitner DW, Buncke HJ, Alpert BS. Partial nail removal after digital replantation as an alternative method of venous drainage. J Hand Surg. 1985;10A:360–4.

39. Han SK, Chung HS, Kim WK. The timing of neovascularization in fingertip replantation by external bleeding. Plast Reconstr Surg. 2002;110:1042–6.

40. Han SK, Lee BI, Kim WK. Topical and systemic anticoagulation in the treatment of absent or compromised venous outflow in replanted fingertips. J Hand Surg. 2000;25A:659–67.

41. Buntic RF, Brooks D. Standardized protocol for artery-only fingertip replantation. J Hand Surg. 2010;35A:1491–6.

42. Koshima I, Soeda S, Moriguchi T, Higaki H, Miyakawa S, Yamasaki M. The use of arteriovenous anastomosis for replantation of the distal phalanx of the fingers. Plast Reconstr Surg. 1992;89:710–4.

43. Kamei K, Sinokawa Y, Kishibe M. The venocutaneous fistula: a new technique for reducing venous congestion in replanted fingertips. Plast Reconstr Surg. 1997;99:1771–4.

44. Koshima I, Yamashita S, Sugiyama N, Ushio S, Tsutsui T, Nanba Y. Successful delayed venous drainage in 16 consecutive distal phalangeal replantations. Plast Reconstr Surg. 2005;115:149–54.

45. Whitney TM, Lineaweaver WC, Buncke HJ, Nugent K. Clinical results of bony fixation methods in digital replantation. J Hand Surg. 1990;15A:328–34.

46. Hahn HO, Jung SG. Results of replantation of amputated fingertips in 450 patients. J Reconstr Microsurg. 2006;22:407–13.

Fingertip Amputations: Coverage, Local and Regional Flaps

David T. Netscher and J. B. Stephenson

Introduction

Armed with the understanding of axial blood supply and perforator sites, the treatment of fingertip amputations has undergone substantial change in the last 40 years. Early innovators such as Kutler [1] and Atasoy [2] proposed local advancement flaps for small defects of the distal fingertip As our knowledge of the axial blood supply to the finger progressed, the principle behind these flaps allowed for the description of multiple local and regional flaps for coverage of finger defects. Today, these flaps serve to enhance the armamentarium of the surgeon when presented with a complex defect of the fingertip.

D. T. Netscher
Division of Plastic Surgery and Department of Orthopedic Surgery, Baylor College of Medicine, Cornell University, 6624 Fannin, Suite 2730, Houston, TX 77030, USA

Weill Medical College, Cornell University, Houston, TX, USA

Deparment of Hand Surgery and Plastic Surgery, St. Luke's Hospital and Texas Children's Hospital, Houston, TX, USA
e-mail: Netscher@bcm.edu

J. B. Stephenson
Hand and Microsurgery, Department of Orthopedic Surgery, Baylor College of Medicine, Houston, TX, USA

The Craniofacial & Plastic Surgery Center of Houston, 920 Frostwood, Suite 690, Houston, TX 77024, USA
e-mail: stephenson.jb@gmail.com

The arterial blood supply to the fingers (Fig. 6.1) comes primarily from the superficial palmar arch and the subsequent common digital arteries. These common digital arteries branch at the level of the metacarpophalangeal (MP) joint to become the proper digital arteries. Other sources of arterial inflow to the finger include distal branches of the deep palmar metacarpal arteries which arise from the deep palmar arch and distal branches of the dorsal metacarpal arteries. Between these sources of arterial inflow are ulnar to radial and palmar to dorsal communications. The ulnar to radial communications are the transverse palmar arches located at the neck of the phalanges deep to the flexor tendon sheath. The palmar to dorsal communications are located at the metacarpal neck and the base and necks of the phalanges. The more distal dorsal communications may actually exist as perforators that replace the contribution of the dorsal arteries. The inherent redundancy in these communications allows for the design and implementation of local flaps of the finger while preserving blood supply to the overall digit.

The Evidence: Literature Review

Many options exist for the treatment of fingertip amputations. These include primary repair, revision amputation, nonvascularized and vascularized composite grafting, skin grafting, and healing by secondary intention. Most of these well-established treatment options are surgically

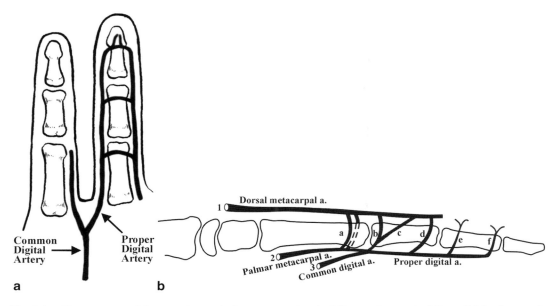

Fig. 6.1 a Transverse arterial connections exist between ulnar and radial digital arteries. **b** There are volar to dorsal arterial connections in the hand and finger (*1* Dorsal car- pal arch, *2* Deep palmar arch, *3* Superficial palmar arch, **a–f** palmar to dorsal connections)

straightforward and are reliable choices for small defects of the fingertip.

Choosing the optimum treatment alternative depends on the goals of treatment. The primary goals of treating a fingertip defect are a functional, pain-free, sensate tip that meets the occupational and avocational needs of the patient. Secondary goals of treatment include restoration of volar pulp contour, avoidance of nail deformities, maintenance of functional length, and quick recovery.

The concept of the "reconstructive ladder" has traditionally been utilized to determine the balance between the reconstructive need of the defect and the reconstructive complexity of the surgery, with the simplest option being the preferred option (Fig. 6.2). However, this concept has been replaced with the "reconstructive elevator," where the best surgical option according to the needs of the patient and the skill of the surgeon may be the more complex option [3]. Bennett and Choudhary stated, "Why climb a ladder when you can take the elevator?" [4]. Hence, the optimum treatment alternative and its surgical complexity will vary according to the goals of treatment and the needs of the patient (Fig. 6.3). Healing by secondary intention may be the ideal choice for straightforward defects of the fingertip. In particular, wounds with minimal bone exposure (<3 mm), no tendon exposure, and less than 1 cm^2 total surface area can be expected to heal within 4 weeks with eventual recovery of normal sensation in the majority of patients [5]. While some have expanded secondary intention to include defects >1 cm^2, this is at the expense of increased time to healing and sometimes a tender and dry scar. A patient with planing injury 2.8×1.8 cm in site and no bone exposed (Fig. 6.4a) is shown. In secondary intention, within hours, phagocytosis of the necrotic tissue at the end of the finger occurs, local blood vessels dilate, and an exudate forms over the wound composed of fibrin clot and inflammatory cells. Phagocytes remove necrotic debris and fibroblasts lay down bridging scar tissue (Fig. 6.4b). Peripheral epithelial cells grow inward to cover the defect. The underlying scar contracts and the defect closes (Fig. 6.4c). New nerve endings subsequently grow into the subdermal layers and sense organs repopulate the newly covered area.

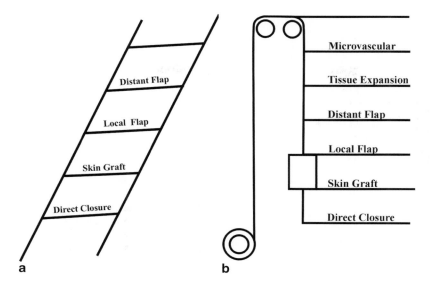

Fig. 6.2 a Reconstructive ladder. **b** Reconstructive elevator

Other advantages of secondary intention healing include low risk of acute infection, minimal long-term stiffness, and satisfactory aesthetics [5, 6]. Long-term complications associated with secondary intention healing include 36% cold intolerance and 26% scar tenderness at 6 months in one study [6]. Skin grafting is another option for coverage of similar fingertip defects. Full-thickness grafts from the hypothenar eminence or a flexion crease are preferred. However, skin grafts typically have poorer sensory recovery and aesthetics than healing by secondary intention.

Revision amputation remains a popular choice for complex defects of the fingertip. In the presence of significant bone loss, tendon loss, or devascularization, revision amputation is preferred over secondary intention or skin grafting. Advantages of revision amputation include less surgical demand and quicker return to work than more complex forms of reconstruction. Complications associated with revision amputation include residual irritating nail remnant, decreased tip sensation, painful neuroma, and cold intolerance.

Nonflap options for coverage of fingertip amputations including healing by secondary intention, skin grafting, and revision amputation remain widely popular and have their established roles and indications. However, secondary inten-

tion is limited to defects of appropriate size without exposure of critical parts. Revision amputation requires shortening of the digit and is limited by poor aesthetics and risk of neuroma formation. Therefore, when secondary intention will not suffice and length preservation is desired, local and regional flaps are preferred.

Indications and Classification

When considering more complex wounds in the appropriate patient, the surgeon should employ the reconstructive elevator and consider local or regional flap coverage. These flaps can be classified as traditional local advancement flaps, staged flaps, and island flaps.

Local Advancement Flaps

An advancement flap is a segment of tissue with an intact blood supply that is advanced forward to fill an adjacent defect. The primary examples of local advancement flaps used in fingertip injuries are the V–Y advancement flaps described by Atasoy [7] and Kutler [8]. Limited fingertip injuries that involve exposed bone are ideal candidates

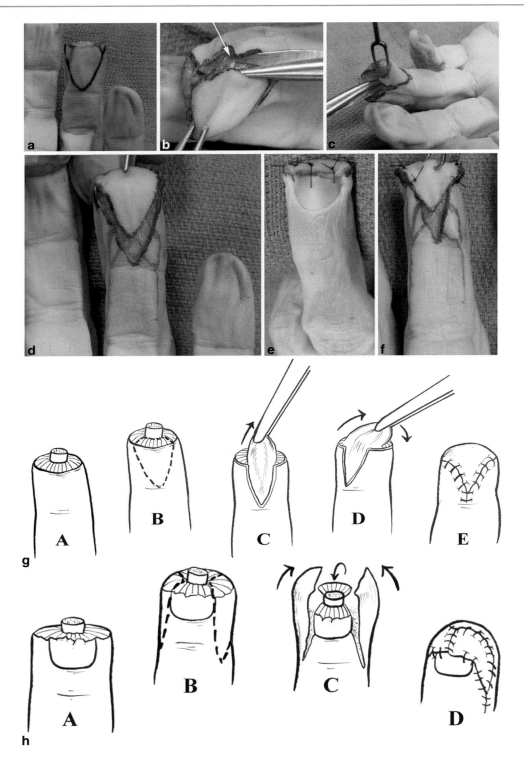

Fig. 6.3 a Preoperative markings of flap for transverse distal tip defect. **b** Fibrous septae (*white arrow*) are carefully identified and released. **c** Flap is elevated directly off the periosteum. **d** Flap is advanced to cover the defect. Note the red markings identifying the preserved oblique arterial vessels. **e, f** Sutures are placed distally through the nail plate to secure the advanced flap. If too much tension is required to close the proximal incisions, then these may be *left* open to heal secondarily. **g** Line drawing of volar V–Y advancement flap. (Atasoy). **h** Line diagram of Kutler flap

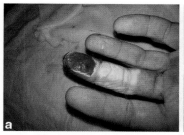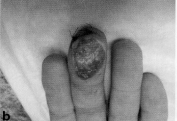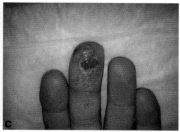

Fig. 6.4 a Acute planing injury of volar pad, no bone exposed **b** At 2 weeks, phagocytosis of the necrotic tissue, dilation of blood vessels, and exudate formation composed of fibrin clot and inflammatory cells. **c** Periph- eral epithelial cells move towards the center to cover the defect, which begins to close by myofibroblast wound contraction.

for V–Y advancement flaps if too much bone debridement is required to allow healing by secondary intention. Patterns of amputation injury determine the most appropriate method of soft tissue advancement. In general, transverse or dorsally angulated amputations of the fingertip are suitable for a volar V–Y advancement flap as described by Atasoy and modified by others. Volarly angulated tip and apical fingertip amputations may potentially be covered by bilateral V–Y advancement flaps as described by Kutler; however, other flaps may be preferred. The advantages of V–Y advancement flaps are the low–moderate technical demand, digit and nail length preservation, and minimal donor-site morbidity.

Staged Flaps

Staged flaps involve two stages for completion of the fingertip reconstruction. The most popular staged flaps are the thenar flap and the cross-finger flap, both random pattern flaps that do not have a specific blood supply. The thenar flap and the cross-finger flap are used for volarly angulated fingertip defects, when local V–Y advancement flaps are not possible. The thenar flap was first described in 1926 by Gatewood [9]. Having undergone modification since its first description, the donor site is typically near the base of the MP joint of the thumb, which reduces the amount of finger flexion and utilizes donor skin redundancy, which reduces the degree of finger flexion and enables primary donor wound closure compared with the

more proximal placement of the thenar donor site that was originally described. At the initial surgery, the flap is elevated and the injured finger is flexed to be inset into the elevated flap. After a period of time, to allow for vascular ingrowth of the recipient bed (typically 14 days), the flap is divided and inset in the volar pulp defect at a second stage. The risk inherent in the thenar flap procedure is that of recipient finger stiffness; hence, this flap is better suited for the pediatric and young adult population.

The cross-finger flap is also used in volar pulp defects with exposed bone or tendon not amenable to secondary intention healing. The dorsal soft tissue over the middle phalanx of the adjacent digit is used to cover the defect while the donor site is covered with a full-thickness skin graft. For skin graft adherence, the paratenon must be left behind on the donor digit. Like the thenar flap, the flap is divided and inset into the recipient bed after a period of time to allow for vascular ingrowth. An advantage of the cross-finger flap over the thenar flap is the ability to provide coverage to multiple traumatized fingertips in a stacked fashion. Additionally, the flap is useful in volar thumb defects where the thumb can rest comfortably against the donor index finger. Cohen and Cronin [10] described a technique for innervating the cross-finger flap to provide better sensibility by utilizing the dorsal branch of the digital nerve. Disadvantages of the cross-finger flap include finger stiffness, cold intolerance, and unacceptable cosmetic deformity of the donor site. The flap may not be suitable for elderly or female patients for these reasons.

Island Flaps

Island flaps are axial pattern flaps that maintain blood flow through a specific vascular pedicle. The idea of island flaps for fingertip coverage was not fully espoused until the principle of axial pattern blood supply to the hand and fingers was better understood. Armed with this understanding, the options for coverage of fingertip defects have flourished. Island flaps allow the surgeon to approach fingertip amputations with respect to the flap options and not the specific pattern of the defect. Island flaps may be classified as homodigital or heterodigital, antegrade or retrograde blood supply, and innervated or noninnervated. Multiple authors [11, 12] have discussed the advantages of island flaps which include:

1. More tissue is available to completely cover large defects.
2. Reconstruction can be completed in a single stage, which allows for early digital mobilization and reduced stiffness.
3. Single-stage coverage minimizes the potential contamination of hardware used for fixation and tendon spacers unlike two-stage procedures.
4. The flap is mobilized to reach the defect, not the fingertip flexed to reach the flap. This prevents immobilization in awkward positions for prolonged periods, which decreases the chance of postoperative stiffness.
5. Island flaps have more bulk and are more similar in texture to the recipient defect than are staged flaps.
6. Innervated island flaps allow the surgeon to provide sensate tissue to the defect with improved long-term sensibility.
7. A greater arc of rotation or advancement can be achieved when not tethered by skin or fascial connections.

When considering the reconstructive elevator, island flaps may be considered the ideal choice for soft tissue coverage and reconstruction of fingertip defects when preservation of length and maximal function are desired and critical structures are exposed or injured.

Techniques

Volar V–Y Advancement Flap

The volar V–Y advancement flap is indicated for transverse or dorsally angulated traumatic amputations of the fingertip involving exposed distal phalanx. The advantage of this flap over revision amputation is the preservation of nail length and the potential for minimizing hook nail deformity. The blood supply of the flap is the oblique terminal branches of the digital arteries arising from the trifurcation at the distal interphalangeal joint. This is, in essence, a subcutaneous pedicle flap.

A triangular flap is designed on the volar pulp of the remaining fingertip (Fig. 6.3 shows cadaver dissection). The width of the flap distally equals the width of the defect. The flap then tapers proximally to a V at the level of the distal interphalangeal flexion crease. Leaving the apex too distal will provide an insufficient flap to advance; leaving the apex too proximal will potentially cause scar contracture at the flexion crease. The volar skin incisions are made with care taken not to incise into the deep subcutaneous tissue. Under loupe magnification, the fibrous septae are released with longitudinal blunt spreading to allow for distal advancement of the flap, while preserving the adjacent oblique vessels. A single hook may be used to grasp the distal flap to create tension and allow for visualization of any tethering septae. The flap is then elevated off the periosteum sharply to release the deep attachments of the terminal pulp fibrous septae and allow distal mobilization. Advancement of up to 1 cm can be expected with adequate release. The distal edge of the flap is typically sutured in place. Proximal sutures may be placed, but if the flap appears ischemic after tourniquet release, then the proximal incision may be left open to heal secondarily. Some have suggested spearing of the distal flap with a longitudinal k-wire as a way to inset the flap without suture and minimize tension. We have not generally recommended this.

Staged Flaps: Cross-Finger Flap and Thenar Flap

Cross-finger flaps are indicated for volar pulp defects with exposed bone or tendon. Multiple "stacked" cross-finger flaps can be used when multiple digits are involved, as is seen in industrial injuries. The blood supply to this flap is considered random.

A dorsal rectangular flap of an adjacent finger is designed over the middle phalanx to match the size of the pulp defect (Fig. 6.5). The flap is elevated off the donor digit just above the paratenon of the extensor mechanism to allow for full-thickness skin grafting of the donor defect. The flap is hinged at the midaxial line on the side of the recipient defect and inset into the defect using interrupted suture. Sensory outcomes of cross finger flaps can be improved by coapting the donor dorsal branch of the digital nerve into the recipient digital nerve stump [13]. A full-thickness skin graft is then placed over the dorsal donor defect. The patient must be splinted postoperatively to prevent shearing of the flap. At 2 weeks postoperative, the flap is divided under local anesthesia. After the second stage, an aggressive range of motion protocol should be instituted to prevent flexion contracture of the digits.

A clinical case example is illustrated in Fig. 6.6. This case is also illustrative of another clinical point as an option when a patient brings in the amputated part of a fingertip amputation. Composite grafts of the amputated part often undergo necrosis. Replantation is difficult because of absence of suitable veins for anastomosis. The perionychial structures may be retained as a full-thickness graft and are supported by a "living" and bulky flap such as a cross-finger flap. The critical perionychial tissues have been preserved.

The thenar flap is indicated in similar volar pulp defects and is particularly well suited for the index and middle fingers of pediatric patients (Fig. 6.7). The affected finger is flexed down to the thenar region to locate the appropriate site of the subcutaneous flap. In children, the flap can often be located near the MP flexion crease, which will provide a well-hidden scar after flap division. The size of the flap is designed about one third larger than the size of the defect. The flap is elevated from the donor site and sutured to the recipient pulp defect. A dressing and splint are applied. Two weeks later, the flap is divided and the remaining raw edge is left to heal secondarily or it is loosely sutured. The donor site is closed primarily or with a small transposition flap. The available soft tissue redundancy at the MP region enables easy donor-site direct wound closure.

Antegrade Homodigital Island Flap

The precursor to antegrade homodigital island flaps was the oblique triangular flap, a local advancement flap popularized by Venkataswami and Subramanian for oblique pulp defects [14]. Island flap modifications were introduced to provide increased mobilization and allow for coverage of defects up to 10×20 mm at the pulp. The flap receives its blood supply from the digital vessel opposite the defect.

The skin pattern for the antegrade homodigital island flap is designed with its midaxis just dorsal to the digit midaxis (Fig. 6.8). The proximal portion of the flap is tapered as a V to the level of the proximal interphalangeal (PIP) joint. A longitudinal incision then extends along the digit's midaxis to the MP joint to allow for proximal dissection of the pedicle. The medial/volar incision is made first, extending through the skin and down to the flexor tendon sheath. The dissection then proceeds laterally/dorsally along this plane until the neurovascular pedicle is visualized within the pedicle on its underside. The dorsal/lateral incision is then made, isolating the neurovascular pedicle within the skin island. After the entire skin island is elevated, retrograde dissection of the neurovascular pedicle with a fibrofatty cuff of tissue is performed with microvascular instrumentation under loupe magnification. The fibrofatty cuff must be generous and handled with care, as this contains the small venae comitantes which provide venous outflow of the flap. Continued proximal dissection will allow for greater flap advancement as the neurovascular pedicle is medialized along the digit. Sufficient mobilization is attained when

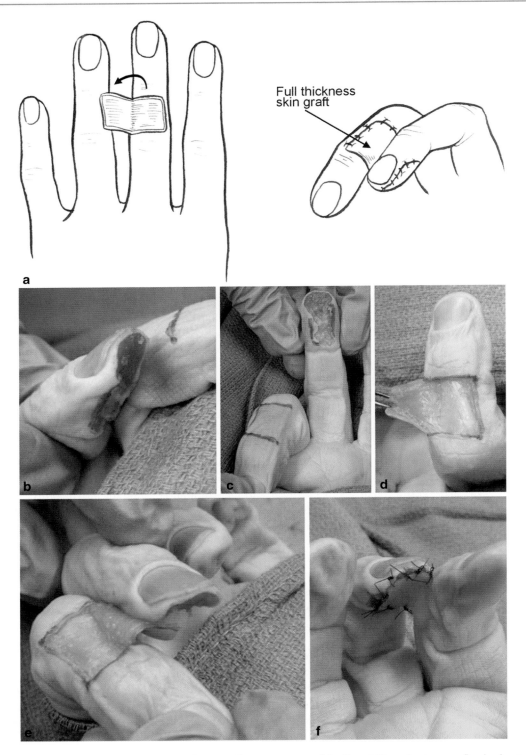

Fig. 6.5 a Line drawing of cross-finger flap. **b** Indications for cross-finger flaps include volar pulp defects. **c** Preoperative markings of dorsal rectangular flap on adjacent finger. Note that the flap is *not* incised on the midaxial line on the side of the recipient defect to allow turnover of the flap. **d** The subcutaneous flap is elevated just above the level of the paratenon to allow skin grafting of the donor site. **e** The flap is turned over to cover the adjacent pulp defect. **f** The cross-finger flap is sutured in place. The donor site is skin grafted (not shown)

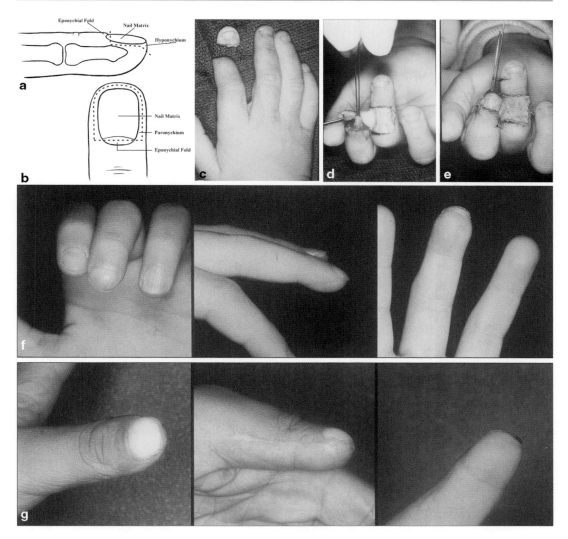

Fig. 6.6 **a** and **b** Perionychial structures are excised from the amputated part. **c** Amputated fingertip. Proximally, germinal matrix is present and will enable future nail plate growth. **d** Cross-finger flap provides volar pulp pad bulk and a vascularized bed for the perionychial graft. **e** Peri-onychial graft sutured in place. **f** and **g** Long-term result in the patient treated with cross-finger flap (*bottom*) and in a patient treated by perionychial graft and advancement Moberg flap for volar pulp support in a thumb

the flap can reach the defect. The defect should never be brought to an inadequately mobilized flap as this can lead to finger flexion contracture. The flap is inset loosely with interrupted sutures and the tourniquet is released to assess adequate vascularity of the skin island. Poor perfusion is remedied by release of suture and possible skin grafting of any donor defect unable to be closed without excessive tension. After initial healing

(7–10 days), range of motion exercises are begun; nighttime extension splints can be used as well to prevent flexion contractures.

Using this flap, Foucher et al. [15] reported 84% of patients achieving sensation with two-point discrimination of 3–7 mm. In patients whose index fingers were treated, 12.5% substituted the middle finger for fine pinch activities. Eighty-three percent of patients achieved full

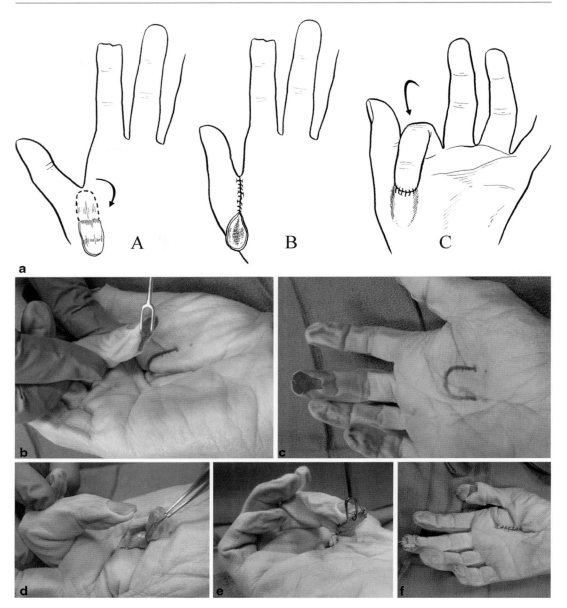

Fig. 6.7 a Line drawing of thenar flap with volar pulp defect. **b** and **c** The affected finger is flexed to the thenar region to locate the proper site for flap placement and design. **d** The flap is elevated in the subcutaneous plane at the level of the palmar fascia. **e** The flap is sutured in place with the finger flexed. **f** At the second stage, the flap is separated from the donor site. Dog ears of the donor site are tailored and the incision is closed

extension, with 17% of patients developing PIP extension deficits (mean 23°, range 10°–70°). Total flap failures occurred in 3% and the mean time off work was 61 days.

Contralateral pulp exchange island flaps have also been described [11] to provide sensate tissue to defects critical for fine pinch (e.g., radial-sided pulp defect of the index and middle fingers). Additional modifications of the antegrade homodigital island flap include a proximal extension of the skin island to the MP joint, a dorsolateral skin

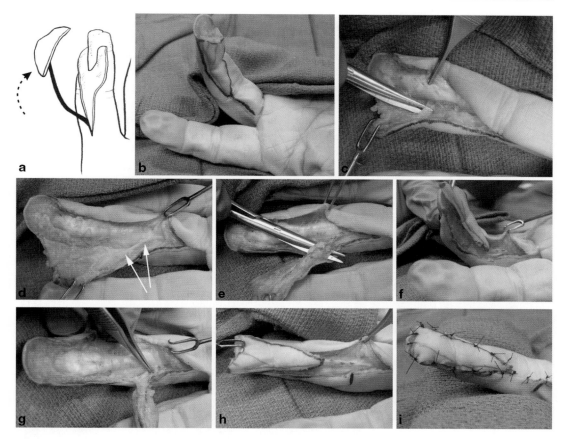

Fig. 6.8 **a** Line drawing of antegrade homodigital island flap for pulp defects. **b** Flap design extending from proximal interphalangeal joint distally to the defect. **c** The volar incision is made and both the flap and ipsilateral neurovascular bundle are elevated off of the flexor tendon sheath. **d** The neurovascular bundle is identified within the flap and dissected proximally (*white arrows*). **e** Once the location of the neurovascular bundle is confirmed within the elevated flap, the dorsal incision is made and the flap is elevated on the neurovascular bundle with a fibrofatty cuff. **f** An attempt is made to bring the flap to the defect, but in this demonstration, the flap is inadequately released and mobilized and so finger flexion is required to bring the defect to the flap. Closure at this point would inevitably lead to postoperative flexion contracture and finger stiffness. **g** Further mobilization of the flap along the neurovascular bundle proximally is warranted. Additional fascial bands are released. **h** Now, after adequate release, the flap can be advanced to the defect without finger flexion. **i** Final inset of the flap with the finger in full extension, minimizing the risk of postoperative contracture and stiffness

pattern to increase the size of the flap, and a step-ladder design to aid in donor-site closure.

Retrograde Homodigital Island Flap

First described to cover exposed PIP joints [16], the retrograde or reverse-flow homodigital island flap can be successfully used to cover both volar and dorsal fingertip defects. The advantages of the retrograde island flap over the antegrade island flap are its greater arc of rotation and potentially larger size. The disadvantages are the need for skin grafting the donor site, the intermediate quality skin compared to the distal glabrous skin captured in the antegrade flap, and the inferior long-term sensation, though the dorsal digital nerve can be retained in the flap and repaired to the digital nerve for improved sensation. The blood supply of the retrograde homodigital island flap is via the transverse communicating arterial arcade of the opposite digital artery. This arcade is located at the condylar neck of the middle phalanx at the base of the flexor tendon sheath.

The retrograde homodigital island flap is designed along the side of the digit overlying the proximal phalanx according to the size of the defect (Fig. 6.9). An additional line is extended longitudinally to allow for distal dissection of the vascular pedicle. Like the antegrade flap, the flap is incised along the volar/medial portion first and dissection proceeds directly down to the flexor tendon sheath. The flap is then elevated laterally/dorsally along this plane until the proximal neurovascular bundle is seen entering the flap. At this point, the flap may remain a noninnervated flap by dissecting the digital nerve from the flap while maintaining continuity of the digital artery with the flap. Some authors have described using either the digital nerve or the dorsal branch of the digital nerve to provide an innervated flap, with neurorrhaphy to the cut distal nerve end within

the defect. The proximal digital artery is ligated and the dorsal/lateral incision is made, isolating the island flap on its distal vascular pedicle. The pedicle is then dissected with a generous fibro-fatty cuff of tissue to preserve the reverse venous outflow to the level of the distal portion of the middle phalanx, where the transverse communicating arterial branch crosses to the opposite digital artery. The flap is inset with interrupted suture and a full-thickness skin graft is placed in the donor site.

Lai et al. [17] reported an overall morbidity rate of 15 % using the retrograde island flap, with a total flap loss rate of 4 %. In a subset of 22 patients in their series, the average two-point discrimination was 3.9 and 6.8 mm in the innervated and noninnervated flaps, respectively. Han et al. reported an update of their experience with the retrograde island flap [18, 19]. They reported that they no longer perform innervated flaps because the long-term results of sensation were no different statistically or clinically compared to nonin-

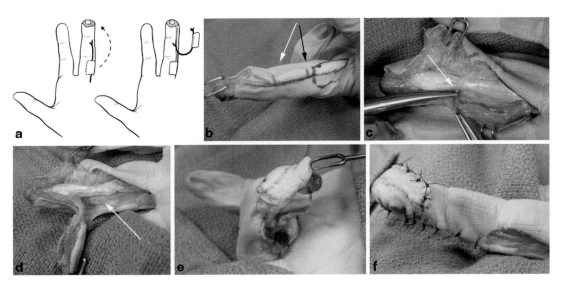

Fig. 6.9 a Line drawing of retrograde homodigital island flap. **b** Flap design along the side of the digit overlying the proximal phalanx. *Red* markings (*arrows*) indicate the transverse communicating arterial arcades at the necks of the proximal and middle phalanges. The flap will receive its retrograde blood supply from the distal arcade at the neck of the middle phalanx (*white arrow*). **c** The volar incision is made and the flap is elevated off of the flexor tendon sheath. The transverse communicating arte-

rial branch at the neck of the middle phalanx is identified proximal to the distal interphalangeal joint (*arrow*). **d** The dorsal incision is made and the flap is elevated with its pedicle. For noninnervated flaps, the digital nerve is dissected away from the artery and preserved (*arrow*). **e** The arc of rotation for the retrograde flap allows coverage of dorsal finger defects. **f** The flap is inset in the volar wound shown. The donor defect on the side of the finger will require skin grafting

nervated flaps. They also prefer to design the flap in a stellate shape to avoid scar contracture.

Figure 6.10 is a clinical case of a patient who had a retrograde island homodigital flap for a large volar pulp fingertip injury.

Heterodigital Island Flap

The heterodigital neurovascular island flap was originally described by Littler to provide a sensate flap to the thumb tip [20]. Concerns regarding donor-site morbidity, decreased long-term sensation and difficulty with cortical sensory reintegration, and acceptable alternatives have substantially decreased its indications and use. The noninnervated heterodigital island flap, however, preserves the donor digital nerve and remains suitable for fingertip defects. In particular, large defects can be covered by the noncritical side of a longer, adjacent digit while preserving the donor digital nerve and donor pulp. The donor digit must be longer than the recipient digit so that donor pulp does not have to be violated in order to obtain sufficient flap size. An ideal scenario involves a large volar avulsion defect of the

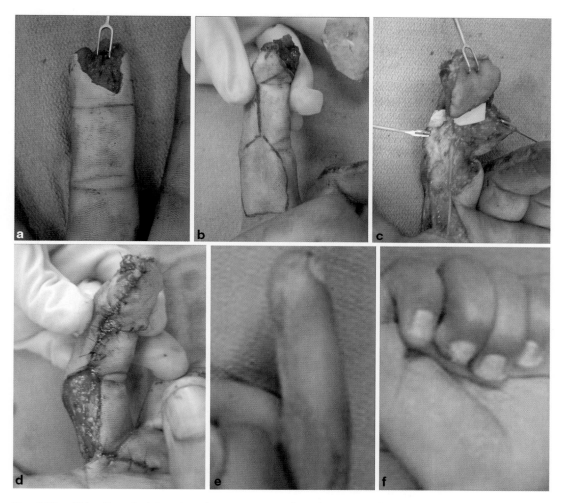

Fig. 6.10 a Volar fingertip injury. **b** and **c** Retrograde flow island flap design and transposition. **d** Insetting of flap. **e** and **f** Long-term outcome showing restoration of fingertip contour, finger is devoid of contractures, and skin-grafted donor site is on side of the finger

tip of the small finger wherein the ulnar side of the ring finger may be used as a donor.

The heterodigital island flap is designed along the noncritical border of the adjacent finger to match the defect (Fig. 6.11). The distal extent of the flap is to the distal interphalangeal joint, thereby avoiding the use of donor pulp tissue. The flap is incised and elevated in a similar fashion to the homodigital island flap. The digital nerve is dissected from the flap to preserve donor digit sensation. The pedicle and its fibrofatty cuff are dissected proximally to the common digital bifurcation and then the flap is transposed to the adjacent, smaller finger and inset into the pulp defect. Full-thickness skin graft is used to cover the donor-site defect.

Figure 6.12 shows a heterodigital island flap used to provide volar distal pulp reconstruction to the middle finger following vascular malformation excision.

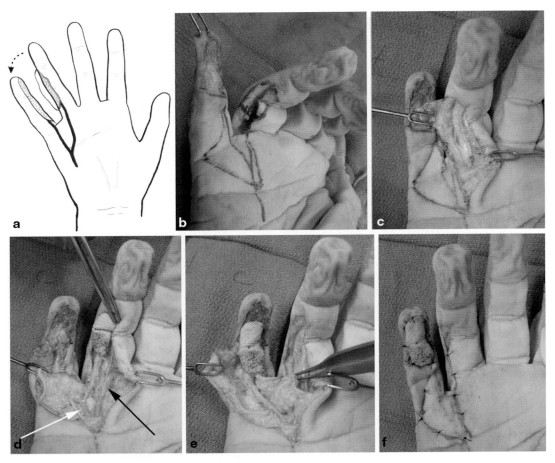

Fig. 6.11 a Line drawing of heterodigital island flap for small finger defects. **b** Flap design on the adjacent ulnar side of the ring finger. Note that the flap design does not involve the pulp of the ring finger. **c** The volar incision is made and the flap is elevated off of the flexor tendon sheath. **d** The digital artery is dissected proximally to the common digital artery bifurcation (*white arrow*). The digital nerve is dissected away from the flap and preserved (*black arrow*). **e** The flap is transposed into the small finger defect. **f** Final flap inset and closure. Note that often a skin graft will be required to close the donor defect

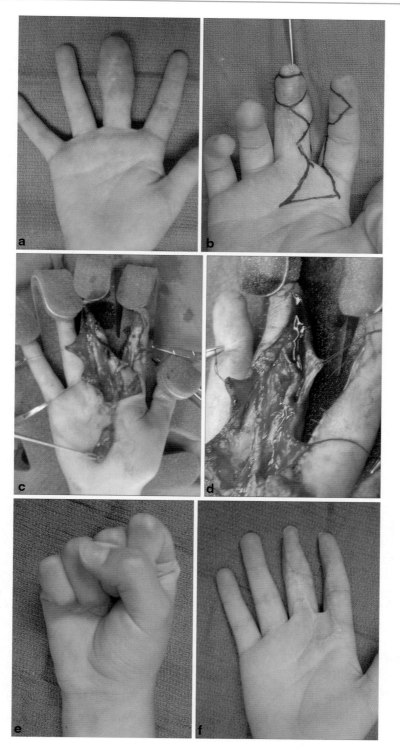

Fig. 6.12 a and **b** Vascular malformation is excised from middle fingertip. **c** and **d** Heterodigital flap is transposed from index and dorsal digital nerve coapted to digital nerve in recipient finger. **e** and **f** Long-term outcome with fully sensate volar fingertip

Author's Preferences

The older, previously axiomatic suggestions of a cross-finger flap for volar oblique wounds and Atasoy volar V–Y advancement flap for dorsal oblique wounds no longer necessarily pertain since we now have intrinsic finger flaps that carry a more generous bulk of tissue and can be advanced or transposed over greater distances. For this reason, our "workhorse" flap has become the antegrade homodigital island advancement flap.

This flap provides sensate tissue with sufficient bulk to cover most defects.

We have found that the Atasoy volar V–Y advancement flap is often insufficient except for smaller defects. When the Atasoy flap is employed, we typically leave the proximal donor portion of the advancement open to avoid a tight wound closure that may compromise the blood supply. Additionally, if a nail plate remnant is still intact, we routinely leave it in place as it provides for secure distal suturing of the Atasoy flap and minimizes later flap retraction.

The cross-finger flap has the disadvantages of more likely resulting in finger contracture and stiffness, being potentially injurious to an additional donor finger, as well as requiring two awkward stages and leaving a possible unsightly visible dorsal finger donor site. For these reasons, we do not routinely perform this operation on older adults or females. However, it is a straightforward dissection and it is still useful when crush injuries or fractures may preclude the use of homodigital flaps. Like the cross-finger flap, the thenar flap has similar disadvantages and is principally useful for index or middle finger volar pulp defects in younger patients.

The primary advantage of the retrograde homodigital island flap is the multiple degrees of freedom for its arc of rotation. It can equally easily cover the dorsum of the fingertip as well as the volar aspect. While the proper digital nerve is typically spared with this flap, a neurorrhaphy of the dorsal oblique sensory branch of the digital nerve can be performed when the flap is transposed to its recipient site. The donor site requires skin grafting and can be unsightly; however, if placed directly in the midaxis, the skin-grafted donor site is less visible.

The traditional heterodigital neurovascular island flap has been maligned for its donor-site morbidity and poor long-term sensory outcomes. However, the noninnervated heterodigital island flap described earlier in this chapter is useful for large finger defects. The ideal indication is for a large volar defect of the small finger with an intact adjacent ring finger. The flap is designed to preserve both the donor digital nerve and the donor pulp. With these modifications, one can use a heterodigital flap without the original disadvantages of the traditional flap design that may result in substantial donor finger morbidity.

Complications

Complications associated with local flaps for fingertip injuries include partial or total flap loss, flexion contracture, decreased sensation, and cold intolerance. Lai et al. [17] reported a partial and total flap loss of 12 and 5 %, respectively. Flap loss related to vascular insufficiency can be addressed by multiple maneuvers. First, the inclusion of a generous cuff of fibrofatty tissue around the digital artery ensures adequate venous outflow. Second, additional proximal dissection of the pedicle can ensure adequate length to allow the flap to reach the defect without undue tension. Third, the release of the tourniquet after flap inset to visualize appropriate capillary refill ensures that the flap is not sewn in too tightly; this can be addressed simply by suture removal.

Flexion contracture is a described complication of thenar and cross-finger staged flaps. As such, these random flaps should be avoided in most adults if a suitable alternative exists. Flexion contractures are reported after island flap reconstruction. However, they are typically better tolerated and can often be stretched out with therapy. It should be emphasized that the risk of flexion contracture is often directly related to the inadequacy of flap mobilization. A defect should never be moved to the flap—the flap should always be mobilized to reach the defect with the finger in full extension. This simple maneuver virtually eliminates the risk of functional flexion contracture.

Cold intolerance remains a problem with any form of reconstruction following fingertip injury. Van den Berg et al. reported 85 % cold intolerance in fingertip injuries regardless of whether healing by secondary intention, bone shortening, or reconstruction [21]. It is likely that cold intolerance is a result of the injury and not the reconstruction.

Lastly, decreased fingertip sensation is reported following local flap coverage of fingertip defects. The best outcomes for sensation following fingertip injury are with healing by secondary intention. However, when secondary intention is not an available treatment option, other forms of reconstruction must be used. In a large series of fingertip reconstruction with reverse digital island flaps, Han et al. reported a static two-point discrimination of 6–11 mm in noninnervated flaps and 4–8 mm in innervated flaps [18]. Takeishi et al. found similar results of innervated reverse island flaps with two-point discrimination of 3–5 mm [22]. Foucher et al. found comparable results for antegrade neurovascular island flaps with 84 % of patients having 3–7 mm static two-point discrimination [11]. Overall, island flaps are well tolerated and have an acceptable complication profile if judicious surgical technique is employed.

Summary

With a better understanding of the axial blood supply to the fingers, the discovery of island flaps has increased the surgical options of the physician treating fingertip amputations. The use of local flaps should be appropriately considered, depending on the nature of the injury and other patient factors. For the patient who desires length preservation and is an acceptable candidate, local flaps such as the antegrade homodigital island flap may be the ideal choice for fingertip coverage following amputation.

References

1. Kutler W. A new method for fingertip amputations. JAMA. 1947;133:29–30.
2. Atasoy E, Ioakimidis E, Kasdan ML, Kutz JE, Kleinert HE. Reconstruction of the amputated finger tip with a triangular volar flap. A new surgical procedure. J Bone Joint Surg. 1970;52A(5):921–6.
3. Gottlieb LJ, Krieger LM. From the reconstructive ladder to the reconstructive elevator. Plast Reconstr Surg. 1994;93(7):1503–4.
4. Bennett N, Choudhary S. Why climb a ladder when you can take the elevator? Plast Reconstr Surg. 2000;105(6):2266.
5. Lamon RP, Cicero JJ, Frascone RJ, Hass WF. Open treatment of fingertip amputations. Ann Emerg Med. 1983;12(6):358–60.
6. Ipsen T, Frandsen PA, Barfred T. Conservative treatment of fingertip injuries. Injury. 1987;18(3):203–5.
7. Atasoy E, Ioakimidis E, Kasdan ML, Kutz JE, Kleinert HE. Reconstruction of the amputated finger tip with a triangular volar flap. A new surgical procedure. J Bone Joint Surg. 1970;52A(5):921–6.
8. Kutler W. A new method for fingertip amputations. JAMA. 1947;133:29–30.
9. Gatewood J. A plastic repair of finger defects without hospitalization. JAMA. 1926;87:1479.
10. Cohen BE, Cronin ED. An innervated cross-finger flap for fingertip reconstruction. Plast Reconstr Surg. 1983;72(5):688–97.
11. Foucher G, Khouri RK. Digital reconstruction with island flaps. Clin Plast Surg. 1997;24(1):1–32.
12. Netscher D, Schneider A. Homodigital and heterodigital island pedicle flaps. In: Rayan GM, Chung KC, editors. Flap reconstruction of the upper extremity: a master skills publication. Rosemont: American Society for Surgery of the Hand; 2009.
13. Cohen BE, Cronin ED. An innervated cross-finger flap for fingertip reconstruction. Plast Reconstr Surg. 1983;72(5):688–97.
14. Venkataswami R, Subramanian N. Oblique triangular flap: a new method of repair for oblique amputations of the fingertip and thumb. Plast Reconstr Surg. 1980;66:296–300.
15. Foucher G, Smith D, Pempinello C, Braun F, Citron N. Homodigital neurovascular island flap for digital pulp loss. J Hand Surg Br. 1989;14(2):204–8.
16. Weeks P, Wray R, editors. Management of acute hand injuries: a biological approach. 2nd ed. St Louis: CV Mosby; 1978. pp. 183–6.
17. Lai C, Lin S, Chou C, Tsai C. A versatile method for reconstruction of finger defects: reverse digital artery flap. Br J Plast Surg. 1992;45(6):443–53.
18. Han SK, Lee BI, Kim WK. The reverse digital artery island flap: clinical experience in 120 fingers. Plast Reconstr Surg. 1998;101(4):1006–11.
19. Han SK, Lee BI, Kim WK. The reverse digital artery island flap: an update. Plast Reconstr Surg. 2004;113(6):1753–5.

20. Littler JW. The neurovascular pedicle method of digital transposition for reconstruction of the thumb. J Bone Joint Surg Am. 1956;38:917.
21. Van den Berg WB Vergeer RA van der Sluis CK ten Duis HJ Werker PMN. Comparison of three types of treatment modalities on the outcome of fingertip injuries. J Trauma Acute Care Surg. 2012;72:1681–7.
22. Takeishi M, Shinoda A, Sugiyama A, Ui K. Innervated reverse dorsal digital island flap for fingertip reconstruction. J Hand Surg. 2006;31A:1094–9.

Reconstruction of the Thumb Tip

7

Margaret A. Porembski, Thomas P. Lehman
and Ghazi M. Rayan

Introduction

Disruption of the anatomy and physiology of the thumb tip by injury can have an adverse impact on hand function. Normal thumb function requires adequate length, normal mobility, with stable, supple, durable, and sensate soft tissue coverage [1, 2]. Inadequately treated thumb-tip injury or disease results in a shortened ray, skin contracture, insensate or hypersensitive pulp, or insufficient soft tissue padding. Reconstruction of acute thumb-tip injuries must be carefully selected in order to restore normal function.

In this chapter, the term thumb tip encompasses some or all the pulp skin up to the interphalangeal (IP) joint crease. Thumb-tip skin loss may be small affecting the distal third, moderate

M. A. Porembski (✉)
Clinical Faculty, Oklahoma Hand Surgery Fellowship Program, OK, USA
e-mail: maporembski@gmail.com

G. M. Rayan
Clinical Professor Orthopedic Surgery, University of Oklahoma, OK, USA
Adjunct Professor of Anatomy / Cell Biology, University of Oklahoma, OK, USA
Director of Oklahoma Hand Surgery Fellowship Program, OK, USA
Chairman, Department of Hand Surgery, INTEGRIS Baptist Medical Center, Oklahoma City, OK, USA
e-mail: OUHSGMR@aol.com

T. P. Lehman
Department of Orthopedic Surgery and Rehabilitation, University of Oklahoma, 920 Stanton L. Young Blvd, Suite WP 1380, Oklahoma City, OK 73104 USA
e-mail: Thomas-Lehman@ouhsc.edu

affecting the distal two thirds, or large affecting the entire pulp. Simple lacerations or tactile pad avulsions involving less than one third of the pulp may be adequately treated with primary closure or allowing wound healing by secondary intention. Nail bed injuries require meticulous repair in order to prevent subsequent nail deformities. For minor thumb-pulp injury, a palmar or lateral V–Y advancement flap, or cross index finger flap may be employed for coverage similar to the other digits. These options offer less than optimal restoration of sensory function. Substantial thumb-tip injuries, i.e., moderate or large skin pulp loss and those involving bone or post-injury complications such as inadequate padding, severe scarring, or insensate pulp, require more complex reconstructions (Fig. 7.1a–d). The three principal reconstructions for these injuries are the Moberg, neurovascular island (NVI), and first dorsal metacarpal artery flaps (FDMA) and will be the focus of this chapter. These options are necessary to achieve the previously mentioned objectives.

Any of these flaps may be employed to provide soft tissue coverage for a thumb tip with a full-thickness skin defect or to restore supple, sensate skin to a thumb that has skin coverage that lacks those qualities. Selection of the appropriate soft tissue reconstruction technique is dependent upon the character of the thumb-tip injury and the patient's goals and expectations.

Management of extensive thumb injuries such as amputations proximal to the IP joint and degloving injuries is beyond the scope of this chapter but will be briefly discussed.

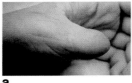 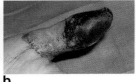 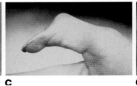 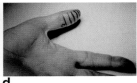

a   b   c   d

Fig. 7.1 **a** Previously treated thumb with inadequate padding. **b** Previously treated thumb with full-thickness skin necrosis of the volar pad. **c** Previously treated thumb in a child with skin graft and a scar contracture of the IP joint. **d** Irreparable nerve damage to both digital nerves of the thumb with loss of sensory function. (Courtesy of G. Rayan MD)

Flaps for Coverage of Thumb-Tip Injuries

Moberg Advancement Flap

The Moberg advancement flap (MAF) is a bi-pedicled, axial-pattern, cutaneous, advancement flap that was first proposed in 1964 by Erik Moberg. The procedure was originally described to restore sensibility to a thumb tip with intact but denervated skin [3]. It is most commonly used to provide skin coverage for amputations or partial degloving of the thumb tip and sometimes for other digits.

Anatomy

Both the radial and ulnar digital arteries of the thumb serve as vascular pedicles to the MAF. It is possible that the flap may survive on a single pedicle, but whenever possible both vascular structures should be present and elevated with the flap to ensure adequate vascular flow. Sensory function is maintained by preserving the paired digital nerves traveling with the arteries.

The dorsal skin of the fingers is supplied by the palmar digital arteries; therefore, using an MAF for fingertip injuries may compromise its circulation. In contrast to the other digits, the dorsal skin of the thumb receives its own blood supply from the dorsal digital arteries. This allows the palmar skin of the thumb to be elevated with both digital arteries as an axial flap without concern about dorsal ischemia.

Indications

The MAF is best suited for pulp tip defects distal to the IP joint and tip amputations measuring 2 cm^2 or less (Fig. 7.2a–f). It is not indicated for larger defects because of potential complications [4]. Palmar, oblique loss of the pulp creates a defect particularly well suited for coverage with an MAF. The flap may also be used to replace scars at the tip or restore sensibility to an insensate digital tip as originally described.

Relative contraindications for the MAF include: elderly patients (especially those with advanced arthritic changes), injury to one or both vascular pedicles of the thumb, soft tissue defect greater than 2 cm^2, and defects proximal to the IP joint.

The use of this flap in the digits has been considered to be a relative contraindication because of the higher risk of dorsal skin necrosis. In fingertip amputations, however, part of the dorsal skin is missing, which lessens the concern about the dorsal skin vascularity. Successful use of Moberg palmar advancement flaps in the fingers, however, has been reported. When this technique is adopted for these digits, the dissection should be modified to preserve the perforating vessels that extend from the palmar to the dorsal aspect of the digit. [5–13]

Surgical Technique

The MAF is typically preformed within a few days of thumb injury, but the timing of coverage is not critical to the outcome. The procedure should be performed as soon as the patient's condition allows. Satisfactory results can be achieved

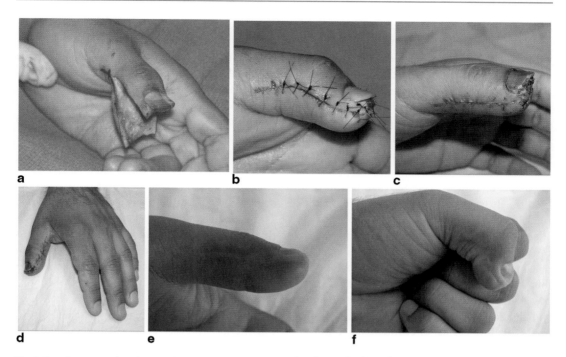

Fig. 7.2 **a** Intraoperative picture of thumb-tip amputation with Moberg advancement flap (MAF) elevation in progress. **b** Flexed thumb IP joint with MAF inset to cover thumb-tip amputation. **c** Thumb appearance at 3 weeks with early healing. **d** Thumb appearance at 3 months showing maintained first web space. **e** Full IP joint extension 4 months following MAF coverage. **f** Satisfactory IP joint flexion 4 months following MAF coverage. (From [35]. Used with permission from the American Society for Surgery of the Hand)

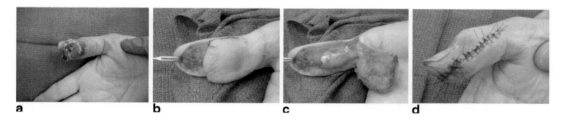

Fig. 7.3 **a** Complex soft tissue injury of thumb pulp. **b** Full-thickness soft tissue defect of thumb tip following debridement. **c** Completed elevation of Moberg advancement flap. **d** The flap after inset with interphalangeal joint flexion to increase distal advancement. (Courtesy of G Rayan MD)

even after several days of delay, provided that the wound is tidy and free of infection at the time of flap coverage.

Prior to flap elevation, the wound should be irrigated and debrided of any foreign material or nonviable tissue. Associated fractures and nail bed injuries should also be addressed prior to flap elevation. The wound margins should be freshened while preserving all viable tissues.

Flap elevation begins with midlateral incisions on the radial and ulnar aspects of the thumb. Dissection should be dorsal to the neurovascular structures towards the flexor tendon sheath (Fig. 7.3a–d). The flap is elevated from distal to proximal. Sometimes the severed digital nerve branches may be divided sharply 5 mm proximal to the skin edge to avoid creating painful neuromas at the thumb tip. The flap is freed of all dorsal attachments and mobilized proximally to the level of the metacarpophalangeal (MP) joint in order to maximize its distal advancement. Proper elevation of the flap should allow advancement of up to 2 cm.

The tourniquet should be deflated, hemostasis obtained, and the wound irrigated prior to flap inset. The flap is advanced distally, which may require flexion of the IP joint and, to some degree, the MP joint to allow maximum coverage of the defect and for the flap to reach the tip of the thumb. The extent of flexion usually does not exceed 30–45°. If additional flexion is necessary for adequate coverage, then one of this flap's modifications described below may be considered.

Complete full-thickness skin coverage of the thumb tip is not essential. A small area of exposed subcutaneous tissue will re-epithelialize and should not have considerable adverse effect on the final functional or cosmetic outcome.

The flap is inset and skin closure is done with 4–0 or, preferably, 5–0 nylon. In children, chromic catgut suture is preferable. Sutures can be placed through the nail plate distally if necessary. The thumb is dressed with non-adherent gauze and immobilized in a thumb spica splint that extends beyond the tip.

Postoperative Care

Splinting is continued for up to 3 weeks depending on concerns about patient compliance or the condition of the flap. Early active range of motion (ROM) is preferred and may begin at 7–10 days postoperatively. The patient is instructed to begin scar massage techniques at 4–6 weeks postoperatively to soften and desensitize the scar. Formal hand therapy may be required if the patient has a great deal of stiffness, especially in the presence of incipient or mild arthritic changes, or scar hypersensitivity.

Technical Modifications

Using this flap requires flexion of the IP joint. This commonly results in mild loss of IP joint hyperextension or stiffness, especially in older patients. Modifications to the MAF have been proposed in order to minimize the degree of flexion necessary to extend the flap to the tip.

Flap advancement may be enhanced to some degree by placement of Burrow's' triangles (Fig. 7.4a–c) or z-plasties (Fig. 7.5a–c) at the proximal aspect of the lateral incisions [4, 13].

O'Brien [9] proposed a transverse incision of the skin flap proximally, preserving the neurovascular structures. This creates a bipedicled island flap and increases the flap reach to the tip, lessening the degree of IP joint flexion (Fig. 7.6). The secondary defect created proximally is covered with a full-thickness skin graft, or with triangular flaps from both sides of the thumb [10]. The island flap concept has been further modified by fashioning the mobilized skin island as a homodigital V flap and performing a V–Y closure at the proximal aspect, eliminating the need for a skin graft [11, 12].

Outcome

Experience with the Moberg flap is typically rewarding (Fig. 7.7a–d). Modifications to extend the reach of the flap are rarely required, and failure of the flap is rare, although limited marginal necrosis may occur. Final ROM is usually near normal, but a small loss of IP joint hyperextension is not uncommon. Sensory function is usually equal or near that of the contralateral thumb, and most patients can return to their normal activities and work after healing is complete.

Complications

Stiffness: Some loss of IP joint hyperextension can be expected, but is unlikely to be dysfunctional. Arthritic changes in the thumb may increase the risk of stiffness. Pinning of the thumb in flexion may also contribute to loss of motion and is not recommended. Although no improvement in outcome has been shown by any of the described modifications, theoretically they enhance flap advancement and decrease the IP flexion required and may improve final ROM [4]. Early ROM exercises help prevent stiffness.

Neuroma: Some risk of digital neuroma formation exists after the use of this flap due to the associated nerve injury. The reported incidence is low however at 0–10% [4, 10]. Sharp transection of the digital nerve branches just proximal to the edge of the skin may help prevent this complication.

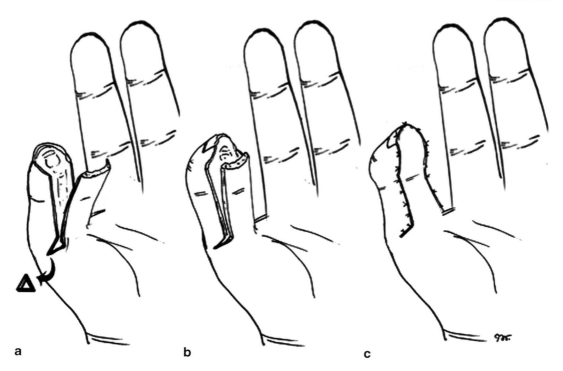

a   b   c

Fig. 7.4 a Burrow's triangles excised at the base of the flap on both sides facilitate distal advancement. **b** The triangular defects are closed increasing the advancement of the flap toward the tip. **c** Final appearance of Moberg advancement flap after advancement. (From: [35]. Used with permission from the American Society for Surgery of the Hand)

Cold Intolerance: This is a common side effect following management of fingertip injuries with any reconstructive procedure. This problem is not necessarily more common after this procedure and it spontaneously resolves with time in most patients In one report, over 30% of patients had severe symptoms of cold intolerance [4]. Therapeutic modalities and topical agents may alleviate some of these symptoms if they are severe. Using thermal, well-padded gloves to keep the hand warm is the most effective treatment measure. Patients should be counseled prior to surgery about this expected consequence.

Pulp Instability: Poor adherence of the flap to the deeper structures at the tip of the thumb may cause instability of the pulp during pinch. This is an uncommon sequela and typically mild in nature, but may be of functional importance.

This may be related to "bowstringing" of the flap that occurs when excessive flexion of the IP joint is required for inset. Using one of the flap modifications to decrease the amount of flexion required to achieve coverage may lessen the risk of this complication.

Nail Deformity: This is not uncommon when the original injury involves a large portion of the nail bed. Careful attention to accepted principles of treatment for fingertip amputations and nail bed injuries will minimize the incidence of this complication.

Dorsal Skin Necrosis: This complication is rarely encountered when the flap is harvested in the thumb without injury or anomaly of the dorsal blood supply. In the other digits, the dorsal skin is at risk for this problem; therefore, care must be taken to preserve the communicating branches from the digital vessels in the flap.

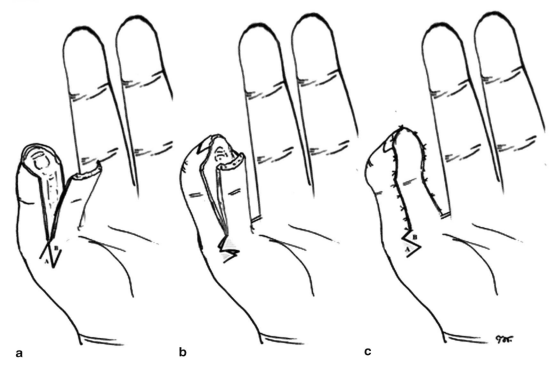

a   b   c

Fig. 7.5 a Z-plasty flaps are raised at the base of the flap on both the radial and ulnar sides. **b** Transposition of the Z-plasty flaps facilitates distal advancement of the flap to-ward the tip. **c** Final appearance of Moberg advancement flap after advancement. (From: [35]. Used with permission from the American Society for Surgery of the Hand)

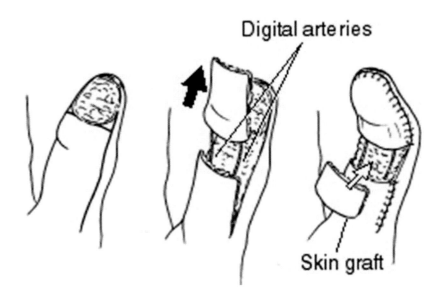

Fig. 7.6 An illustration of island modification of Moberg advancement flap. (From: [35]. Used with permission from the American Society for Surgery of the Hand)

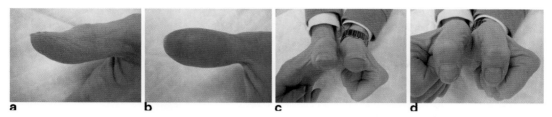

a   **b**   **c**   **d**

Fig. 7.7 a, b Full restoration of soft tissue coverage of thumb tip was achieved with a Moberg advancement flap with adequate soft tissue padding and near normal sensory function. **c, d** There is no residual flexion deformity and the patient returned to work and hobbies without limitations. (Courtesy of G Rayan MD)

Neurovascular Island Flap

The NVI flap is an axial flap transferred on a pedicle consisting of a digital artery, sensory nerve, accompanying veins, and fascia. It was first described by Littler in 1960 to restore sensory function or coverage of a thumb defect [14]. The classic NVI flap is a fasciocutaneous flap transferred from the ulnar side of the long or ring finger to the thumb pulp [15–17].

Indications
The NVI flap is indicated for coverage of full-thickness thumb-tip defects of greater size or a pattern which is not amenable to Moberg flap coverage. It may also be used to resurface a severely scarred thumb pulp, and restore sensory function to an insensate thumb [15–17]. Finally, it can be used as an adjunct flap to provide sensibility after an insensate soft tissue resurfacing procedure such as a groin or other tubed flap or in osteoplastic thumb reconstruction of more extensive injuries [15, 17] (Fig. 7.8a–e).

Relative contraindications for NVI flap reconstruction include a history of heavy smoking, atherosclerosis, diabetes, connective tissue diseases, or vasospastic disorders. Since the flap sacrifices a portion of a healthy digit, the benefits of correcting the thumb defect should outweigh the deficit created in the donor digit [15].

Surgical Technique
Selection of the donor site should be done before the patient is brought to the operating room. The donor finger must have normal innervation in an area that is less essential to hand function. Sensibility is essential on the palmar aspect of the thumb and the radial sides of the index and long fingers during opposition and fine manipulation. Sensibility on the ulnar side of the small finger is important in protection of the hand. The ulnar sides of the ring or long fingers are less essential to hand function and may be suitable donor sites for this flap [16]. Since it is supplied by the ulnar nerve, the ulnar side of the ring finger is the preferred donor in cases where there is median nerve damage [15].

The donor finger must also have a robust blood supply. The digit that shares the web space with the donor flap digit must have an intact digital artery on its unshared side. The proper digital artery to this neighbor digit shares a common digital arterial origin with the flap pedicle and will be divided during flap harvest. A digital Allen's test or handheld Doppler is used to assess the status of the digital arteries to the donor and neighboring digits. If the history or physical examination raises concerns about arterial patency, preoperative digital arteriography may be required. However, this is rarely necessary. The final assessment of adequacy of perfusion is made during dissection of the pedicle.

In the operating room, and under tourniquet control, the soft tissue defect should be irrigated and debrided of any nonviable tissue or foreign debris; it should be clean and free of contamination or evidence of infection. If the flap is used to provide sensation to a thumb with intact skin, a primary defect must be created. Ideally, this defect is created on the ulnar thumb pulp with its most distal aspect 3 or 4 mm proximal to the thumb tip. This full-thickness skin defect is

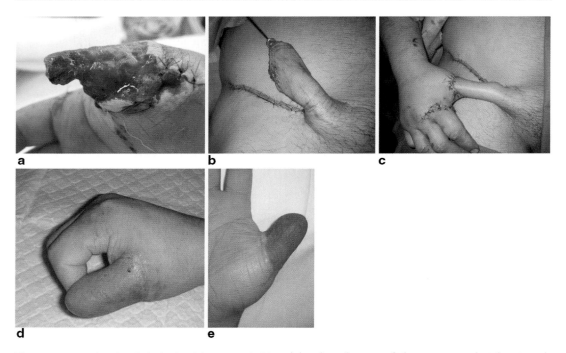

Fig. 7.8 **a** Extensive thumb degloving injury not suitable for Moberg advancement flap coverage. **b** Elevated groin flap. **c** inset groin flap **d**, **e** healed groin flap. Degloving injury has adequate soft tissue coverage, but absent sensibility. **a**, **c**, **d**, **e**. (From: [36]; Figs. 44.3a, b, c. Used with permission from Thieme. **b** Courtesy of G Rayan MD)

raised with a knife, keeping the volar fat pad intact underneath. The skin can be preserved as a skin graft for donor-site resurfacing if possible. Any painful neuromas can be resected and buried within the thenar or adductor muscles at this time. A zigzag incision is marked on the volar aspect of the thumb from the defect to the MP flexion crease. The volar zigzag incision flaps are raised to expose the bed for the transferred pedicle. As such, they should be free of constriction points. Alternatively, the skin proximal to the thumb defect can be left intact to tunnel the flap beneath it after it is raised.

A template of the thumb defect and its pedicle is made from a sterile suture pack or piece of Esmarch bandage. The approximate location of the superficial palmar arch is marked as the pivot point for the proposed flap. The template is then used to mark the donor site. If necessary, the flap can include a skin paddle extending as far proximally as the web space. A mid-axial incision for pedicle access is marked on the donor finger and continued in a zigzag manner into the palm to the

level of the palmar arch. Dissection begins from proximal to distal to identify the palmar arch and confirm normal anatomy of the planned donor pedicle structures. The neurovascular pedicle is freed within a cuff of peri-neurovascular fat to ensure that the volar digital veins are included. As the dissection is carried out distally, the radial digital artery to the adjacent finger is identified and divided to allow mobilization of the pedicle. The dissection then continues distally via the mid-axial incision on the donor finger. Thin skin flaps are raised along each side of the pedicle in the finger. The island itself is raised as a thick flap to ensure that the terminal branches of the neurovascular bundle are included. The fine draining veins adjacent to the neurovascular bundle are also included in the dissection. The pedicle is sharply elevated off the fibro-osseous sheath from distal to proximal to the point that it branches from the superficial palmar arterial arch. Internal neurolysis and separation of the common digital nerve to the 4th web space into its radial and ulnar digital nerve components allows for complete mobilization of the pedicle. The use of microsurgical instruments is recommended for the dissection (Fig. 7.9).

A subcutaneous tunnel is created via blunt dissection to connect the primary defect to the harvest site. This tunnel can be made in the subcutaneous or subfascial plane. Smooth passage of the flap through the tunnel can be achieved by using a Penrose drain. The drain is passed through the tunnel from the thumb defect to the palm wound. The flap is then placed inside the drain which is then gently backed out through the tunnel to be delivered. Alternatively, a zigzag incision can be created to connect the volar thumb and midpalmar incisions. This approach is recommended if the soft tissues of the palm have been previously scarred or injured. Care must be taken to prevent any twisting or excessive tension on the neurovascular pedicle. The flap should be inspected for tethering or kinking with the thumb both fully abducted and hyperextended.

The tourniquet is released and the flap is allowed to reperfuse. Hemostasis should be achieved before flap inset and wound closure with interrupted nylon sutures. Individual sutures can be removed if they cause flap blanching. The donor finger mid-axial and zigzag palmar incisions are also closed with interrupted nylon sutures. A vessel loop placed beneath the flap can be used as a passive drain to prevent hematoma formation, but this is often unnecessary. If used, this drain is removed within 24–72 h. A full-thickness skin graft is then used to resurface the secondary defect. This should be harvested from a site which provides an adequate amount of glabrous skin. Potential harvest sites include the volar wrist and hypothenar eminence, or any skin raised from the thumb itself (Fig. 7.10).

The skin paddle should be left partially exposed. A thumb Spica splint is applied with care taken not to compress the pedicle. The splint is worn until the sutures are removed at 2 weeks. A removable splint is used for an additional 2 weeks and a therapy program is initiated to include active ROM and sensory reeducation. Therapy is directed at both the donor and recipient sites. Resisted exercises to regain grip strength may begin at 6 weeks.

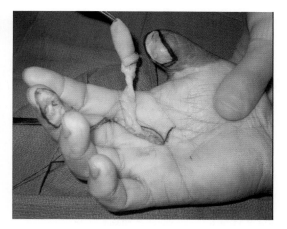

Fig. 7.9 A neurovascular island flap has been raised from the ulnar side of the long finger and is ready to be tunneled to the primary defect at the tip of the thumb. (Courtesy of G Rayan MD)

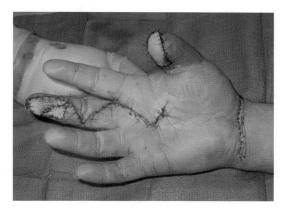

Fig. 7.10 The flap has been transferred, and the secondary defect in the middle finger is covered with a full-thickness skin graft from the volar wrist. (Courtesy of G Rayan MD)

Outcomes

Most authors report satisfactory outcomes and flap survival with the NVI flap. In the early postoperative period, a stimulus to the flap is perceived as originating at the donor digit. After a variable period of time, the same stimulus is perceived to arise from both the donor and recipient digits—a phenomenon known as double sensibility [15, 16]. Ideally, this should progress to perception of the stimulus as only at the thumb. A frequent criticism of the NVI flap is poor sensory reorientation of

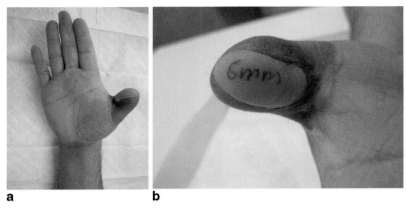

Fig. 7.11 a, b The flap has healed and incorporated and has a 6-mm two-point discrimination. (Courtesy of G Rayan MD)

flap perception from the donor to the recipient site [15]. Tubiana and Duparc reported the ultimate sensibility of the flap was comparable in quality to normal. However, 40 % of the patients were not able to reorient sensibility to the recipient finger. They did observe sensibility in the thumb pulp surrounding the flap increased from its preoperative level [16]. Other authors have reported complete sensory reorientation rates from 0 to 59 %. However, complete reorientation is probably not essential for functional success of the transfer.

Regardless of reorientation, the return of two-point discrimination has varied considerably. Outcomes from absent two-point discrimination to near normal have been documented [16–19]. Some authors have also reported deterioration to protective sensation only over time. [15] (Fig. 7.11a, b).

Technical Modifications

Puckett described a "quartering technique" of island harvest to allow primary closure of the entire donor site. This is accomplished by excising the island as a wedge where the widest dimension does not exceed 25 % of the total digital circumference. Careful mobilization of the ulnar wedge and subperiosteal elevation of the radial side allows primary closure. This does decrease the overall volume and circumference of the donor digit but reportedly avoids the morbidity of cold intolerance, skin color changes, and lack of sensation associated with skin grafting [20]. This modification is not often used but may be feasible for resurfacing a small thumb defect.

A modification of the NVI flap in which the divided nerve of the transferred island flap is sutured to one of the digital nerves in the thumb, the "disconnection/reconnection technique," has been advocated to overcome the potential problems of poor sensory reorientation, residual paresthesia, and deterioration of two-point discrimination over time [18, 19]. The nerve and vessels in the transferred flap are separated and the donor nerve is cut in the palm and embedded in the lumbrical, [18] or thenar muscle, or subcutaneous fat [19] to avoid neuroma. The original digital nerve of the thumb is sutured to the stump of the donor nerve in the flap. To reduce the reinnervation time, the neurorrhaphy should be as close to the flap as possible [15, 18, 19].

Comparison studies of the modified and standard techniques have reported all of the modified technique patients perceived tactile stimulus on the flap as coming from the thumb where only 35 to 61 % of the standard technique patients were able to do so. There were no differences in two-point discrimination in the study groups. However, the modified technique did increase overall operative time [15] and there is the concern about incomplete axonal regeneration. In an invited critique, Foucher reported cold intolerance in 83 % of his series of donor fingers, decreasing his indications for this technique considerably. His main indication for use of this technique is acute injuries in young patients where spare skin can be moved as an island from an injured finger to an injured thumb [21].

Complications

Complications of the NVI flap can occur in the flap, the donor, neighbor, or recipient digit. Early flap loss may be related to poor inflow or outflow due to either poor intrinsic quality of the donor vessels or technical errors during dissection or transfer. Donor-digit complications include cold intolerance, joint stiffness, scarring, poor sensibility or hyperesthesia, flexion contracture, nail deformity, [15, 20] skin graft dryness, or fissuring. Complications in a neighboring digit may occur in instances of multi-digit injury where an occult zone of injury is not fully appreciated leading to potentially devastating vascular compromise.

First Dorsal Metacarpal Artery Flap

The concept of the dorsal metacarpal artery flap was first introduced by Holevich in 1963, and first implemented by Foucher and Braun in 1979. The FDMA flap is frequently used for providing coverage to the injured thumb. Creation of the flap is uncomplicated. It is performed in a single stage and does not require meticulous dissection, [22] nerve repair, or direct microvascular anastomosis, [23, 24] making it a good choice in emergent cases. When appropriately harvested, it can provide sensate skin coverage to the tip of the thumb without the need for bone shortening. It can be used as an island, reversed-flow, or pedicle flap. If needed, periosteum or tendon can be incorporated into the flap. There is minimal donor-site morbidity and early postoperative ROM can be initiated [1, 22, 23].

The flap is a composite fasciocutaneous island flap supplied by the FDMA and its ulnar branch, drained by one or two associated veins, and innervated via terminal dorsal branches of the radial nerve to the index finger. Anatomical studies have demonstrated the FDMA as constant at its origin in the base of the first web space. Its ulnar branch courses along the aponeurosis of the first dorsal interosseous muscle, with few collateral branches, and it reliably supplies the skin at the dorsal aspect of the index finger proximal pha-

lanx [24]. A skin island up to 1.5×4.5 cm based on a pedicle up to 7 cm long can be harvested [23, 25] (Fig. 7.12).

Indications

Indications for use in the thumb include resurfacing thumb-tip amputations with tissue loss from the palmar, dorsal, or lateral aspect. It can provide coverage of a large pulp or dorsal defects (>2 cm) with exposed tendon, bone, and/or joint or amputation or other defects proximal to the IP joint. A history of prior open fractures to the index finger metacarpal or proximal phalanx or soft tissue damage is a contraindication for FDMA use. Relative contraindications include medical comorbidities, advanced age, peripheral vascular disease, or an ongoing infection [23].

Surgical Technique: Island Flap

First, a Doppler is used to map the course of the FDMA and its main ulnar branch along the index metacarpal. A "lazy S" incision is then marked along the first web space and over the dorsal radial

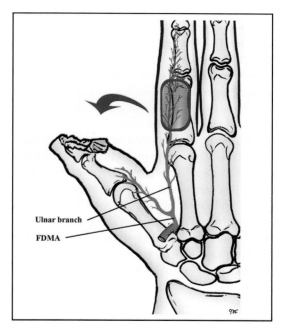

Fig. 7.12 Anatomic diagram of the first dorsal metacarpal artery flap. (From: [23] Figure 3. Used with permission from the American Society for Surgery of the Hand)

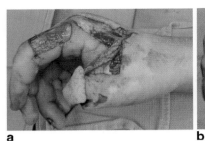
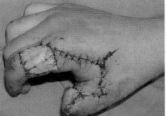
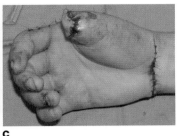

a   b   c

Fig. 7.13 a First dorsal metacarpal artery flap has been raised and pivoted to the defect. **b, c** The flap has been inset, and the secondary defect in the index finger covered with a full-thickness skin graft from the volar wrist. (Courtesy of T Lehman MD)

aspect of the index metacarpal extending towards the anatomic snuffbox. Next, a template of the defect is made and used to outline the flap over the dorsum of the index finger proximal phalanx. The flap should preserve the dorsal skin of the MP and proximal interphalangeal (PIP) joints, whenever possible. If a larger flap is required, the skin over the PIP joint can be incorporated. The flap width should not extend beyond the radial and ulnar mid-axial lines. The flap pivot point is marked at the origin of the FDMA from the radial artery. The incision is then made along the borders of the flap and extended proximally. The radial artery and the FDMA origin are exposed at the proximal end of the incision. The flap is raised from distal to proximal and ulnar to radial with care taken to remain superficial to the extensor paratenon. This preserves vascularity to the donor-site bed for the full-thickness skin graft and improves gliding of the extensor mechanism. The pedicle is isolated subdermally along the radial border of the index metacarpal and it may be raised with the periosteum. The pedicle should include the perivascular fat and fascia of the first dorsal interosseous muscle. If the flap is to provide sensory innervation, cutaneous branches of the radial nerve can be identified superficially and included in the vascular pedicle. To avoid damage, the neurovascular structures within the pedicle itself are not dissected [22, 23] (Fig. 7.13a).

Once the flap is raised, the tourniquet is released to confirm adequate blood flow to the flap. A generous subcutaneous tunnel extending to the thumb is created with hemostat dissection. The flap is then transferred to the defect. Care is taken to avoid torsion, excessive traction, or compression of the neurovascular pedicle. To avoid compression of the pedicle at the thumb IP joint, the skin portion of the flap is elongated proximally and the lateral side of the thumb opened [22]. The flap is inset into the defect and secured to the adjacent skin. The donor area is covered with a full-thickness skin graft [22, 23] (Fig. 7.13b, c).

When raising a pedicle flap, the approach is similar except the skin overlying the neurovascular pedicle is included in the dissection. The flap is transposed and inset directly to the defect without creation of a tunnel. This flap can be used for thumb defects, but is probably most often used in defects of the first web space or reconstructing first web space contracture.

A well-padded and non-constricting thumb Spica splint that allows a portion of the flap to remain visible for monitoring is applied. The splint is worn for 2 weeks. Sutures are then removed and a therapy program for ROM initiated.

Modifications

The FDMA flap may also be raised as a reversed-flow flap. When using this modification, the course of the FDMA is mapped and a defect template made as in the island flap technique. The template is used to mark the skin on the hand dorsum over the arterial pedicle. The fasciocutaneous island flap is harvested by raising a paddle including the interosseous muscle fascia. Next, the FDMA is ligated near its origin in the radial artery. The vascular pedicle and fascial dissection continues distally to the level of the metacarpal neck. Dissection to this level avoids injury to perforating vessels originating from the palmar supply that emerges between the second and third metacarpal heads to anastomose with the FDMA terminal branches. The flap is secured to the primary defect. The secondary defect usually requires a skin graft, but sometimes direct closure may be possible especially when used as pedicled flap [23].

Paneva-Holevich has described a bipedicled NVI flap from the dorsoradial surface of the index finger for thumb coverage. The flap includes a palmar pedicle supplied by the index finger digital artery and dorsal branch of the palmar digital nerve. A dorsal pedicle is supplied by the FDMA and the dorsoradial digital branch of the radial nerve. A skin island up to 7 cm length and 1.5 cm width can be raised with this technique [26].

An island flap based on the dorsoradial branches of the radial digital neurovascular bundle of the thumb has been reported for thumb-pulp resurfacing. This flap avoids sacrifice of skin on a normal finger as in an FDMA or the classic NVI flap from the middle finger. Since the flap is taken from the distal thumb, it avoids the advancement limitations posed by the Moberg flap. However, it does require an intact dorsal radial thumb surface [27].

Outcomes
Satisfactory outcomes are often expected after using this flap including adequate coverage of durable skin and maintaining length without further shortening. When used to restore sensibility to the damaged digit, two-point discrimination is typically greater than 10 mm [1, 23]. There is no significant difference in sensibility results in the FDMA flap based on patient age according to one study [1].

Complications
Marginal flap loss is more common than complete loss. Complete loss can be attributed to errors in flap design where there is excessive tension or torsion on the pedicle [23]. Neuroma of the original thumb nerves or difficulty with precision grip without visual control has been report-

ed. Cold intolerance of either the flap or donor area, and diminished ROM of the index finger can also occur [1, 23]. Finally, hair growth over the palmar surface of the thumb or an unsightly scar may result [22].

Comparisons Among Flaps

Based on published series with long-term follow-up, satisfactory results are to be expected when the MAF is employed [4, 10]. Normal and near-normal sensory recovery have been reported with at least 75 % of patients achieving two-point discrimination of 5 mm. Three-point pinch strength was slightly decreased, but grip and key pinch strength were near normal. The patients who underwent MAF coverage of a soft tissue defect had better outcomes than patients who had the procedure to close an amputation site.

Delikonstantinou et al. reported a group of 14 patients who underwent thumb-pulp reconstruction with either an FDMA or Littler NVI flap. They assessed healing, sensibility, and functional outcome. They found both flaps were reliable and the reconstructed thumbs had full ROM and stability. Differences reaching statistical significance were decreased ROM at the donor site (two of six patients) and increased operative time (mean of 139 vs. 94 min) in the Littler NVI flap. Static two-point discrimination was increased in the FDMA group (mean of 12.4 vs. 7.5 mm), also statistically significant. At 1 year postoperatively, all patients in the FDMA group achieved cortical reorientation whereas 50 % in the Littler NVI group were reoriented [28].

Both the FDMA and NVI flaps are regional innervated fasciocutaneous axial flaps. Each has its advantages and disadvantages. The NVI flap is solely an island flap, whereas the FDMA is much more versatile and can be harvested as an island, pedicle, or reversed-flow flap to cover the thumb and other areas in the dorsum of the hand and first web space. Sensory function is better preserved in the NVI flap [23, 28] than the FDMA flap but cortical reorientation is less likely to be disrupted with the FDMA flap [28]. The NVI flap offers a better tissue match and can cover a larger defect than the FDMA flap [1, 28]. However, the more demanding dissection can lead to longer operative time and has been associated with more donor-site morbidity [28].

Flaps for Coverage of Extensive Thumb Injuries

More distant flaps are available for coverage of larger thumb deficits. These are more frequently used for soft tissue and/or bony reconstruction of the entire thumb, but may be employed to address larger complex wounds that include the tip of the thumb. These are not the focus of this chapter and will be discussed briefly.

Reverse Radial Forearm Flap

When used to cover deficits in the hand, the radial forearm flap is designed as a retrograde flow flap based on the radial artery distally. The flap can be used to cover defects including the thumb and part of the hand. It is typically raised as a fasciocutaneous flap but may also be raised as an osteofasciocutaneous or fascial flap depending on what is required [29, 30]. The flap prerequisite is a patent palmer arterial arch and ulnar artery so that flow is maintained in the radial artery after it is divided proximally. When skin is harvested, the resulting secondary defect requires skin grafting and may be unsightly. Fascial flaps result in only a linear scar at the harvest site, but require skin grafting for coverage in the digit [30].

Posterior Interosseous Flap

This flap is similar to the radial forearm flap but is based on the posterior interosseous artery. It is a fasciocutaneous or fascial flap that can be rotated distally to cover deficits in the proximal portion of the thumb and digits, particularly dorsally. Depending on the exact location of the rotation point, which is the distal communication between the anterior and posterior interosseous vessels, it may not extend beyond the IP joint of the thumb [31, 32].

Groin Flap

The groin flap can provide fasiocutaneous tissue for transfer and coverage of large defects, especially in the dorsum of the hand with exposed tendons when local or regional flaps are not available [33, 34]. It can be a good option for coverage of an extensive degloving injury to the thumb. When used in the thumb it is transferred as a staged pedicle interpolation flap based on the superficial circumflex iliac artery. A sufficient flap may be raised allowing closure of the secondary defect. The medial portion of the flap is not divided in the first stage, but the free edges are sewn together to form a tube and the lateral portion is inset to cover the thumb primary defect. Division of the medial portion of the flap with final inset is performed 2 weeks after the first stage (Fig. 7.8a–e). This flap provides very reliable coverage. However, the thick layer of subcutaneous fat present in some patients may make this flap unsuitable for use in the digits [34]. A neurovascular island flap can then be used to supplement the groin flap and provide sensate tissue at the thumb tip [15, 17].

Conclusion

The most frequently used flaps for coverage of thumb-tip injuries are the Moberg advancement, neurovascular island, and FDMA flaps. Each offers a unique solution to a specific thumb-tip injury scenario. Knowledge of the vascular anatomy of each flap combined with careful surgical technique is expected to maintain thumb length, offer durable soft tissue padding, restore sensory function, and achieve excellent outcomes and patient satisfaction.

References

1. Tränkle M, Sauerbier M, Germann G. Restoration of thumb sensibility with the innervated first dorsal metacarpal artery island flap. J Hand Surg Am. 2003;28(5):758–66.
2. Eski M, Nisanci M, Sengezer M. Correction of thumb deformities after burn: versatility of first dorsal metacarpal artery flap. Burns. 2007;33(1):65–71.

3. Moberg E. Aspects of sensation in reconstructive surgery of the upper extremity. J Bone Joint Surg. 1964;46A:817–25.
4. Baumeister S, Menke H, Wittemann M, Germann G. Functional outcome after the Moberg advancement flap in the thumb. J Hand Surg. 2002;27A:105–14.
5. Posner MA, Smith RJ. The advancement pedicle flap for thumb injuries. Br J Plast Surg. 1999;52:64–8.
6. Macht SD, Watson HK. The Moberg volar advancement flap for digital reconstruction. J Hand Surg. 1980;5:372–6.
7. Aarons M. Fingertip reconstruction with a palmar advancement flap and free dermal graft: a report of six cases. J Hand Surg. 1985;10A:230–2.
8. Kinoshita Y, Kojima T, Matsuura S, Hayashi H, Miyawaki T. Extending the use of the palmar advancement flap with v-y closure. J Hand Surg. 1997;22B:212–8.
9. O'Brien B. Neurovascular island pedicle flaps for terminal amputations and digital scars. Br J Plast Surg. 1968;21:258–61.
10. Foucher G, Delaere O, Citron N, Molderez A. Long-term outcome of neurovascular palmar advancement flaps for distal thumb injuries. Br J Plast Surg. 1999;52:64–8.
11. Bang H, Kojima T, Hayashi H. Palmar advancement flap with v-y closure for thumb tip injuries. J Hand Surg. 1992;17A:933–4.
12. Elliot D, Wilson Y. V-Y advancement of the entire volar soft tissue of the thumb in distal reconstruction. J Hand Surg. 1993; 18B:399–402.
13. Germann G. Principles of flap design for surgery of the hand. Atlas Hand Clin. 1998;3:33–57.
14. Wallace AB editor. Transactions of the international society of plastic surgeons: second congress. Edinburgh: E & S Livingstone; 1960.
15. Schlenker JD, Trumble TE. Neurovascular Island flap. In: Rayan GM, Chung KC, editors. Flap reconstruction of the upper extremity. Rosemont: American Society for Surgery of the Hand; 2009.
16. Tubiana R, Duparc J. Restoration of sensibility in the hand by neurovascular skin island transfer. J Bone Joint Surg Br. 1961;43-B:474–80.
17. Campbell Reid DA. The neurovascular island flap in thumb reconstruction. Br J Plast Surg. 1966;19:234–44.
18. Adani R, Squarzina PB, Castagnetti C, Laganá A, Pancalidi G, Caroli A. A comparative study of the heterodigital neurovascular island flap in thumb reconstruction, with and without nerve reconnection. J Hand Surg Eur. 1994;19(5):552–9.
19. Oka Y. Sensory function of the neurovascular island flap in thumb reconstruction: comparison of original and modified procedures. J Hand Surg Am. 2000;25(4):637–43.
20. Puckett CL, Howard B, Concannon MJ. Primary closure of the donor site for the Littler neurovascular island flap transfer. Plast Reconstr Surg. 1996;97(5):1062–4.
21. Kumta SM, Yip KMH, Pannozzo A, Fong SL, Leung PC. Resurfacing of thumb-pulp loss with a heterodigital neurovascular island flap using a nerve disconnection/reconnection technique. J Reconstr Microsurg. 1997;13(2):117–23.
22. Sherif MM. First dorsal metacarpal artery flap in hand reconstruction. II. Clinical application. J Hand Surg Am. 1994;19(1):32–8.
23. Rayan GM. First dorsal metacarpal artery flap. In: Rayan GM, Chung KC, editors. Flap reconstruction of the upper extremity. Rosemont: American Society for Surgery of the Hand; 2009.
24. Foucher G, Braun JB. A new island flap transfer from the dorsum of the index to the thumb. Plast Reconstr Surg. 1979;63(3):344–9.
25. Sherif MM. First dorsal metacarpal artery flap in hand reconstruction. I. Anatomical study. J Hand Surg Am. 1994;19(1):26–31.
26. Paneva-Holevich Y. Further experience with the bi-pedicled neurovascular island flap in thumb reconstruction. J Hand Surg Am. 1991;16(4):594–7.
27. Pho RWH. Local composite neurovascular island flap for skin cover in pulp loss of the thumb. J Hand Surg Am. 1979;4(1):11–5.
28. Delikonstantinou IP, Gravvanis AI, Dimitriou V, Zogogiannis I, Douma A, Tsoutsos DA. Foucher first dorsal metacarpal artery flap versus Littler heterodigital neurovascular flap in resurfacing thumb pulp loss defects. Ann Plast Surg. 2011;667(2):119–22.
29. Kaufman MR, Jones NF. The reverse radial forearm flap for soft tissue reconstruction of the wrist and hand. Tech Hand Up Extrem Surg. 2005;9(1):47–51.
30. Rogachefsky RA, Mendietta CG, Galpin P, Ouellette EA. Reverse radial forearm fascial flap for soft tissue coverage of hand and forearm wounds. Br J H Surg. 2000;25(4):385–9.
31. Chemma TA, Lakshman S, Cheema MA, Durraini SF. Reverse-flow posterior interosseous flap—a review of 68 cases. Hand. 2007;2(3):112–6.
32. El-Sabbagh AH, Zeina AAE, El-Hadidy A, El-Din AB. Reversed posterior interosseous flap: safe and easy method for hand reconstruction. J Hand Microsurg. 2011;3(2):66–72.
33. Button M, Stone IJ. Segmental bony reconstruction of the thumb by composite groin flap. J Hand Surg. 1980;5(5):488–91.
34. Trzcinski D, Rayan GM. Groin flap. In: Rayan GM, Chung KC, editors. Flap reconstruction of the upper extremity. Rosemont: American Society for Surgery of the Hand; 2009.
35. Lehman TP, Rayan GM. Moberg advancement flap. In: Rayan GM, Chung KC, editors. Flap reconstruction of the upper extremity: a masters skills publication. Rosemont: American Society for Surgery of the Hand, 2009. pp. 74–9.
36. Rayan G, Trzcinski D. Groin flap. In: Slutsky D, editor. The art of microsurgical Hand reconstruction. New York: Thieme; 2013.

Free Tissue Transfer for Fingertip Coverage

Luis R. Scheker, Fernando Simon Polo
and Francisco J. Aguilar

Introduction

Amputation of the pulp of the fingers and thumb is a frequent injury in a hand surgeon's daily clinical practice. The hands are the second most vascularized and innervated region of the body after the face, thus allowing for multiple flaps to treat them. However, sometimes, because of the size, sensitivity, and aesthetic characteristics, pulp defect reconstructions need specific tissue supply from a region other than the hand. Due to its similar characteristics, the foot is the most suitable donor site for these tissue transfers.

Treatment of Fingertip Injuries

The basic objectives for the treatment of fingertip injuries are preserving the length of the digit when possible, and providing soft tissue coverage with protective sensation at a minimum and a painless fingertip [1]. There is a wide diversity of treatment options based on the characteristics and nature of the lesion (one of the most important is the size), the physical demands and preferences

of the patient, and the expertise of the treating surgeon and the health-care system. Management varies from healing by secondary intention to complex reconstruction or even replantation.

For lesions with pulp loss and no distal bone exposure, management options include primary closure, healing by secondary intention, skin grafting, and even completion amputation. When adequate soft tissue coverage is available volarly, primary closure or healing by secondary intention is preferable. Recovery of sensation after the latter has been found to be superior to other surgical methods, and two-point discrimination (2PD) approaches normal after healing, but the lesion needs several months for complete cicatrization. [1]

When there is bone exposure and no volar soft tissue coverage available, these injuries are candidates for pulp reconstruction, as long as 5 mm of nail bed distal to the lunula is preserved (as this amount of nail remains both aesthetic and functional) [2]. The use of flaps in such instances provides an important tool for coverage when more simple measures are inadequate [3].

Depending on the size of the defect, the pulp can be reconstructed using local, regional, distant flaps, or free tissue transfers. Local flaps restrict donor morbidity to the same injured digit, and furnish tissue coverage nearly identical in quality to the lost tissue, so sensation, aesthetic, and functional recovery are optimal; but they are limited in size and distance of transfer. For transverse or dorsal oblique amputations that need less than 1 cm of tissue advance, the Atasoy–Kleinert V–Y flap [4] is the best option for all digits.

L. R. Scheker (✉) · F. S. Polo · F. J. Aguilar
C. M. Kleinert Institute for Hand and Microsurgery,
225 Abraham Flexner Way Suite 700, Louisville,
KY 40202, USA
e-mail: lscheker@kleinertkutz.com

L. R. Scheker
University of Louisville School of Medicine,
Louisville, USA

L. M. Rozmaryn (ed.), *Fingertip Injuries*, DOI 10.1007/978-3-319-13227-3_8,
© Springer International Publishing Switzerland 2015

The Kutler lateral V–Y flap [5] is better suited for volar oblique amputations that have more tissue loss volarly than dorsally, but also it can be used for transverse amputations [1] as long as the advancement needed is less than 3–4 mm.

In the case of the thumb, one flap that has demonstrated good sensation recovery, but inferior aesthetic recovery is the Moberg flap [6]. This can be used when a defect is <2 cm and a V–Y advancement flap cannot provide adequate coverage.

It is true that other advancement flaps such as the step-advancement island flap and/or the oblique triangular neurovascular advancement flap allow more distance of advancement and they are also sensate flaps, but these are based on only one neurovascular pedicle, wherewith the sensation recovery would not be as good as other options that provide two pedicles. Some authors have reported what, in their opinion, are good results using homodigital transposition flaps such as the reverse digital artery island flap [7]. However, these flaps sacrifice one digital artery, involve extensive dissection, are prone to congestion, and result in abnormal sensation [8] since they are not neurosensory flaps.

When local flaps are inadequate, it is popular to use regional flaps such as the cross-finger flap and the thenar flap, or distant flaps such as the groin flap, chest flap, and cross-arm flap.

One must differentiate between the basic objective of the treatment and the best treatment. The fact that one treatment is technically easier, more reliable, or saves time or money does not make it the best option.

These very popular regional and distal flaps, because of their simplicity and reliability, have major drawbacks that should not be obviated: The cross-finger flap is a two-stage procedure, insensate nonglabrous skin is used, fingers are held in an awkward position and immobilized for 2–3 weeks, and a second digit is violated as a donor site. The thenar flap provides glabrous skin cover but otherwise shares the same problems as the cross-finger flap [8]. The same occurs with distant flaps, that in addition to being insensate flaps, rely on donor-site blood supply while the flap incorporates and can lead to stiffness sec-

ondary to the prolonged period of immobilization required for healing [1].

An excellent alternative to these flaps is the free flap or free tissue transfer, a procedure in which soft tissue with or without bone is harvested with its vascular pedicle and transferred to a recipient site, where the pedicle is anastomosed to local vessels, thus vascularizing the tissue [9].

Although using free tissue transfer flaps can involve breaking the guidelines of the reconstructive ladder, it is justified in select cases since the ideal objectives of fingertip coverage can be reached: highest sensory, functional, and aesthetic recovery, and avoiding the aforementioned disadvantages of simpler flaps. In addition, it has been demonstrated that free tissue transfer success rate in experienced hands approaches 99%, whereas local or regional flaps can be less successful because of initial damage to regional soft tissues. [10] We concur as Dr. Levin [10] reported in 2008, that frequently local flaps are used by individuals without microsurgical skills when a free flap is the best treatment. Local flaps are often damaged because of compromised inflow and outflow, therefore these patients will need a second and more complex operation, morbidity will be prolonged and will compromise the finger which finally often needs to be salvaged by free tissue transfer.

The interest in transplanting autologous tissue peaked and the earliest free flaps were described in the 1970s. However, the failure rate was high due to the complexity of the anatomy and that the field of autologous tissue transplantation was in the early stages of development. Pioneers such as Buncke, Acland, Shaw, and Tamai popularized the free tissue transfer for use in extremity trauma. Over the next 10 years, a variety of composite flaps evolved. But it was in the 1980s and 1990s when, with microsurgical evolution, new skin flaps were identified based on defined vascular territories, the evolution of perforator flaps, and the increased success of flaps. This expanded horizons for extremity reconstruction [10].

For fingertip repair, not every free flap can be used. Standard free flaps are too bulky, or not durable or sensate enough. Only flaps that allow ideal outcomes of fingertip reconstruction should be used, like the ones that [4]: restore grasping function without slippage [11], restore the contour of the pulp with glabrous skin and no bulging mass [12], are strong enough to withstand friction [13], provide sufficient soft tissue for a cushion effect [14], and have sufficient sensory acuity for fine manipulation (discriminating sensibility) [15]. To accomplish these goals, several small free flaps have been developed in the last few years, although not all of them meet expectations. The most popular small flaps for fingertip coverage are:

- Thenar free flap
- Free flap from the flexor aspect of the wrist
- Arterialized venous flap (AVF)
- Posterior auricular free flap
- Free medialis pedis flap
- Free medial plantar artery perforator flap (MPAP)
- Great and second toe pulp neurovascular flaps

All provide glabrous or hairless skin coverage. The aesthetic similarity and functional capacity of tissue transfers from the foot are unrivaled. However, when patients refuse a flap from the foot, or they are not indicated (i.e., athletes), the other flaps offer acceptable outcomes.

The Thenar Free Flap

The free thenar flap combines a good match of the skin components (thick skin of similar glabrous texture and color to that of the digits) with the freedom of a free flap transfer when patients will not accept any transfer of tissue from the foot and local flaps are not indicated. It can be nourished by the radial digital artery of the thumb, as it was first used as a free flap by Tsai in 1991 [16], by the radial artery [17], or by the superficial palmar branch of the radial artery (SPBRA) [17–19], as is the free flap from the flexor aspect of the wrist. The most frequently used artery is the SPBRA, which offers a perfect match size for anastomosis to the digital artery.

Venous drainage is based on the volar superficial veins of the thenar eminence or the venae co-mitantes of the artery itself. The sensibility of this area is mainly provided by the sensory branch of the radial nerve, which may be overlapped by the antebrachial cutaneous nerve [19].

Operative Technique

The first step consists of identification of the radial artery and the origin of its volar branch. This branch can be confirmed preoperatively by using a Doppler flowmeter. To locate them intra-operatively, the skin must be incised for 2–3 cm in a slightly angled fashion at the wrist crease. Sometimes, a perforator rising from the radial artery, distinct from the volar artery and supplying directly the thenar region, can be found. In this situation, the flap can be based exclusively on this perforator. Its origin is about 3 cm proximal to the wrist crease. For this reason, the initial incision is addressed to first find this branch [19].

If it is not available or the diameter is too small, we recommend moving 1–2 cm distally to isolate the SPBRA with one or two venous branches that run parallel to or across the SPBRA toward the thenar eminence. In addition, there are several branches of the antebrachial nerve radial to the SPBRA and they distribute to the thenar eminence. The design of the flap can be adapted so that the flap includes the terminal part of these branches [18]. Other authors do not include sensory branches in their dissections or include other nerve branches such as the palmar branch of the superficial radial nerve. After dissection of all these structures the flap can be elevated and then the SPBRA is sutured to the digital artery, the veins sutured to the dorsal digital veins and the nerve to the digital nerve in an end-to-end fashion.

The main indication for the thenar free flap is for the patient who would rather not sacrifice soft tissue from the foot when other local flaps are not usable.

Advantages of this flap are that it requires minimal dissection, the sacrifice of a nondominant artery, and the thickness and glabrous texture offer an optimal stability in palmar pinch. [17]

The main disadvantages are the possibility of an enlarged scar in the donor area, potentially unpleasant, and the variability of sensory recovery. For small skin defects, it has been reported that even without neurorrhaphy, the pedicled thenar has high possibilities to recover spontaneous reinnervation better than very popular regional flaps (i.e., cross-finger flaps). This is supposed to be a consequence of the higher presence of sensory receptors in the thenar area [20].

Free Flap from the Flexor Aspect of the Wrist

The distal portion of the flexor aspect of the forearm has been used as the donor site of several kinds of flaps. Sakai [21] described a free flap harvested from the flexor aspect of the wrist based on the SPBRA, with the intention of providing a thin, pliable, and hairless coverage for the fingertip without sacrificing the radial artery (what other traditional flaps from the forearm do).

This flap can incorporate a portion of palmaris longus and/or the palmar cutaneous branch of the median nerve to be used as a vascularized tendon and/or nerve graft for other defects of the hand and digits, but it is a non-innervated flap. This must be taken into account while reconstructing fingertips.

Results in sensibility obtained in the pulp using this flap have been compared with other frequently used nonglabrous local flaps, and seem to be similar (between 9 and 11 mm). The explanation for these acceptable outcomes given by some authors is that this flap is very thin and is applied to a sensitive area [22].

The operative technique for harvesting the flap follows Sakai's instructions: The flap is drawn transversely, with its palmar side along the distal wrist crease, so that the donor site can be closed easily and primarily. As for the draining vein, one or two subcutaneous small veins of sufficient length are marked from the flap to the proximal portion of the forearm. First, the skin incision is made down to the level of the radial artery to confirm the origin of the SPBRA. The skin incision is then deepened to the muscles and tendons along the margins of the flap. On the proximal side of the forearm, one or two subcutaneous veins of adequate size and length are

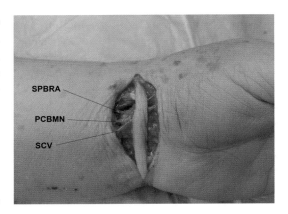

Fig. 8.1 Free flap from the flexor aspect of the wrist. *SBPRA* superficial palmar branch of the radial artery, *PCBMN* palmar cutaneous branch of the median nerve, *SCV* subcutaneous vein

chosen for drainage, and others are ligated. The flap is then raised over the muscles and tendons. At the distal wrist region or the thenar site, the SPBRA running into the palm is ligated and cut to the length that will be needed. The flap is then ready to be elevated and transferred. The donor defect is closed primarily.

The wrist flexor aspect free flap can be an interesting alternative for treatment, although lack of sensation and donor-site scar characteristics (which should be left in the distal wrist crease, otherwise it may suggest the wound is self-inflicted) are important drawbacks [21] (Fig. 8.1).

Arterialized Venous Flaps

Venous flaps are those in which the primary blood supply enters and exits the flap through the venous system. The exact vascular circuit or mechanism of physiologic nutrition, however, remains unclear [23].

There are several clinical applications for them in the reconstruction of hands and fingers when conventional flaps are limited or unavailable [24]. They can be used as pedicled venous flaps, free venous perfusion flaps, free arterial perfusion (arterialized) venous flap, and innervated AVF for different goals such as resurfacing soft tissue defects, skin and vascular defects, reconstruction of circumferential injuries, and, of course, for fingertip reconstruction.

Several classifications of the venous flaps have been described in literature based on: vessels that enter and leave the flap as well as the direction of flow within these vessels [25], presence of an intravenous valve, the venous network of the donor site, the location, and the number of veins at the recipient site [26]. Probably the most commonly used venous flaps in plastic and microsurgery surgery are the three classification types of Thatte et al. [25] which are type I, unipedicled venous; type II, bipedicled; and type III, AVFs, which are perfused by a proximal artery anastomosed with a cephalad end vein and drained by a distal vein. The most reliable of these is the type III [27] and that is why clinical use has mostly focused on it.

Success in reconstructing skin defects of the digits with AVFs seems to be influenced by the donor site and size of the flap [27]. The influence of donor site on the survival of AVFs has been attributed to the configuration of the venous network of different donor sites. The most frequent donor sites for venous flaps are: the distal volar forearm, the dorsum of the foot and medial aspect of lower leg, and the thenar and hypothenar eminences [28]. The configuration of the dorsal skin of digits and hypothenar or thenar eminence is more favorable than that of the volar forearm, while the donor site of the lower leg, in which there is a poor venous network, is considered the last choice for venous flaps. Kakinoki et al. [29] showed that the size of the flap was the factor that correlated statistically with a successful result. AVFs with a surface area less than 767 mm^2 were less likely to develop necrosis of the skin (Fig. 8.2).

For fingertip reconstruction, the most indicated AVFs are the thenar and hypothenar flaps, first described by Iwasawa et al. [28], since the volar forearm and dorsum of the foot skin are not glabrous skin, have poor skin texture for volar surface reconstruction, and result in instability with pinching.

The operative technique of the AVF from thenar and hypothenar eminences was described this way in the original paper:

The donor site is the lateral side of the metacarpophalangeal joint for the thenar venous flap and the lateral side of the hypothenar region for the hypothenar flap. A branch of the dorsal cutaneous vein is located in either the thenar or the hypothenar region. When elevating the flap, a segment of the branch of the dorsal cutaneous vein, the subcutaneous tissue and deep fascia of the thenar or hypothenar muscles are included. At the recipient site, a proper digital artery and dorsal vein are prepared at the interphalangeal joint level and microvascular anastomoses are performed between these vessels [28].

The skin of the thenar and hypothenar regions is not completely glabrous. However, it has a thick keratosis layer and deep fascia of the thenar and hypothenar muscles that provide durability for mechanical stress and good stability. None of these is a sensory flap. Nevertheless, good sensory recovery has been reported with thenar and hypothenar flaps by Iwasawa et al. The authors explained this recovery is due to the fact that palmar tissue has many sensory receptors [28].

Innervated AVFs have been described from the dorsum of the foot preserving sensation by anastomosing branches of superficial peroneal nerves with the digital nerves [30] but they are nonglabrous flaps. The authors explain that, "ideally, the volar side of the finger should be reconstructed with glabrous skin such as palm or instep. Although small arterialized venous flaps that use medial plantar skin are useful for finger pulp reconstruction it is difficult to harvest a thin and pliable arterialized venous flap from medial plantar skin. It is also not easy to include enough long cutaneous veins and cutaneous branches of medial plantar nerve in the instep venous flap."[31]

Compared with conventional arterial flaps, the advantages of venous flaps are that they provide non-bulky and good-quality tissue, ease of design, and harvest without the need to perform deep and tedious dissection, no sacrifice of a major artery at the donor site, no limitation of the donor sites, and less donor-site morbidity with optimal postoperative contour. They could be a good option for reconstruction of small defects of the fingers, but it should be noted they are either insensate or nonglabrous skin flaps or both. Also, they have an unstable postoperative course and are difficult to monitor. They are not very reliable

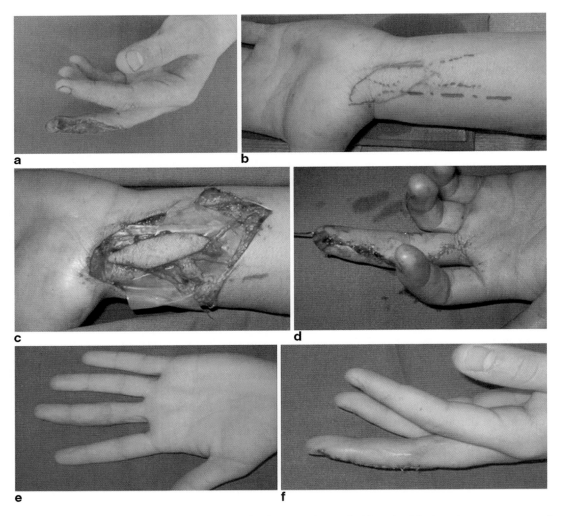

Fig. 8.2 Arterialized venous flap from the distal volar forearm. The terminal branch of the lateral cutaneous nerve of the forearm is included in order to provide a sensate flap. (Courtesy: Dr. Thomas Giesen)

due to their inconsistent survival and possible partial loss, but these problems may be solved by techniques such as surgical delay procedure, pre-arterialization technique, surgical expansion, and application of growth factors after meticulous preoperative planning. [23].

Posterior Auricular Artery Sensate Flap

This flap provides wound coverage while retaining sensation and negligible donor-site morbidity. It is used for fingertip radial-side pulp reconstruction and is based on the posterior

auricular artery. The first clinical success for the free retroauricular skin flap was reported by Wada and coworkers in 1979 [32], and it has been popular for intraoral and facial reconstruction for years. It was in 2009 when Hsieh et al. [33] first described this flap for fingertip reconstruction.

The posterior auricular sensate free flap is not simple but some authors consider it cost-effective because the sensation recovery is good and primary closure of the donor site is possible. The donor-site scar is located in the posterior auricular area, and it provides good aesthetic appearance of finger reconstruction area with no joint stiffness.

Surgical Technique

The posterior auricular vessels over the posterior auricular sulcus must be detected preoperatively using a Doppler probe. The posterior auricular vessel is identified after incision over the posterior auricular sulcus and meticulous dissection. A skin island in the posterior auricular area is designed over the entry area of the posterior auricular vessel. The flap is elevated from the layer beneath the posterior auricular vessel. The great auricular nerve is also identified in the posterior auricular area. The pedicle of the posterior auricular flap is anastomosed to the radial digital artery and dorsal vein, and the great auricular nerve is anastomosed to the radial side digital nerve. Primary closure of the posterior auricular donor site can be accomplished with no morbidity [33] (Fig. 8.3).

Widespread utilization of the posterior auricular free flap has yet to become popular due to a considerable amount of technical challenges, although previous success has been reported and can be promising. Technical challenges include a short vascular pedicle, a superficial venous system that is not always present, extremely small vena comitantes, anatomic variation [34] (for instance, sometimes posterior auricular vessels are too small to transfer in a free flap), tendency of the flap based on the superficial temporal vessels to become congested, and limited flap size (although this is not usually a problem when treating pulp injuries).

Since there are few reports of this flap as far as pulp coverage is concerned in the literature, it is difficult to draw reliable conclusions about its indications and true functional and aesthetic results. Hsieh et al. [33] report 7 mm of static 2PD and good aesthetic recovery and consider this flap an alternative to foot tissue transfers.

Inversely, there are other flaps such as the posterior interosseous artery flap [35] or the temporoparietal free fascial flap with a split-thickness skin graft [36] that are mentioned in the literature as useful for fingertip coverage. The former gives excellent cover but it is a nonglabrous skin flap, and the latter, even though it provides a pseudo-glabrous surface, is relatively insensate. These reasons are more than enough not to consider them ideal options for the replacement of pulp injuries.

Glabrous Skin Flaps

Defects on the volar surface of the fingers require replacement with specialized sensory cells that can only be found in the hand itself, on the toes, or on the sole area of the foot, what is generally known as glabrous tissue [37]. The best way to accomplish this replacement is by microneurovascular transplantation of glabrous skin from the foot [38].

The most widespread free flaps that can provide glabrous skin on a consistent vascular pedicle are the free medialis pedis flap, free MPAP flap, and great toe and second toe pulp neurovascular island (NVI) flaps. Free medialis pedis flap and free MPAP flap are interconnected and share anatomy and some properties. The complex vascular anatomy of the medial plan-

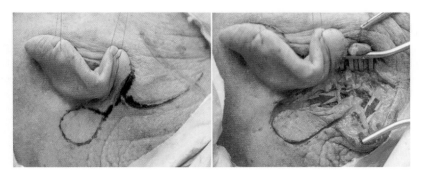

Fig. 8.3 Posterior auricular artery sensate flap. Cadaver dissection. *Arrows* show the vascular pedicle and the great auricular nerve. (Courtesy: Dr. Shih-heng Chen)

tar system was reported in 1990 by Masquelet and Romana [39]. The medial plantar artery is divided into the superficial and deep branches of the medial plantar artery. The deep branch of the medial plantar artery in turn subdivides into lateral and medial branches. The medial branch runs dorsally between the tibialis posterior tendon and the abductor hallucis muscle, after which it courses distally along the medial margin of the foot, proximal to the tubercle of the navicular bone. The artery is usually accompanied by one or two venae comitantes.

The medialis pedis flap receives its blood supply from the medial branch of deep division of the medial plantar artery. In contrast with this, the MPAP flap is nourished by superficial division of the medial plantar artery [40] (Fig. 8.4).

The *free medials pedis flap* for resurfacing skin defects of the hand and digits was first reported by Ishikura et al. [22] based on Masquelet and Romana's studies [39] for soft tissue defects of the foot in which a thin and supple skin cover was needed. The advantages of this flap are: It is very thin in comparison with other standard free flaps; it can be used for small repairs; it possesses two draining venous pathways, the vena comitantes and the subcutaneous veins; the diameters of its vessels are similar to those of the fingers; it provides a good color and texture match for the

repair; and according to Ishikura, a good recovery of protective sensation is achievable.

This latter point is questionable since one of its main disadvantages is that it is an insensate flap. Other drawbacks are that skin grafting is usually necessary for donor-site closure and that in cases where the posterior tibial artery represents the dominant or singular inflow source to the foot, the harvesting of this flap could potentially compromise the circulation to the foot. Although it can be an appropriate flap for volar hand and digit injuries given that it provides glabrous skin coverage, its use is discouraged for fingertip lesions since it is not a sensory flap (Fig. 8.5).

The *free medial plantar artery perforator flap*, despite its anatomical proximity to the medialis pedis flap, has several positive differences: It is thicker, providing adequate cushioning surface; donor site can close primarily if flap width is less than 2 cm, and it can be sensate including the cutaneous branch of medial plantar nerve or saphenous nerve for anastomosing to the digital nerve [41].

Before 1986, when Hidalgo described favorable results using it for palm coverage [42], its utilization was limited for resurfacing feet and heel defects since Mir and Mir presented it in 1954 [43]. However, the first report of this flap as a neurovascular flap for pulp reconstruction was published by Inoue 2 years later [44] (Fig. 8.6).

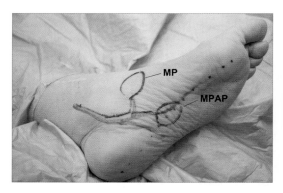

Fig. 8.4 Free medialis pedis (*MP*) flap and free medial plantar artery perforator (*MPAP*) flap schematic design. The *red line* indicates the posterior tibial artery trajectory with the medial plantar artery branch for MP flap and superficial division of the medial plantar artery branch for MPAP flap. Cadaver dissection

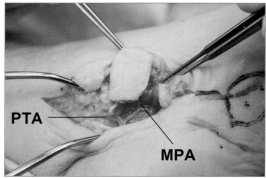

Fig. 8.5 Free medialis pedis flap. Cadaver dissection. *PTA* posterior tibial artery, *MPA* medialis pedis artery

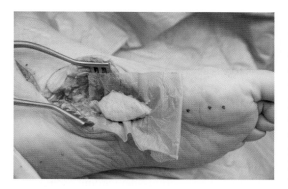

Fig. 8.6 Free medial plantar artery perforator flap. Cadaver dissection

Operative Technique

The posterior tibial artery can be located by palpation posterior to the medial malleolus and followed downward to the instep groove between the abductor hallucis muscle and the flexor digitorum brevis muscle. The perforator can be easily identified by marking the septum between the abductor hallucis and the flexor digitorum brevis with a straight line. From this line, a perpendicular line is drawn to the navicular tubercle and the perforator will be located in a 2-cm-radius area from this line [40] and adjacent to the first cuneiform bone. This can be confirmed by Doppler.

The medial plantar flap is designed on the axis of the plantar surface of the first metatarsal with the perforator in the central area [38]. The plantar incision is made and the suprafascial plane is dissected until the perforators are identified. To expose the medial plantar vessels, a dissection between the abductor hallucis muscle and the flexor digitorum muscle is performed. Then, the lateral incision is made and the vein draining into the saphenous system is preserved, in case the comitantes veins of medial plantar artery are too small for anastomosis. The saphenous vein branch is also isolated with the saphenous nerve to innervate the flap. After releasing the tourniquet, flap circulation is evaluated and if there is no problem, the flap is harvested and inset on the finger. Inflow is provided by a digital artery and outflow is established via dorsal vein. The digital nerves are repaired to the saphenous nerve branch.

The advantages of this flap were well detailed by Huang et al. [40]: (a) It can be up to 7 cm long and 2 cm wide, providing a large surface area; (b) medial plantar vessels remain intact, therefore there is no compromise of the foot's blood supply; (c) provide cushioning and glabrous skin, (d) flap elevation can be performed quickly in experienced hands because a short pedicle does not require a tedious dissection; and (e) size and length of pedicle are compatible with the digital vessel.

It also presents disadvantages: Preserving small perforators without causing further injury is difficult and delicate surgical skills and sometimes microscope-assisted procedures are needed. When the donor area is more than 2 cm wide, it is necessary to use split-thickness skin graft to close. And mainly, there is some lack of good 2PD recovery although it is a sensate flap [45]

Great Toe Pulp Neurovascular Island Flap

Of all the free flaps utilized for digital pulp reconstruction, the free neurovascular toe flap provides a particularly efficient solution for loss of cutaneous substance [46, 47]. It not only restores the finger with a solid and well-cushioned cover but also with a dense population of specific sensory end organs attached to the flap [45]. That is the main advantage of these flaps in comparison with any other flaps, as they comply with one of the major surgical principles described by Sir Harold Gillies, the father of modern plastic surgery: "replace like to like" [48].

With the free neurovascular toe flap we not only provide tissue with the same unique mechanical and aesthetic characteristics of the finger and thumb pulp but also provide their same specific sensory functional pattern. From the mechanical and aesthetic point of view, the palmar aspect of the hand is gifted with anatomical characteristics of skin, subcutaneous tissue and appendages, suitable for carrying out its principal functions of pinching and grasping [49]. It is devoid of hair and the epithelium is of thick cornified stratified squamous epithelium, rich in ridges and grooves that become thicker with usage [50]. Also, the epidermis is thick compared with that on other body areas and has abundant sweat glands but not sebaceous glands [49]. The connective tissue forms a dense array of tissue with numerous fibrous septa interconnecting the volar digital skin, periosteum, and synovial sheaths, and the connective tissue of dermis is more compact and less elastic. The subcutaneous tissue exists in many compartments in between these fibrous septa, adding a cushion effect and durability to an area constantly exposed to friction forces [41]. The pulp of the toes is the unique area of the body that has the same characteristics, so there can be no better option for replacement in case of this tissue loss.

As far as the sensory function is concerned, it is known that sensory endings can be divided into three general patterns: free sensory endings, sensory endings with expanded tips, and encapsulated sensory endings. Free nerve endings are encapsulated and are responsible for pain and temperature sensation. Sensory endings with expanded tips are the so-called Merkel's cell and the Ruffini complexes. Merkel's cell neurite complexes are only present in glabrous skin and are responsible for transmitting sensation of constant touch, pressure, and static tactile gnosis whereas Ruffini complexes are only present in hairy skin. The encapsulated sensory endings are found exclusively in glabrous skin. They are the Pacinian corpuscles and Meissner's corpuscles, highly sensitive converters of mechanical stimuli. Also, Meissner's corpuscles seem to provide the ultimate degree of sensitivity for tactile gnosis and discrimination. Both corpuscles are fast-adapting fiber mechanoreceptors that mediate sensory relays concerning moving touch, fluttering, vibration, and moving tactile gnosis [37, 38].

It is logical to assume that replacing specifically these specialized sensory endings by the same kind of sensory endings, we will be able to get the best critical sensory recovery. It has been observed that there is a correlation between the return of functional sensibility and the total number of Meissner's corpuscles in the transplanted tissue [51], which would demonstrate the necessity of using selectively glabrous skin tissue to replace glabrous skin loss if we want to achieve the best sensory result. Despite these apparent logical advantages, the application of this flap has been typecast only for selective cases and patients.

Classically, it has been differentiated between manual laborers in whom fast functional recovery is the main purpose; thus, easy, quick recovery and reliable procedures are recommended (simple revision amputation, skin grafting, island flap, etc.) and sensitivity-demanding professions such as musicians, in whom sensitivity recovery is the priority and who need specific solutions to reach that goal.

The toe pulp NVI flap is typecast in literature as the ideal and almost exclusive indication for those latter patients. However, in our opinion its indications should be expanded for any patient when preserving functional and aesthetic appearance of the injured digit is the priority and the size of the defect contraindicates the use of local flaps.

History

Reconstruction of pulp defects with toe pulp NVI flap was described for the first time in 1978 by Buncke and Rose [46]. In their paper, they propose a new technique that offered durable skin cover which becomes innervated by the sensory nerve of the recipient finger itself, and does not result in deformity or anesthesia of an adjacent finger nor require cortical reorientation of stimuli, unlike Littler's technique [52].

Although only four out of six flaps they presented survived, they showed an innovative idea that has been applied by surgeons for pulp reconstruction all over the world. Precisely, this low flap survival rate at the beginning questioned this technique's reliability, and literary tradition has retained this idea for the last century without taking into account more recent results that show flap survival rates up to 99.7% in the largest series [53]. In fact, the current average survival rate has been shown to be 98% [54]. Undoubtedly, the development of microsurgery and technique refinement since the first reports have contributed to making this flap very reliable.

Another argument of the authors who criticize the reliability of toe to pulp NVI flap is its anatomy variability, which can complicate the dissection of the flap and the fact of sacrificing a major artery, which may adversely affect foot circulation during old age [33].

It is true that neurovascular anatomy of the foot is quite complicated and a significant amount of variations have been described. The first dorsal metatarsal artery (FDMA) originates from the dorsalis pedis artery when the latter dives plantarward at the base of the first intermetatarsal space. As described by Poirier and Charpy [55], the artery courses over the dorsum of the first dorsal interosseus muscle and divides into two branches—medial and lateral—at the level of the metatarsophalangeal joint of the big toe. The medial branch provides two dorsolateral collaterals to the big toe. The lateral branch terminates as the dorsomedial branch of the second toe. Distally, in the web space, the FDMA plunges plantarward and bifurcates into its terminal branches, both medial and lateral. The medial plantar branch forms the plantar hallucal arteries, both fibular and tibial, whereas the lateral branch terminates as the medial plantar artery of the second toe. The lateral branch of the first plantar metatarsal artery (FPMA) joins the FDMA at the level of its plantar bifurcation. The plantar tibial hallucal artery crosses transversely between the mid-segment of the proximal phalanx and the flexor hallucis longus tendon to reach the medial plantar aspect of the big toe, where it is joined by the medial bifurcation branch of the FPMA. Poirier and Charpy clearly state that it is the FDMA and not the FPMA that provides the three inner plantar collaterals of the first and second toes. The FPMA is considered a branch of the dorsalis pedis or a terminal branch of the lateral plantar artery. It arises at the level of the inferior border of the second metatarsal from the dorsalis pedis arterial area during its vertical course in the first intermetatarsal space. It is directed medially and anteriorly, separated from the FDMA by the first dorsal interosseous muscle. It is located deep to the level of the oblique head of the adductor hallucis and the flexor hallucis brevis. Initially applied against the lateral surface of the first metatarsal,

the artery passes between the bone and the flexor hallucis brevis muscle. At the level of the distal bifurcation triangle of this muscle, the FPMA divides into two branches: lateral and medial. The lateral branch courses between the two heads of the flexor hallucis brevis and then passes plantar to the lateral head of the short flexor. It turns around the lateral sesamoid, pierces the deep lateral sagittal septum of the plantar aponeurosis for the big toe, courses on the plantar aspect of the deep transverse metatarsal ligament, and joins the FDMA at the point of bifurcation in the first web space. The medial branch of the FPMA also emerges between the two heads of the short flexors of the big toe, passes around the medial sesamoid or between the two sesamoids, and terminates in the tibial plantar hallucal artery. This medial branch is joined by a thin branch from the medial plantar artery [56].

This thorough description given by Poirier and Charpy has suffered corrections or addenda and a significant amount of variations of the FDMA has been described in reference to: (a) the origin and principal source of supply (Gilbert [57], May Jr [58]), (b) the relationship with the first dorsal interosseous muscle and to the insertion of the adductor of the big toe (Murakami [59]), and (c) the relationship with the first dorsal interosseous muscle and to the deep transverse metatarsal ligament (Gilbert [57], Leung [60]). Also, variations of the FPMA, the tibial hallucal artery, and the dorsomedial hallucal artery have been described.

As far as the venous system is concerned, dorsal and plantar veins form in the toes and freely intercommunicate in the subcutaneous tissue of the web space. These veins drain deeply into venae comitantes accompanying the FDMA and FPMA and, in addition, subcutaneously into one or more large dorsal veins leading from each web space. These join and continue proximally as a single large vein (1.5 mm in diameter) to cross over the extensor hallucis longus tendon and join the medial greater saphenous system [58].

Nerve branches of the superficial peroneal nerve over the first metatarsal space are very small and terminate in the skin at the base of the toes in most cases. The larger deep peroneal nerve accompanies the FDMA and courses beneath the extensor hallucis brevis tendon but remains superficial to the interosseus muscle and fascia. The nerve appears as two trunks, approximately 1 mm in diameter at or before the mid-metatarsal level, and each continues distally into either side of the first web adjacent to the dorsal digital artery to the region of the nail bed. The plantar digital nerves are separate structures, approximately 1.4 mm in diameter, as they course distally with the FPMA plantar to the transverse metatarsal ligament and the tendon sheath of the flexor hallucis longus. Each digital nerve remains plantar to its respective plantar digital artery as it continues distally toward the region of the tuft of the toe [58].

After seeing this, the criticism of some authors can make sense but we think that a good knowledge of the anatomy of the foot can guarantee a safe harvesting of the flap in caring and experienced hands.

Indications

This technique has two major indications: (1) the acute loss of the fingertip pad in the thumb and index finger and (2) the posttraumatic distal insensibility, with pulp atrophy, and distal neuroma, without any possibility of nerve anastomosis [47].

Operative Technique [38]

The NVI flap from the pulp of the great toe is a sensory cutaneous flap of glabrous skin. In general, it is preferable to use the homolateral foot as a donor site for the thumb and the contralateral foot for the index as this lines up better when using the ulnar digital artery of the thumb and the radial digital artery of the index as recipient arteries.

It is important to know whether the toe arterial supply is plantar or dorsal dominant, since this would condition the dissection. When the dorsal system is dominant, which occurs in 60% of cases, the dissection is simpler and a longer pedicle can be included with the flap, and a shorter incision is needed on the plantar surface of the foot. A Doppler examination will help to demonstrate the dominance.

The flap is designed as an oval with the long axis along the midaxial line of the lateral aspect of the great toe with 1–4 cm in length and 1–2.5 cm in width. The first incision should be done near the proximal end of the marked oval flap, extending proximally to find small tributaries in the subcutaneous tissue that may drain from the flap area. Once the venous tributaries are identified, then dissection can be carried out more proximally, identifying the major draining vein. When the vein has been identified, an incision continues into the web space and dissection is taken down through skin and subcutaneous tissue into the web space, identifying the lateral digital nerve to the great toe. This usually is on the plantar side of the digital artery. Once the digital nerve is identified, the artery supplying the toe will then be identified, and dissection of the artery is carried out proximally until finding communication between the dorsal and plantar systems. Care is taken at this juncture to identify either a plantar-dominant or a dorsal-dominant arterial system. If there is a dorsal-dominant system, then dissection is carried out proximally to whatever length is needed at the hand. If on the contrary, there is plantar-dominant system, which occurs in 40% of the time, the incision must be carried out more onto the plantar surface of the foot in between the first and second metatarsals, and dissect the plantar artery through this area. In this case, dissection can be difficult and tedious and this is one of the main causes of several authors' criticism to this flap.

If a long arterial pedicle is needed and dissection of the plantar digital artery is difficult, it is possible to just ligate the plantar artery and extend the arterial pedicle with a vein graft between the recipient artery and the plantar artery of the flap. Once the plantar artery, vein, and nerve are identified and dissected proximally, the rest of the incision can be carried out both dorsal and plantar around the previous markings. Dissection of the flap should be carried out through skin and subcutaneous tissue, identifying the major branches that go into the skin from the lateral digital artery supplying the flap.

Once the flap is elevated and adequate perfusion has been demonstrated, both of the flap and the toe, the artery, and then the vein can be ligated, and the digital nerve divided. The artery is then repaired preferably end to end with the digital artery of the finger; then the vein is repaired end to end to a branch of the cephalic vein of the dorsum of the thumb or index and finally the digital nerve is repaired after circulation has been established. The skin is carefully closed using nylon 4/0 nylon threads, which cause limited irritation to soft tissue [45], although we usually follow Dr. Kleinert's recommendation and close the skin with 6/0 nylon in order to improve the aesthetic outcomes of the scar (Fig. 8.7).

There have been published technical refinements of this flap based on different pedicle types in order to facilitate the harvesting and simplify the operation, making the flap more reliable. Sun et al. [61] used a communicating branch of toe web veins as a venous return pathway of the free toe pulp, that is, a pathway from the accompanying veins of the plantar digital artery (small tributaries veins) to the communicating branch between the deep and superficial toe web veins to the superficial dorsal metatarsal veins. Accompanying veins are taken as return veins of free flap and the relatively larger dorsal metatarsal vein

is taken as the one for anastomosis. Direct anastomosis of thin accompanying veins is avoided; thus, the operation is simplified.

In addition, this flap admits a significant number of modifications in order to increase its indications. For instance, second toe pulp to hand flap, first web space flap, toe wrap-around flap, second toe-wrap around flap, combined lateral aspect of great toe flap and medial aspect of second toe flap, and combined lateral great toe and web space and medial second toe flap.

The second toe pulp is the next best choice for pulp reconstruction after the great toe flap. The great toe is larger and has a higher 2PD than the second (7–18 mm over 10–25 mm) [47], hence our predilection.

The first web space flap also has many similarities with the great toe pulp neurosensory flap in both its anatomic dissection and clinical application, but is usually used for larger defects.

The other ones have different indications than the pulp repair and are used, for example, for degloving injuries distal to the metacarpophalangeal joint with skeleton and tendons intact and complete amputations at the first distal phalanx of the thumb; therefore, they will not be discussed here.

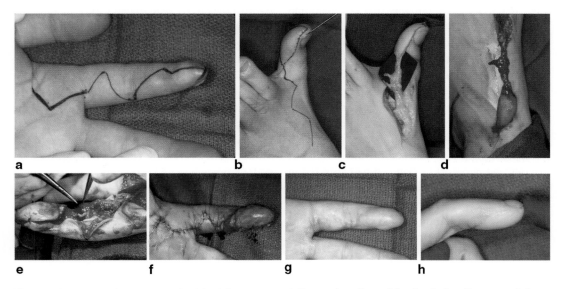

Fig. 8.7 Great toe pulp neurovascular island flap. **a** Postop painful index fingertip amputation with neuroma formation and unstable skin. **b** Design of the flap. **c** Flap's vascular pedicle. **d** Intraoperative confirmation of good inflow and outflow of the flap before ligature and elevation. **e** Neurovascular anastomosis. **f** Immediate postoperative aspect of the flap. **g, h** Excellent aesthetic and functional recovery

Second Toe Pulp Neurovascular Flap

The second toe pulp neurovascular flap is a modification of the great toe pulp flap and shares with it all the anatomical and technical characteristics, except for the flap's design which is performed as an oval with the long axis along the midaxial line of the medial aspect of the second toe.

Usually it is used for small pulp defects, specifically in fingers other than the thumb because, as mentioned before, its 2PD is lower than the great toe, although the sensation recovery is also excellent.

In 2008, Lee et al. [53] developed an alternative technique for harvesting partial second toe pulp for transfer by means of a short pedicle. This technique uses the medial digital artery of the toe and subcutaneous veins as the pedicle instead of the dorsal metatarsal artery and veins as in most of the traditional cases for anastomosis, and avoids the more extensive dorsalis pedis artery harvest, facilitating a markedly deceased operative time with a >99 % success rate.

First Web Space Flap

The first web space flap was first designed and studied by May and colleagues [58]. The first web space of the foot receives its arterial supply from the four digital arteries that arise from the first dorsal and the plantar metatarsal artery. It has a dual sensory innervation from the two dorsal digital nerves, which originate from the deep peroneal nerve, and two plantar digital nerves from the medial plantar nerve [58].

Based on this unique anatomic distribution of arteries and nerves, this flap can be harvested in diverse shapes and sizes and can been useful for larger defects and for other injuries of the fingers and the hand in addition to the pulp (first web of the hand contractures, volar defects of the hand up to 12 × 3 cm, pulp defects in two adjacent fingers). These larger injuries would be the best indication for the use of this flap.

According to this diversity of flap design and clinical application, some authors have tried to classify the first web space flap to ease the clinical decision making facing a hand injury. An interesting paper was written by Woo et al. in 1999 [62] that classified it into four types: type I: web skin flap; type II: two-island skin flap; type III: fill-up web flap; and type IV: adjuvant web flap. But, although this classification is useful for other injuries, it is not very transcendent as far as selective pulp defects are concerned. (Fig. 8.8)

The outcomes of the toe pulp neurovascular island flap published in the most up-to-date reports are excellent in both function and aesthetic terms. Currently, it is the preferred option for digital pulp reconstruction for a significant number of authors, including ourselves.

The main drawbacks of this flap are related with the donor site. It has a considerable morbidity and hypertrophic scarring, partial skin necrosis, partial loss of toe, problems with walking, and postsurgical deformities have been reported. Also, it has to be noted that it is an operation on two distant areas and, as mentioned before, a major artery is sacrificed.

Another argument of detractors is that this is a lengthy procedure to perform, is technically demanding, and supposedly not very reliable. But new studies show that, at present, its reliability is no longer an issue and is comparable to that of any other free tissue transfer [54]. In addition, using easy flaps only to achieve flap survival is an old-fashioned idea from the early days of reconstructive microsurgery. Nowadays, the emphasis must be put in optimizing function and appearance [9], and that is what toe pulp NIV flap can guarantee, although minimizing donor-site morbidity should be also considered.

It is also true that there is a learning curve and much practice is required before making it a worry-free procedure [54], but good microsurgery training can minimize risks.

Conversely, the advantages of this procedure are numerous. As mentioned, it obtains excellent functional and aesthetic results with durable and glabrous skin, almost normal pulp contour (even including fingerprint), satisfactory sensory restoration, not only protective but also critical sensory restoration (static 2PD range 4–7 mm), and no need for cortical reorientation [54].

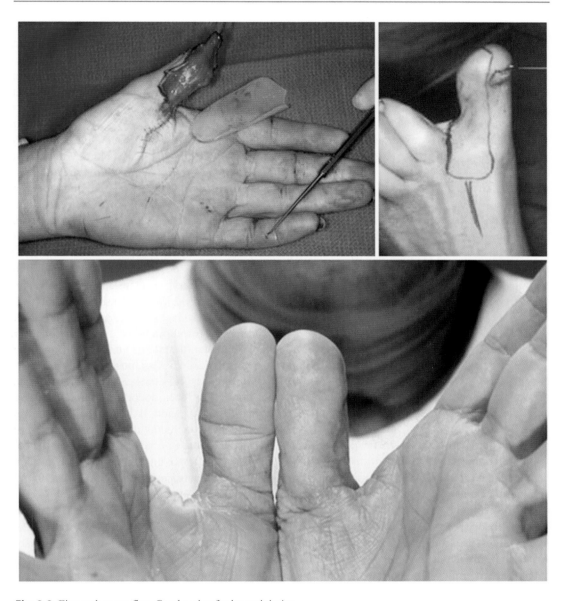

Fig. 8.8 First web space flap. Good option for larger injuries

It is interesting to mention that it has been shown that recovered sensation is more precise in the recipient site than at the donor site. Although several possible explanations exist, this phenomenon is probably best explained by cortical reeducation and adaptation with continuous, repetitive use postoperatively. Needless to say, an aggressive rehabilitative program is essential for this achievement [62]. This explanation has been supported by several investigators [47, 54, 63]

and especially Morrison et al. [64], who demonstrated that discriminative sensibility regresses to a state of mere protective sensation in the part of the body that is immobile.

Of course, as with any other procedure, the toe pulp neurovascular flap has contraindications and cannot always be used. Pulp defects shorter than 1.5 cm, concomitant injuries to the donor toe, concomitant acute infection, injury to the flap pedicle, and life-threatening associated injuries are the absolute contraindications for using this flap [45]. There are also relative contraindications if there is need for rapid recovery regardless of the aesthetic or functional result, in which case simpler treatments should be suggested. The surgeon's inexperience or facility limitations could be a contraindication, in which case the patient should be referred to other surgeons or facilities.

Conclusion

Amputation of the pulp of the fingers and thumb is a frequent injury in the hand surgeon's daily clinical practice. There is a wide diversity of treatment options from healing by secondary intention to complex reconstruction. When local flaps are inadequate, if we want to offer the best treatment option for certain injuries and demands of patients, free tissue transfer is an option.

The most popular small flaps for fingertip coverage that provide glabrous or hairless skin coverage are the thenar flap, the free flap from the flexor aspect of the wrist, AVFs, posterior auricular artery sensate flap, and glabrous skin flaps.

The thenar flap is indicated for patients who would rather not sacrifice any soft tissue component from the foot. It requires minimal dissection and sacrifices a nondominant artery, but it can cause a potentially unpleasant scar in donor area and the sensory recovery is variable.

The free flap from the flexor aspect of the wrist can be an interesting alternative to glabrous skin flaps when they are contraindicated or not available. It is a versatile flap because it can incorporate a portion of palmaris longus and/or the palmar cutaneous branch of the median nerve as grafts and can be used for different defects in hand or digits, but being an insensate flap is one of its main drawbacks.

The AVF from the thenar and hypothenar eminences is an interesting reconstructive tool, despite the fact that it is not a complete glabrous flap or a sensory flap. Also, they have an unstable postoperative course, but when conventional arterial and glabrous flaps are not available its use should be considered.

The posterior auricular artery sensate flap is used for fingertip radial-side pulp reconstruction. Although good results have been reported, the fact of having a short vascular pedicle, extremely small vena comitantes, anatomic variation, and limited flap size has avoided its widespread utilization.

The best way to accomplish replacement with glabrous tissue of the defects on the volar surface of the fingers is by microneurovascular transplantation from the foot [38]. The most proven free flaps to provide glabrous skin on a consistent vascular pedicle are the free medialis pedis flap, free MPAP flap, and great toe pulp and second toe pulp NVI flaps.

Free medialis pedis flap and free MPAP flap are interconnected and share anatomy and some properties. But the former's use, even though it can be used for small repairs, is usually discouraged for fingertip lesions since it is not a sensory flap. The latter, despite its anatomical proximity to the medialis pedis flap, possesses several positive differences: It is thicker, providing adequate cushioning surface; donor site can be closed primarily if flap width is less than 2 cm; and it can be sensate including the cutaneous branch of the medial plantar nerve or saphenous nerve for anastomosing to the digital nerve [41]. However, though it is a sensate flap, some lack of 2PD recovery must be expected [45].

Of all the free flaps utilized for digital pulp reconstruction, the free NVI toe flap provides the most efficient solution for loss of cutaneous substance [46, 47]. It not only restores the finger with a solid and well-cushioned cover but also with a dense population of specific sensory end organs attached to flap [45]. The two major indications for this flap are the acute loss of the fingertip pad in the thumb and index finger and the posttraumatic distal insensibility, with pulp atrophy, and distal neuroma, without any possibility of nerve anastomosis [47]. Its variable anatomy, the donor-site morbidity, the sacrifice of a major artery, and surgical technical demands are its main drawbacks, but the excellent results make them worth it.

In addition, the free NVI toe flap admits a significant number of modifications that can increase its indications. The second toe pulp NVI flap, the next best choice for pulp reconstruction after the great toe, is one of these modifications. It is used for small pulp defects, especially in fingers other than the thumb. Another modification is the first web space flap, which is usually indicated for larger defects than pulp.

In our opinion, although classically the free NVI toe flap has been typecast in literature as ideal and an almost exclusive indication for patients with high-demanding professions, its indications should be expanded for any patient when preserving functional and aesthetic appearance of the injured digit is the priority and the size of the defect contraindicates the use of local flaps, since in those terms this flap is shown to be unrivaled.

References

1. Lee DH, Mignemi ME, Crosby SN. Fingertip Injuries: an update on management. J Am Acad Orthop Surg. 2013;21:756–66.
2. Rosenthal EA. Treatment of fingertip and nailbed injuries. Orthop Clin North Am. 1983;14:675–97.
3. Foucher G, Boulas HJ, Braga Da Silva J. The use of flaps in the treatment of fingertip injuries. World J Surg. 1991;15(4):458–62.
4. Atasoy E, Iokimidis E, Kasden ML, Kutz JE, Kleinert HE. Reconstruction of the amputated fingertip with a triangular volar flap: A new surgical procedure. J Bone J Surg. 1979;52A(5):921–6.
5. Kutler W. A new method for fingertip amputation. JAMA. 1947;133:29–30.
6. Moberg E. Aspects of sensation in reconstructive surgery of the upper extremity. J Bone Joint Surg. 1964;46A:817.
7. Han SK, Lee BI, Kim WK. The reverse digital artery island flap: clinical experience in 120 fingers. Plast Reconstr Surg. 1998;101:1006–13.
8. Lim GJS, Yam AKT, Lee JYL, Lam-Chuan T. The spiral flap for fingertip resurfacing: short-term and long-term results. J Hand Surg. 2008;33A:340–7.
9. Lawson R, Levin LS. Principles of free tissue transfer in orthopaedic practice. J Am Orthop Surg. 2007;15:290–9.
10. Levin LS. Principles of definitive soft tissue coverage with flaps. J Orthop Trauma. 2008;22:S161–6.
11. Foucher G, Braun JB. A new island flap transfer from the dorsum of the index to the thumb. Plast Reconstr Surg. 1979;63:344–9.
12. Venkataswami R, Subramanian N. Oblique triangular flap: A new method of repair for oblique amputations of the fingertip and thumb. Plast Reconstr Surg. 1980;66:296–300.
13. Sokol AB, Berggren RB. Finger tip amputations. Review of procedures and applications. Calif Med. 1973;119:22–8.
14. De Lorenzi F van der Hulst RR den Dunnen WF Vranckx JJ Van- denhof B Francois C Boeckx WD. Arterialized venous free flaps for soft-tissue reconstruction of digits: a 40-case series. J Reconstr Microsurg. 2002;18:569–74; discussion 575–567.
15. Huang SH, Wu SH, Lai CH, Chang CH, Wangchen H, Lai CS, Lin SD, Chang KP. Free medial plantar artery perforator flap for finger pulp reconstruction: report of a series of 10 cases. Microsurgery. 2010;30:118–24.
16. Tsai TM, Sabapathy SR, Martin D. Revascularization of a finger with a thenar mini-free flap. J Hand Surg Am. 1991;16:604–6.
17. Omokawa S, Ryu J, Tang JB, et al. Vascular and neural anatomy of the thenar area of the hand: its surgical applications. Plast Reconstr Surg. 1997;99:116–21.
18. Kamei K, Ide Y, Kimura T. A new free thenar flap. Plast Reconstr Surg. 1993;92:1380–4.
19. Sassu P, Lin CH, Lin YT, Lin CH. Fourteen cases of free thenar flap. A rare indication in digital reconstruction. Ann Plast Surg. 2008;60:260–6.
20. Barbato BD, Guelmi K, Romano SJ, et al. Thenar flap rehabilitated: a review of 20 cases. Ann Plast Surg. 1996;37:135–9.
21. Sakai S. Free Flap from the flexor aspect of the wrist for resurfaciong defects of the hand and fingers. Plast Reconstr Surg. 2003;111(4):1412–20.
22. Ishikura N, Helshiki T, Tsukada S. The use of a free medialis pedis flap for resurfacing skin defects of the hand and digits: results in five cases. Plast. Reconstr. Surg. 1995;95(1):100–7.
23. Yan H, Brooks D, Ladner R, Jackson WD, Gao W, Angel MF. Arterialized venous flaps: a review of the literature. Microsurgery 2010;30(6): 472–478.
24. Yan H, Zhang F, Akdemir O, Songcharoen S, Jones NI, Angel M, Brook D. Clinical applications of venous flaps in the reconstruction of hands and fingers. Arch Orthop Trauma Surg. 2011;131(1):65–74.
25. Thatte MR, Thatte RL. Venous flaps. Plast Reconstr Surg. 1993;91:747–51.
26. Woo SH, Kim KC, Lee GJ, Ha SH, Kim KH, Dhawan V, Lee KS. A retrospective analysis of 154 arterialized venous flaps for hand reconstruction: an 11-year experience. Plast Reconstr Surg. 2007;119(6):1823–38.
27. Inoue G, Maeda N. Arterialized venous flap coverage for skin defects of the hand or foot. J Reconstr Microsurg. 1988;4:259–66.
28. Iwasawa M, Ohtsuka Y, Kushima H, Kiyono M. Arterialized venous flaps from the thenar and hypothenar regions for repairing finger pulp tissue losses. Plast Reconstr Surg. 1997;99:1765–70.
29. Kakinoki R, Ikeguchi R, Nankaku M, Nakamua T. Factors affecting the success of arterialised venous flaps in the hand. Injury. 2008;39(Suppl 4):18–24.
30. Takeuchi M, Sakurai H, Sasaki K, Nozaki M. Treatment of finger avulsion injuries with innervated arterialized venous flaps. Plast Reconstr Surg. 2000;106(4):881–5.

31. Nakazawa H, Nozaki M, Sasaki K, Sakurai H. Utility of arterialized venous flap for the reconstruction of soft tissue defects of the finger tip. Jpn J Plast Reconstr Surg. 1999;41:1011.

32. Wada M, Fujino T, Terashima T. Anatomic description of the free retroauricular flap. J Microsurg. 1979;1:108–13.

33. Hsieh JH, Wu YC, Chen HC, YB Chen. Posterior auricular artery sensate flap for finger pulp reconstruction. J Trauma. 2009;67(2):E48–50.

34. Kobayashi S, Nagase T, Ohmori K. Color Doppler flow imaging of postauricular arteries and veins. Br J Plast Surg. 1997;50:172–5.

35. Costa H, Pinto A, Zenha H. The posterior interosseous flap, a prime technique in hand reconstruction. The experience of 100 anatomical dissections and 102 clinical cases. J Plast Reconstr Aesthet Surg. 2007;60:740–7.

36. Hirase Y, Kojima T, Bang HH. Secondary reconstruction by temporoparietal free fascial flap for ring avulsión injury. Ann Plast Surg. 1990;25:312.

37. Halbert CF, Wei FC. Neurosensory free flaps. Hand Clinics. 1997;13(2):251–62.

38. Buncke GM, Buntic RF. Glabrous skin flaps. In: Wei FC and, Mardini S, editors. Flaps and reconstructive surgery. Taipei: Elsevier Inc.; 2009. p. 457–472.

39. Masquelet AC, Romana MC. The medialis pedis flap: a new fascio- cutaneous flap. Plast Reconstr Surg. 1990;85:765–72.

40. Huang SH, Wu SH, Lai CH, Chang CH, Wangchen H, Lai CH, Lin SD, Chang KP. Free medial plantar artery perforator flap for finger pulp reconstruction: report of a series of 10 cases. Microsurgery. 2010;30:118–24.

41. Lee HB, Tark KC, Rah DK, Shin KS. Pulp Reconstruction of fingers with very small sensate medial plantar free flap. Plast Reconstr Surg. 1998;101(4):999–1005.

42. Hidalgo DA, Shaw WW. Anatomic basis of plantar flap design. Plast Reconstr Surg. 1986;78:627.

43. Mir y Mir L. Functional graft of the heel. Br J Plast Surg. 1954;14:444.

44. Inoue T, Kobayashi M, Harashina T. Finger pulp reconstruction with a free sensory medial plantar flap. Br J Plast Surg. 1988;41:657.

45. Gu JX, Pan JB, Liu HJ, Zhang NC, Tian H, Zhang WZ, Xu Tao, Feng SH, Wang JC. Aesthetic and sensory reconstruction of finger pulp defects using free toe flaps. Aesth Plast Surg. 2014;38:156–63.

46. Buncke HJ, Rose EH. Free toe-to-fingertip neurovascular flaps. Plast Reconstr Surg. 1979;63(5):607–12.

47. Foucher G, Merle M, Maneaud M, Michon J. Microsurgical free partial toe transfer in hand reconstruction: a report of 12 cases. Plast Reconstr Surg. 1980;65(5):616–27.

48. Gillies H, Millard DR. The principles and art of plastic surgery. Boston: Little, Brown; 1957.

49. Southwood WFW. The thickness of the skin. Plast Reconstr Surg. 1955;15:423.

50. Barron JN. The structure and function of the skin of the hand. Hand. 1970;2:93.

51. Wei FC, Carver N, Lee YH, Chuang DCC, Chen SL. Sensory recovery and Meissner corpuscle number after toe-to-hand transplantation. Plast Reconstr Surg. 2000;105:2405.

52. Littler JW. Neurovascular pedicle transfer of tissue in reconstructive surgery of the hand. J Bone Joint Surg. 1956;38A:917.

53. Lee DC, Kim JS, Ki SH, Roh SY, Yang JW, Chung KC. Partial second toe pulp free flap for fingertip reconstruction. Plast Reconst Surg. 2008;121(3):899–907.

54. Yan H, Ouyang Y, Chi Z, Gao W, Zhang F, Fan C. Digital pulp reconstruction with free neurovascular toe flaps. Aesth Plast Surg. 2012;36:1186–93.

55. Poirier P, Charpy A. Traité d'anatomie humaine. Paris: Masson; 1899.

56. Sarrafian SK, Kelikian AS. Angiology. In: Kelikian AS, Sarrafian SK, editors. Sarrafian's anatomy of the foot and ankle: descriptive, topographic, functional (3rd ed). Philadelphia: Lippincott Williams & Wilkins. 2011;302–380.

57. Gilbert A. In Tubiana R, ed. Chirugie de la main. Paris; Masson et Cie; 1976.

58. May JW Jr, Chait LA, Cohen BE, ÓBrien BMcC. Free neurovascular flap from the first web of the foot in hand reconstruction. J Hand Surg. 1977;2(5):387–93.

59. Murakami T. On the position and course of the deep plantar arteries, with a special reference to the so-called plantar metatarsal arteries. Okajimas Folia Anat Jpn. 1971;48:295.

60. Leung PC, Wong WL. The vessels of the first metatarsal web space. J Bone Joint Surg Am. 1983;65(2):235.

61. Sun W, Wang Z, Qiu S, Li S, Guan S, Hu Y, Zhu L. Communicating branch of toe web veins as a venous return pathway in free toe pulp flaps. Plast Reconstr Surg. 2010;126(5):268e–9e.

62. Woo SH, Choi BC, Oh SJ, Seul JH. Classification of the first web space free flap of the foot and its applications in reconstruction of the hand. Plast Reconst Surg. 1999;103:508.

63. Deglise B, Botta Y. Microsurgical free toe pulp transfer for digital reconstruction. An Plast Surg. 1991;266(4):341–6.

64. Morrison WA, ÓBrien B, Hamilton RB. Neurovascular free foot flaps in reconstruction of the mutilated hand. Clin Plast Surg. 1978;5(2):265–72.

Fingertip Burns

9

Kevin J. Malone, Roderick B. Jordan and Bram Kaufman

Thermal Injury

Much is written regarding management of thermal burns to the hand. Significant attention has been given to the evaluation, classification, and treatment of dorsal hand burns due to the issues related to the thin dorsal skin and the vulnerability of the extensor tendons and bones once the dorsal skin has been compromised. Little to no attention has been given to thermal burns of the fingertips. Hand burns are common because of the role that the hand plays with regard to our interaction to the surrounding environment. With that in mind, it makes sense that the fingertips are often involved in thermal burns because of their use as sensory appendages. However, finger and hand burns are often given low priority in the setting of a burn to a large percentage of the body surface. Management of hand burns may have a low impact on patient survival in this situation but can have a huge impact on long-term

outcomes and the patient's ability to regain functional independence [1, 2].

Thermal burns are graded based on the depth of the injury. This classification can give some prognostic information and help direct treatment. First-degree burns involve the superficial dermal layers. The skin is often erythematous and hyperesthetic. These burns respond well to conservative treatment with wound care and are expected to heal within 2–3 weeks from injury. Second-degree burns involve deeper layers and are further divided into superficial and deep. In the superficial group, the skin will often develop blisters but remain erythematous and hyperaesthetic. This group of injuries also responds well to local wound care. The deep group presents with skin blistering and a white/pale skin surface. The skin is typically hypoaesthetic. Some of these burns may require debridement and possibly skin grafting for healing. Third-degree burns are full thickness. The skin is hard, dry, and necrotic appearing. The skin is insensate. These injuries universally require surgical intervention, as they will not heal satisfactorily by secondary intention. Fourth-degree burns are full-thickness burns that also involve other tissues including bone, muscle, or tendon. This group of injuries requires more complex reconstruction if salvage is to be attempted. This level of burn in the palm or the digits may result in immediate arterial thrombosis and limb or digit salvage may not be possible [3, 4].

A majority of fingertip burns are scalding injuries from kitchen accidents. These tend to be first- or second-degree burns due to the quick

K. J. Malone (✉)
Department of Orthopaedic Surgery, MetroHealth Medical Center, Case Western Reserve University School of Medicine, 2500 MetroHealth Drive, Cleveland, OH 44109, USA
e-mail: kmalone@metrohealth.org

R. B. Jordan · B. Kaufman
Department of Surgery, Division of Plastic Surgery, MetroHealth Medical Center, 2500 MetroHealth Drive, Cleveland, OH 44109, USA
e-mail: rjordan@metrohealth.org

B. Kaufman
e-mail: bkaufman@metrohealth.org

pain/withdrawal reflex. More significant burns occur with higher-temperature objects and if the hand cannot be removed from the insulting agent due to patient impairment. Special attention should be given to children. This group of patients may be more prone to reach and touch something hot resulting in thermal injury. Additionally, the thinner dermal layer in children may predispose these patients to a higher degree of thermal injury. Finally, wound care and compliance with post-injury therapy may be more challenging in younger patients [4].

Thermal injury results in impairment of the capillary basement membrane. This leads to protein leakage into the interstitial space. The oncotic pressure gradient becomes reversed resulting in tissue edema and the development of inflammatory changes. These effects of thermal injury can be seen outside of the zone of injury. The edema occurs early, often within an hour of the injury and will peak at approximately 24 h. Due to the anatomy of the hand, the edema is often dispersed dorsally and immobilization of the burned hand can lead to more significant edema. Contamination of the injured tissue can lead to further edema development as well as inflammation and scarring that can increase the amount of tissue injury and convert a partial-thickness burn into a full-thickness burn and what begins as a skin problem can quickly affect all tissues of the hand including tendon, muscle, bone, and articular cartilage [1, 4].

Patient management begins with appropriate evaluation of the injury. This includes obtaining an accurate history regarding the source of the burn and mechanism of the injury. Assessment of the depth and the extent of the burns is critical. There are no universally accepted means to measure burn depth. This may be easier to determine on the dorsal aspect of the finger and hand than on the thicker palmar skin. Vascular integrity of the injured finger should be evaluated. This can be done by assessment of the speed of capillary refill. Third- and fourth-degree burns will not demonstrate capillary refill and will not bleed when cut. If the finger burn is part of a whole body burn, vascular shunting away from the distal extremities may make vascular evaluation of the hand and digits challenging until adequate resuscitation has occurred. Vascular integrity of the

digits is of particular importance in the setting of circumferential burns where swelling may cause external vessel compression and escharotomy may be appropriate to relieve this pressure. Sensation assessment can help determine the grade of the burn but this can be hard to assess acutely. Radiographs of the injured hand should be considered based on the etiology of injury [1, 4].

Appropriate burn treatment is far simpler than treatment of the complications of a poorly treated burn. Many isolated burns to the hand and fingers can be treated as an outpatient and the majority of these are first- and second-degree burns that can be effectively treated by nonoperative means. Principles of treatment include wound care, antibiotics, splinting to avoid intrinsic minus contracture formation if hand is involved, elevation, and range of motion to address edema formation. Wounds should be cleaned and dressed with impregnated gauze. Blisters that have ruptured should be debrided. Intact blisters should be protected unless their location and size block joint motion. In this situation, they should be ruptured and debrided. Experienced hand therapists can administer much of this treatment. First- and second-degree burns typically heal within 14 days. Third-degree burns may need later excision and grafting. Topical agents like silvadene can help debridement of nonviable tissue and bacteria. These agents are not typically necessary in the superficial burns. Deeper burns allowed to heal by secondary intention can often form hypertrophic scars and contractures that impair hand function and motion. Careful monitoring of joint motion is imperative and one should consider excision and grafting if progressive motion loss is appreciated. Intermediate-thickness non-meshed split-thickness skin grafts are typically appropriate for dorsal hand burns but may not be durable enough for replacement of the volar skin on the palm or digits [1, 2, 4].

Hand burns that are of higher degree or that are a part of a whole body burn are often treated as an inpatient. Consideration should be made to transfer these patients to a regional medical center that has a group of dedicated physicians, therapists, and nurses for burn care. As mentioned previously, hand and finger burns are often given lower priority in care when burns of the proximal extremities, chest, abdomen, back, face, and neck are present. The principles of care for the burned hand are same here as for those treated as an outpatient. The more significant hand and finger burns may also need surgical intervention. If digital vascularity is compromised early, one must consider amputation or escharotomy based on the depth, location of the burn as well as the portion of the body involved in the burn. There is some debate about the role of digital escharotomy as this may commit the patient to later skin grafting of the fingers. If escharotomy is to be performed in the digit, it is important to avoid exposure of the neurovascular bundles in an effort to avoid late desiccation of the digital nerves. Due to the thin dorsal skin and the vulnerability of the dorsal digital venous plexus, the finger may be subjected to venous congestion with moderate swelling and escharotomy in this setting can potentially result in digital salvage [1, 2, 4].

Deep or contaminated burns require debridement. This can be done surgically or enzymatically with topical agents. Early and appropriate debridement can reduce the edema and contamination that could otherwise lead to progressive tissue loss. This may also allow for earlier skin grafting. It is important to avoid application of enzymatic debridement agents to exposed tendons due to the risk of desiccation of these structures. One can consider temporary interphalangeal joint extension pinning and/or metacarpophalangeal joint pinning in the setting of full-thickness burns in the region of these joints to prevent nonfunctional contracture formation. When possible, early treatment, coverage, and initiation of motion is critical to the maintenance of the gliding surfaces within the hand and fingers. Deep burns involving the digital pulp or fingernail complex will often result in insensate deformed and painful fingertips. There are few viable reconstructive options in this situation and fingertip amputation should be considered, particularly when the burn is isolated to the fingertip [1, 2, 4, 5].

Successful treatment of finger burns is dependent on the accurate and early assessment of the burn and initiation of appropriate treatment as outlined above. Experienced hand therapists play a vital role in improving patient outcomes. Similarly, consideration should be given to trans-ferring burned patients to centers with dedicated resources to the management of these injuries.

Electrical Injury

Electrical burns may be classified as high-voltage or low-voltage electrical burns. The generally accepted distinction is that a current of more than 1000 V causes high-voltage electrical burns and a current of less than 1000 V causes low-voltage electrical burns. High-voltage electrotrauma is characterized by widespread, devastating injuries that involve the deep structures of the extremity. The electrical energy imparted to the victim is converted in the body to heat, a phenomenon known as the Joule effect, and accounts for the majority of the injury to the tissues. The extent of the burn depends not only on the size and nature of the voltage and current (direct current, DC, or alternating current, AC) but also on the length of exposure, the location of the exposure, and the resistance of the tissues. The greatest resistance is offered by the bone tissue, followed in descending order by the tendons, adipose tissue, skin (depending on humidity), muscle, blood vessels, and nerve tissues. In a general sense, tissues with a greater resistance will suffer more injury [6]. In addition, cross-sectional area is indirectly related to the tissue damage such that the smaller the cross-sectional area across which current travels, the greater the injury. Joints, in particular, have a small cross-sectional area and a high proportion of high-resistance bone [7].

Clinically, high-tension electrical injuries result in cutaneous injury at the entry or exit point of the current that is minor compared with massive necrosis of deeper structures. Without outward cutaneous signs of injury, the deep tissue destruction is often underestimated at initial assessment. Repeated, extensive debridements are necessary and frequently result in a nonfunctional or non-salvageable limb. Electrical burn is still a major risk factor for amputations [8]. Only after the extremity has been adequately debrided can reconstruction be contemplated. Reconstruction of high-voltage injuries most often involves, amputations, various local, regional, and distant flaps as well as microvascular reconstructions [9–12].

In contrast to high-voltage electrical burns, low-voltage injuries present with a local point of contact. Low-voltage injuries generally fall into one of three groups: electrotrauma with passage of electric current, electric arc, and secondary burns caused by flames from clothing [13].

Low-voltage injuries are less destructive of the local tissues but proportionately affect the upper extremities almost twice as often as high voltage. Low-voltage (110–220 V) 60-Hz AC current may induce ventricular fibrillation more frequently than high-voltage injuries. Low-voltage injuries are similar to thermal burns and have zones of injury oriented in a bull's-eye pattern with a central zone of coagulation necrosis, an indeterminate zone of stasis, and a viable outer zone of hyperemia [14]. Initial management must include careful monitoring and treatment for cardiac arrhythmias, which occurred in 41 % of 91 patients in one review. Management of low-voltage and electrical arc injuries primarily includes local wound care and reconstruction if needed, although distal fingertip and even amputations through the distal interphalangeal (DIP) joint have been reported [15].

Low-voltage burns are most often minor injuries with flash burns comprising the majority. In one study, nearly 70 % of 124 patients with low-tension injuries suffered flash burns. These often had significant tattooing but were superficial dermal burns. Of the flash burns, 58 % were treated operatively with tangential debridement and autograft while the other 42 % healed spontaneously. Typically, the injury in low-voltage burns demarcates within 48 h setting the stage for complete healing or reconstruction within 5 days of the injury [16].

Surgical reconstruction of the fingertip for electrical burns includes local skin grafts (full or split thickness), local flaps (volar V–Y, bilateral V–Y), regional flaps (e.g., thenar, cross finger), island flaps (reversed homodigital island flap) [17], and rarely microvascular (e.g., toe pulp or first web space flap) [18–20]. Figures 9.1, 9.2, 9.3 and 9.4 illustrate a case of staged reconstruction for electrical burns to the thumb and index finger with debridement, microvascular free tissue transfer, and ultimately thumb reconstruction with the second toe.

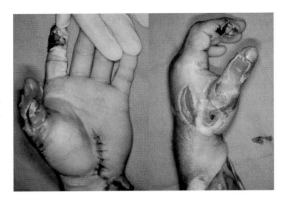

Fig. 9.1 Image of electrical burn to left hand immediately following debridement of nonviable tissue and escharotomy on the day of injury

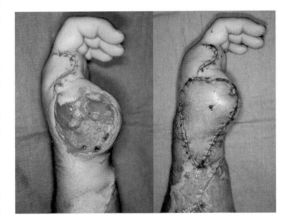

Fig. 9.2 Post injury day five following amputation of nonviable thumb and index finger with microvascular free tissue transfer for wound coverage

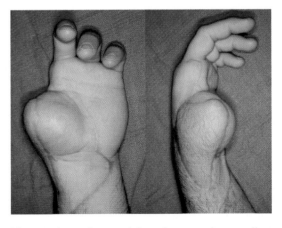

Fig. 9.3 3 months post injury demonstrating excellent wound healing

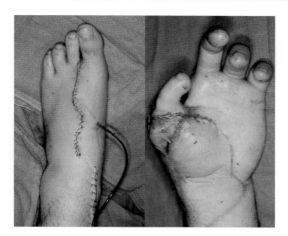

Fig. 9.4 Immediate postoperative images following transfer of second toe for thumb reconstruction

Chemical Burns

According to the *American Burn Association National Burn Repository (2013 report), chemical burns account for 3 % of admissions to burn centers* [21]. Chemicals cause from 2 to 11 % of all burns and contribute to as many as 30 % of burn-related deaths [22]. Improper handling of materials and/or use of exposure protection clothing in both the industrial workplace and residential environment are associated with these injuries. The hand and fingers are particularly at risk when proper protection is not employed. One review showed that the hands and upper extremities are the most frequently injured areas from chemical burns exceeding all other sites combined [23]. Fingertips are at no greater risk than the hand in general to chemical injury. However, as in other burns, chemical burns of the fingertips may result in a longer functional recovery due to the interference with tactile sensation and prehension.

The ability of a chemical to produce a burn injury is dependent on its concentration, amount exposed to the tissue, and the duration of contact. Chemical burns can be caused by numerous substances most of which are a strong base, a strong acid, or a halogenated hydrocarbon. Prolonged exposure to less noxious substances can also lead to a significant chemical burn. All chemicals capable of producing a burn do so by specific chemical reactions with tissue. In general, exposure to acids results in coagulation necrosis of the tissue while alkalis produce tissue liquefaction. Other chemicals are vesicants that result in necrosis from ischemia due to release of inflammatory mediators. The burn injury from exposure to a chemical continues until it is washed off, neutralized, or exhausted by the interaction with tissues [24]. For the majority of chemical burns, immediate and continuous water irrigation is the most critical initial treatment. The hands and fingers can easily be positioned under a water tap. The continuous flow of water not only dilutes the chemical but also dissipates any heat from a chemical reaction. Studies have shown that chemical burns not receiving irrigation within 10 min of exposure have a greater incidence of full-thickness injury. The only exception to water irrigation is exposure to elemental sodium, potassium, or lithium which will ignite with exposure to water [25].

Acid Burns

The appearance of an acid burn ranges from mild erythema of a superficial injury to the leathery appearance of a full-thickness skin loss. Acid burns are typically severely painful. As noted above, the most important step to mitigate injury is to begin copious irrigation of the affected part within 10 min of exposure. Additionally, a dilute solution of sodium bicarbonate may be used with the irrigation. After irrigation, the wounds are treated similarly to other burn wounds [24].

Hydrofluoric (HF) acid is an inorganic acid with multiple uses in industry. This acid is highly corrosive, injuring tissue by two different mechanisms. First, the high hydrogen ion concentration typical for all acid burns erodes the cutaneous barrier. Second, soluble free fluoride ions penetrate the damaged skin barrier causing liquefaction necrosis of the soft tissue, desiccation of the wound, and if deep enough will erode the bone. The free fluoride ion binds with intracellular calcium and magnesium producing cell death with rerelease of the fluoride ion. Death has been reported from exposure of 1 % of total body surface area to HF acid, secondary to a rapid and severe hypocalcemia. Cutaneous exposure to a dilute concentration of HF acid may have delayed onset of symptoms but will ultimately produce tissue necrosis with severe pain. A more concentrated solution may produce a painful lesion with a minimal apparent initial injury. Once a HF acid exposure is diagnosed, treatment must be initiated early. Prompt irrigation with water is the first modality. Fingernails should be trimmed to remove the possibility of acid being trapped beneath them. The next line of treatment is aimed at binding the free fluoride ions. Application of calcium gluconate burn gel is the only effective topical agent for HF acid burns. Massaging the gel into more superficial exposures will mitigate the pain of the burn as well as progression of the injury. Injection of a 10% calcium gluconate solution into the affected area is the most often used method to stop the progression of injury, mitigate pain, and prevent systemic fluoride toxicity. Small-volume injections are given using a 30-gauge needle. Pain relief is dramatic and guides both the number of injections and need for repeat treatment. Injection into pulp spaces of the fingertips should be done cautiously to avoid vascular embarrassment from pressure in a closed space. For more extensive HF acid burns of the hands, intra-arterial calcium gluconate infusion can be used. Pain relief is usually quite rapid and the infusion stops systemic effect of HF acid burns. Injections of calcium gluconate are also avoided [24, 26].

Alkali Burns

In addition to being used in industrial settings, alkali chemicals are prevalent in the residential setting, being an ingredient in drain cleaners, oven cleaners, fertilizers, and cement products. In general, alkali exposures have less immediately apparent tissue damage but ultimately result in a deeper injury. The high pH of alkalis results in saponification of tissue fats resulting in necrosis. Alkali molecules are then available to produce the damage to deeper tissues. The pH change in tissue associated with an alkali injury is more dramatic and prolonged than seen with acid burns and requires longer irrigation (an hour or more) to mitigate injury.

Cement burns are common, particularly in individuals not familiar with the caustic quality of wet cement. "Do-it-yourselfers" are more prone to handle wet cement without appropriate skin protection, particularly impermeable gloves. Wet cement has a pH greater than 12 and is capable of producing a full-thickness alkali burn. Symptoms may not appear for several hours after exposure. Erythema, pain, and a burning sensation ultimately appear. Prolonged irrigation is the early treatment modality. Mild exposures will lead to superficial desquamation (particularly glabrous skin) followed by a period of skin hypersensitivity until normal epidermal thickness is achieved. More severe exposures can result in full-thickness skin loss [24, 27].

Gasoline/Hydrocarbons

Gasoline, hydrocarbons, and solvents primarily irritate skin but prolonged exposure may result in a cutaneous burn. Treatment is removal of the compound from skin contact and prolonged irrigation. Topical treatment of the resultant cutaneous injury is similar to that of thermal injuries [25].

Phosphorus Burns

While more commonly associated with injury from munitions explosion exposure in military personnel, white phosphorus burns can occur in the civilian sector from exposure to fireworks, insecticides, and fertilizers. Phosphorus ignites with exposure to air and is controlled by wetting. However, re-drying results in the exothermic oxidation of the phosphorus. Until definitive treatment can be delivered, the affected area should be covered with mineral oil to prevent exposure to air. Treatment requires both irrigation of the affected skin and removal of the phosphorus particles. The latter is facilitated by the use of a Wood's lamp. Alternatively, the affected area may be washed with a 1% copper sulfate solution that results in black cupric phosphate particles that are more visible. The copper sulfate solution must be washed off to prevent copper toxicity [25].

Cold Injuries

Much of our knowledge of and appreciation for cold injuries is from military experiences in harsh weather environments dating back to the Spartan times and through World War II. Now, these injuries are more frequently seen in nonmilitary populations, specifically those without resources or mental capacity to seek refuge in cold temperatures. Intoxication also plays an important role in cold injuries as the body's shivering response to keep warm may be blunted and cutaneous vasodilation may result in cold injuries at relatively warmer temperatures. In response to the cold exposure, the body directs blood away from the skin and away from the extremities. This leaves the skin and subcutaneous tissues, particularly of the distal extremities, vulnerable to freezing. Any other factors or conditions that reduce circulation, including cigarette smoking and peripheral vascular disease can increase the effects of cold injury. Hand and feet injuries account for 90 % of the reported episodes of frostbite [28–30].

The presence of wind can accelerate the effect of cold weather. An increase in wind speed from 10 to 20 mph at 0 °F can reduce the time of freeze injuries in exposed skin from 60 to 30 min. A windchill temperature of −40 °F can lead to a freeze injury of exposed skin in minutes. The extent of the injury is more closely related to the duration of cold exposure, rather than the temperature itself. Cold injuries exist within a spectrum of severity based on the rate of cooling and the presence of ice crystals in the tissues. Frostbite is the result of slow rate of cooling which leads to the formation of ice crystals. These are potentially reversible injuries [31].

There are two potential phases of cellular death in frostbite injuries. The first occurs during the freezing when ice crystals change the osmotic gradient in the tissues resulting in water being drawn out of the cells. This alters the cell's stability and function. Additionally, capillary blood flow is diminished as the blood viscosity increases and this results in hypoperfusion and hypoxia. Fortunately, the diminished metabolic activity of the tissue in response to the cold temperature may have some protective function for the cells such that the cells may survive the freezing phase. However, when the freezing occurs rapidly intracellular and extracellular ice crystals can cause immediate cell lysis and death. The second phase of the injury occurs during the tissue rewarming. Once the person has been removed from the cold environment, vasospasm lessens and limb perfusion increases. However, the effects of the cold exposure have damaged the microcirculation vasculature and intravascular thrombosis can occur. Prostaglandin and thromboxane are released during this course of freezing and thawing can potentiate vasoconstriction, platelet aggregation, and thrombosis. This process can result in further tissue ischemia in an apparently well-perfused limb with good pulses. Rapid rewarming can lessen this phase of the injury. As tissue reperfusion progresses, blisters form in the skin. Hemorrhagic blisters suggest significant injury to the dermal arterial supply and carry a poor prognosis. Additionally, skin that does not show blistering after rewarming suggests poor blood flow and also carries a poor prognosis. It is important to be aware that as the vasospasm to the cold limb is diminished during the rewarming phase, cold venous blood from the extremities is returned to the chest and can lower the body's core temperature [3, 32].

Clinically frostbite injuries are graded in terms of severity. First-degree frostbite is a superficial injury that is manifested by hyperemia and no blister formation on rewarming. Sensation is generally preserved and tissue loss is unlikely. Second-degree frostbite injury is a more severe superficial injury. Nonhemorrhagic blistering occurs with potentially significant swelling. Wound care to the ruptured blisters can prevent infection and tissue loss. Third-degree frostbite involves some of the deeper tissues. Hemorrhagic blisters can occur in the deeper dermal layers. The skin is initially insensate but can progress to long-term paresthesias and neuropathic pain. Fourth-degree frostbite involves deeper tissue like bone and muscle. There is no reperfusion of the damaged tissue during rewarming. The involved digits will mummify and require amputation. Classification of these injuries may not be possible acutely. An involved extremity or digit may have multiple degrees of frostbite simultaneously with higher degrees of severity present more distally [3, 32].

Treatment of patients with frostbite injuries includes rapid rewarming in water baths of 104–108 °F. This process can be quite painful and narcotic medications are often necessary. Affected body parts can develop significant edema. Splinting, elevation, and range-of-motion exercises can be effective in reducing the swelling. Patients should receive tetanus prophylaxis if they have not received a booster within 5 years. Nonsteroidal anti-inflammatory medications can augment pain relief and also help with wound healing by diminishing prostaglandin synthesis and the potentially cytotoxic inflammatory response to rewarming, and by preventing the microvascular thrombosis from occurring. Topical aloe vera applied to the wounds has also been shown to improve healing. There is debate regarding the role of blister debridement or blister aspiration to remove the high concentrations of toxic metabolites that have been found in blister fluid that have been shown to potentiate an inflammatory response and dermal ischemia. There is some evidence that administration of tissue plasminogen activator (tPA) during the rewarming phase can reduce the incidence of amputation. Bruen et al. demonstrated that patients with abnormal digital perfusion as seen on digital angiography experienced a reduction in the incidence of digital amputation from 41 to 10 % when tPA was administered following frostbite injury [32, 33].

Hyperbaric oxygen (HBO) therapy for the treatment of frostbite injuries has been reported in several cases, dating back to 1963, with good anecdotal results. HBO increases local tissue oxygen tension and can increase the revascularization and viability of damaged tissue. Favorable results have been reported even when initiating this treatment 2 weeks or more after injury. It has been proposed to initiate this treatment early, during the rewarming phase, to minimize the reperfusion component of the injury. Currently, HBO treatment for frostbite injuries is considered investigational in the USA [34].

Surgical intervention is indicated when clinical infection has been identified for wound debridement. Also, in the deep frostbite injuries amputation will often be required but the timing of amputation is based on demarcation of the area of necrosis and can take up to several weeks post

injury before this has been established. Technetium-99m (^{99m}Tc) scintigraphy has been proven to be a reliable diagnostic tool in determining prognosis following frostbite injury as well as the level of amputation that can expedite this process. Cauchy et al. demonstrated that ^{99m}Tc-bone scan can be used to establish the likelihood (positive predictive value, 0.84) of amputation at approximately day three following injury [35]. This information is valuable in patient education as well as in expediting appropriate care and possibly hospital discharge. When amputations are to be performed, it is recommended to amputate proximal enough for primary tension free wound closure. Skin grafts are not recommended in the digits as they are prone to cold intolerance and have limited sensibility. Sympathectomy has shown some ability to lessen future cold intolerance issues but appears to have minimal impact on recovering from a frostbite injury [32].

Patients with frostbite injuries typically are left with long-term sequelae including cold intolerance, pain, abnormal sensation, and skin color changes. Deeper structures like articular and physeal cartilage can also be affected which can promote the development of osteoarthritis and growth arrest which are dependent on the age of the patient and the severity of the injury [36].

Complications Following Finger Burns

Secondary Nail Deformities

Fingernail deformities after burn injury to the hand are common. Burns that do not result in loss of nail matrix can still result in a distortion of the nail plate. A normal nail is the product of an uninjured germinal matrix, dorsal nail matrix (dorsal roof of the nail fold), and sterile matrix. A burn injury may alter any combination of these components and result in a deformed fingernail, but a common problem is proximal scar retraction of the nail fold. In normal nail growth, the dorsal nail matrix produces the dorsal nail lamina that results in a smooth and shiny nail appearance. When the nail fold is everted, the dorsal nail lamina is lost. The resultant nail is dull, rough, grooved, and appears elongated. Pain/tenderness may occur due to the exposure of the dorsal nail matrix. In more severe deformities, the distal nail may be thin and unstable hindering fingertip fine manipulation.

The key concept is that in many cases the structure of the nail fold is not lost but only displaced by proximal scar "unfurling" the fold. Release of the scar and restoration of the dorsal nail matrix to the roof of the nail fold will improve the appearance and function of the nail. Various procedures have been described to allow correction of the nail fold. Achauer and Welk published a one-stage reconstruction utilizing bilateral triangular proximally based skin flaps harvested from the lateral finger pulp. The flaps are inset into the transverse dorsal incision that is made 2–3 mm proximal to the distal margin of the eponychium. The donor sites are primarily closed with no narrowing of the tip pulp reported. Skin grafts are not needed. The authors reported uniform improvement in the nails with no complications or recurrence of the deformity [37]. Donelan and Garcia reported good results with the use of a distally based bipedicled skin flap with full-thickness skin grafting of the resultant donor defect. Improvement in the nail appearance and function was reported with no instances of flap loss [38]. Figures 9.5, 9.6 and 9.7 illustrate a case in which the nail plate and nail bed were damaged from a thermal injury requiring soft tissue coverage of the exposed phalanx with a homodigital island flap.

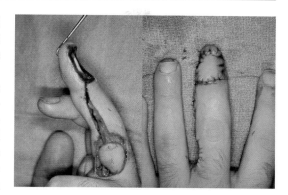

Fig. 9.6 Soft tissue coverage with the use of a homodigital island flap

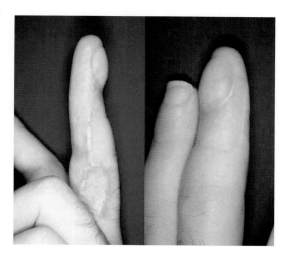

Fig. 9.7 Final clinical results

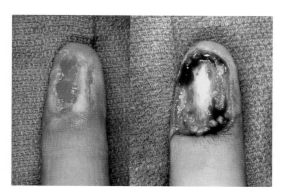

Fig. 9.5 Nail bed damage following thermal injury with exposed phalanx after initial debridement

Mallet Deformity

The mallet deformity is a loss of continuity of the conjoined lateral bands as they approach the distal phalanx. The disruption of the extensor apparatus at this location is most often due to a sudden forceful flexion applied to the extended digit. The deformity can be classified into four types, loosely based on the anatomic perturbation and mechanism of injury [39]. Type I is the result of a closed or blunt trauma with loss of extensor tendon continuity only. Type II involves a laceration over the dorsum of the DIP, which divides the tendon. Type III is a deep abrasion with loss of skin, subcutaneous cover, and tendon. Type IV injuries result from an intra-articular fracture of the dorsal distal phalanx upon which the extensor tendon inserts.

The burned fingertip that results in a mallet deformity almost always approximates the type III injuries, unless the mechanism of injury involves a concomitant trauma. The significance of this distinction is that the management of type III mallet injuries is significantly more complicated than that of the other types. The injury in these patients with burns involves the obvious injury to the skin, but also some degree of extensor tendon loss and often an open DIP joint. Once discontinuity of the distal extensor tendon occurs, the entire extensor apparatus becomes unbalanced and shifts proximally, ultimately placing greater than normal extension force on the proximal interphalangeal (PIP). This can result in a delayed swan neck deformity.

The techniques available for repair of type I, II, and IV mallet deformities assume a stable and pliable soft tissue envelop. In the case of type III mallet finger from burns, this is rarely the case where the skin and tendon have likely been lost to the burn. Usually, such an extensive burn is not isolated to one or even a few digits and more extensive burns and injures take precedence in treatment priorities. By the time the mallet deformity presents for definitive treatment the open joint has either ankylosed or become infected leading to a therapeutic amputation.

In the rare case of a delayed mallet finger presentation in the setting of a burn, there are few options. The lack of resilient skin on the dorsum of the digit through which one can address the underlying cause of the mallet most often leads to a nonoperative treatment and expectant management with prolonged splinting in extension. One alternative to nonoperative treatment is arthrodesis of the DIP joint, but this approach also requires a stable soft tissue envelope. Thus, if the hand surgeon is to attempt salvage of an impending open DIP joint or proceed with joint fusion, some soft tissue coverage procedure is necessary.

The reconstructive options for the dorsal aspect of the burned DIP are confined to skin flaps. Skin grafts alone will not provide the stability necessary for underlying tendon or joint reconstruction. Regional flaps such as cross-finger flaps, thenar flaps, and hypothenar flaps are good options for skin coverage. More elegant reconstructions include the homodigital or heterodigital island flaps, which can provide excellent coverage with the advantage of maintaining a perfused flap and the benefits of a more robust blood supply [40]. If there has been loss of extensor tendon proper then any of these options still require additional intervention to address the extensor tendon proper.

Kostopoulos et al. studied the arterial blood supply of the extensor apparatus and found that the supply was segmental through the paratenon and through a common trunk originating from the proper digital artery. The network nourished not only the extensor apparatus but also the dorsal digital skin and periosteum [41]. This arterial anatomy is the basis of a unique and elegant approach in the reversed homodigital island flap that incorporates extensor tendon into the flap, which can be used to repair the tendon defect [42]. Also, the dorsal metacarpal artery flap, distally based with incorporation of the extensor indicis proprius has been described to reconstruct dorsal digital defects of the index finger over the PIP and DIP joints [43].

The limiting factor with all of these options is that often the burn is extensive and has injured many or all of the potential flap donor sites. In addition, burns of sufficient severity to obliterate the extensor apparatus over the DIP are rarely due to local trauma and much more extensive, and even life threatening, burns take precedence in terms of treatment and rehabilitation. As such, often the burn mallet deformity is left untreated.

References

1. Luce EA. The acute and subacute management of the burned hand. Clin Plast Surg. 2000;27(1):49–63.
2. Barillo DJ, Harvey KD, Hobbs CdL, Mozingo DW, Cioffi WG, Pruitt BA Jr. Prospective outcome analysis of a protocol for the surgical and rehabilitative management of burns to the hands. Plast Reconstr Surg. 1997;100:1442–51.
3. Smith P. Injury. In: Smith P, editor. Lister's the Hand diagnosis and indications. Philadelphia: Elsevier; 2002. p. 1–140.
4. Salisbury RE. Acute care of the burned hand. In: McCarthy JG, May JW, Littler JW, editors. Plastic surgery. Philadelphia: Saunders; 1990. p. 5399–417.
5. Boswick JA. Rehabilitation of the burned hand. Clin Orthop. 1974;104:162–74.

6. Kaloudová Y, Sín R, Rihová H, Brychta R, Suchánek I, Martincová A. High voltage electrical injuries. Actga Chir Plast 2006;48(4):119–22.

7. Garcia-Sanchez V, Morell PG. Electric burns: high- and low-tension injuries. Burns. 1999;25:357–60.

8. Tarim A, Ezer A. Electrical burn is still a major risk factor for amputations. Burns. 2013;39(2):354–7.

9. Foucher G, Nagel D, Briand E. Microvascular great toenail transfer after conventional thumb reconstruction. Plast Reconstr Surg. 1999;103(2):570–6.

10. Lin PY, Sebastin SJ, Ono S, Bellfi LT, Chang KW, Chung KC. A systematic review of outcomes of toe-to-thumb transfers for isolated traumatic. Hand. 2011;6(3):235–43.

11. Raveendran SS, Syed M, Shibu M. Toe-to-hand transfer in a severely burned upper limb: a surgical dilemma. J Plast Reconstr Aesthet Surg. 2009;62(11):e463–5.

12. Zhang J, Xie Z, Lei Y, Song J, Guo Q, Xiao J. Free second toe one-stage-plasty and transfer for thumb or finger reconstruction. Microsurgery. 2008;28(1):25–31.

13. Lipový B, Rihová H, Kaloudová Y, Suchánek I, Gregorová N, Hokynková A. The Importance of a multidisciplinary approach in the treatment of mutilating electrical injury: a case study. Acta Chir Plast. 2010;52(2):61–64.

14. Jackson DM. The diagnosis of the depth of burning. Br J Surg. 1953;40(16):588–96.

15. Hussmann J, Kucan JO, Russell RC, Bradley T, Zamboni WA. Electrical injuries- morbidity, outcome and treatment rationale. Burns. 1995;21(7):530–5.

16. Laberge LC, Ballard PA, Daniel RK. Experimental electrical burns: low voltage. Ann Plast Surg. 1984;13:185–90.

17. Foucher G, Smith D, Pempinello C, Braun FM, Citron N. Homodigital neurovascular island flaps for digital pulp loss. J Hand Surg, Br. 1989;12(2):204–8.

18. Kim HD, Hwang SM, Lim KR, Jung YH, Ahn SM, Song JK. Toe transfer for reconstruction of damaged digits due to electrical burns. Arch Plast Surg. 2012;39:138–42.

19. Deglise B, Botta Y. Microsurgical free toe pulp transfer for digital reconstruction. Ann Plast Surg. 1991;26(4):341–6.

20. Foucher G, Nagle DJ. Microsurgical reconstruction of fingers and fingertips. Hand Clin. 1999;15(4):597–606.

21. American Burn Association, National Burn Repository® 2013. Version 9.0. http://www.ameriburn.org/2013NBRAnnualReport.pdf.

22. Hardwicke J, Hunter T, Staruch R, Moiemen N. Chemical burns-an historical comparison and review of the literature. Burns. 2012;38(3):383–7.

23. Curreri PW, Asch MJ, Pruitt BA. The treatment of chemical burns: specialized diagnostic, therapeutic and prognostic considerations. J Trauma. 1970;10(8):634–42.

24. Murray JF. Cold, chemical, and irradiation injuries. In: McCarthy JG, May JW, Littler JW, editors. Plastic surgery. Philadelphia: Saunders; 1990. p. 5436–7.

25. Chick LR, Lister GD. Emergency management of thermal, electrical, and chemical burns. In: Kasdan ML, editor. Occupational hand and upper extremity injuries and diseases. Philadelphia: Hanley and Belfus; 1991. p. 265–9.

26. Dibbell DG, Iverson RE, Jones W, Laub DR, Madison MS. Hydrofluoric acid burns of the hand. J Bone Joint Surg. 1970;52(5):931–6.

27. Wilson GR, Davidson PM. Full-thickness burns from ready-mix cement. Burns Incl Therm Inj. 1985;12(2):139–45.

28. Bracker MD. Environmental and thermal injury. Clin Sports Med. 1992;11(2):419–36.

29. Christenson C, Stewart C. Frostbite. Am Fam Physician. 1984;30(6):111–22.

30. Murphy JV, Banwell PE, Roberts AH, McGrouther DA. Frostbite: pathogenesis and treatment. J Trauma. 2000;48(1):171–89.

31. McCauley RL, Heggers JP, Robson MC. Frostbite: methods to minimize tissue loss. Postgrad Med. 1990;88(8):67–77.

32. Mohr WJ, Jenabzadeh K, Ahrenholz DH. Cold injury. Hand Clin. 2009;25:481–96.

33. Bruen KJ, Ballard JR, Morris SE, Cochran A, Edelman LS, Saffle JR. Reduction of the incidence of amputation in frostbite injury with thrombolytic therapy. Arch Surg. 2007;142:546–53.

34. McCrary BF, Hursh TA. Hyperbaric oxygen therapy for a delayed frostbite injury. Wounds. 2005;17(12):321–31.

35. Cauchy E, Marsigny B, Allamel G, et al. The value of technetium 99 scinitgraphy in the prognosis of amputation in severe frostbite injuries of the extremities: a retrospective study of 92 severe frostbite injuries. J Hand Surg. 2000;25A:969–78.

36. Nakazato T, Ogino T. Epiphyseal destruction of children's hands after frostbite: a report of two cases. J Hand Surg (Am). 1986;11(2):289–92.

37. Donelan MB, Garcia JA. Nailfold reconstruction for correction of burn fingernail deformity. Plast Reconstr Surg. 2006;117:2303–8.

38. Achauer BM, Wel RA. One-stage reconstruction of the postburn nailfold contracture. Plast Reconstr Surg. 1990;85(6):937–40.

39. Doyle JR. Extensor tendons - acute injuries. In: Green DP, Hotchkiss RN editors. Operative Hand Surgery, 3rd edition. New York: Churchill Livingstone. 1993. p 1934.

40. Schuind F, Van Genechten F, Denuit P, Merle M, Foucher G. Homodigital neurovascular island flaps in hand surgery. A study of sixty cases. Ann Chir Main. 1985;4(4):306–15.

41. Kostopoulos E, Casoli V, Verolino P, Papadopoulos O. Arterial blood supply of the extensor apparatus of the long fingers. Plast Reconstr Surg. 2006;117:2310–8.

42. Rahmanian-Schwarz A, Schiefer J, Amr A, Schaller HE, Hirt B. Vascularized tendon incorporated in reverse homodigital and heterodigital island flaps for the reconstruction of dorsal digital defects. Microsurgery. 2012;32:178–82.

43. Schiefer JL, Schaller HE, Rahmanian-Schwarz A. Dorsal metacarpal artery flaps with extensor indices tendons for reconstruction of digital defects. J Investig Surg. 2012;25:340–3.

Pediatric Fingertip Injuries

10

Matthew E. Koepplinger

Introduction

Fingertip injuries in children occur from a variety of mechanisms. These commonly involve the fingertip becoming entrapped under the weight and force of a closing door. Other mechanisms may involve the fingertip being injured in machinery or along sharp edges from prying, inquisitive exploration. Still other less common mechanisms involve overuse from excessive video game controller usage. The severity of these injuries ranges from simple soft tissue involvement that may be managed conservatively, or with simple wound closure management, to more complex injuries that include loss of soft tissue, open fracture injuries that may involve growth plate disruption, or nail bed injury that should be managed surgically.

The difficulty underlying these injuries stems from the complexity of the anatomy of the fingertip and the involvement of injury to many important structures that, if not managed properly, may result in compromised growth and development of the digit, complicated infectious processes, compromised function of the digit, and undue worry and distress on the part of the surgeon, parent, and patient alike. Little consensus exists on the most appropriate methods of management of these complex injuries. Many surgeons are

uncomfortable managing these injuries due to their complexity and the possibility of unknown outcome of function over the long term resulting from growth restriction, joint stiffness, or neurovascular compromise.

Literature Review

Crush injuries of the fingertip are the most common hand injuries seen in children [1]. Many injuries may involve fracture of the distal phalanx, soft tissue injuries to the nail bed, or loss of soft tissue in the way of an amputation. These injuries can be debilitating, adversely affecting daily living activities, and resulting in undesirable cosmetic consequences. The growth and development of the child may also be affected with impaired tactile sensation or the inability to pick up small objects.

Fingertip injuries occur as a result of a variety of mechanisms, most commonly as a crush in a door jam, in addition to various associated blunt crush injuries [1]. Most injuries occur in children and adolescents with the long finger being most commonly involved. Almost 50 % of these injuries are associated with a tuft fracture of the distal phalanx. Many involve simple lacerations in the nail bed with varying patterns of injury: straight, stellate, and tearing [2–4]. In addition to crush mechanisms, it is estimated that 25,000 emergency department visits per year in the USA involve hand injuries sustained by home exercise equipment. Of these 25,000, about 8700 occur between

M. E. Koepplinger (✉)
Department of Orthopaedic Surgery, University of Texas Health Science Center, 6400 Fannin, Suite 1700, Houston, TX 77030, USA
e-mail: matthew.e.koepplinger@uth.tmc.edu

L. M. Rozmaryn (ed.), *Fingertip Injuries,* DOI 10.1007/978-3-319-13227-3_10,
© Springer International Publishing Switzerland 2015

the ages of infancy and 5 years [5, 6]. Stationary bicycles and treadmills contributed to more injuries than any other piece of home exercise equipment, with the stationary bicycles causing an estimated 8300 cases of injury [6].

Seemingly innocuous devices have also been suggested as responsible for repetitive stress injury to fingers of children, inducing pain and blistering. Cell phone use for text messaging and excessive television video game play have been implicated in an increase in repetitive stress injury in teenagers and children, enabling new diagnostic eponyms as "cell phone thumb" or "PlayStation thumb" [7, 8]. Posttraumatic punctate hemorrhages have been described on the fingertips associated with excessive manual activity. The papillary blood vessels rupture, with extravasation of blood into the stratum corneum [8, 9].

Crush Injuries to the Fingertip

Treatment of crush injuries to the fingertip creating a subungual hematoma is not standardized, and is often based on individual physician preference. The need for nail removal and nail bed repair is a matter of debate. Nail bed repair has been advocated for subungual hematomas involving greater than 25 % of the nail area, and particularly in the presence of a fracture [10, 11]. Trephination of the nail plate may adequately alleviate pressure of moderate to large hematomas, and allow healing of the nail bed [10–15]. The nail bed is highly vascular, and prone to developing hematoma after compression of the nail bed

between the nail and the underlying bone. This hematoma under pressure of an intact nail plate can be the source of terrific discomfort for the patient. Simple trephination of the nail plate, or another technique that is designed to alleviate pressure of the hematoma, often provides substantial pain relief and may minimize the need for dangerous, unnecessary narcotic pain medications. Irregular lacerations of the nail bed or those greater than 3 mm in size may benefit from repair (Fig. 10.1), particularly with concomitant fracture of the distal phalanx [16]. The interconnection of the nail bed matrix with the periosteum renders larger lacerations or those associated with fracture worthy of repair, according to some authors. However, this is not supported sufficiently in the literature [1, 16].

There is a lack of quality evidence from randomized controlled trials to guide key treatment decisions for the management of fingertip injuries in children regarding whether or not prophylactic antibiotics should be given following surgical treatment or the superiority of paraffin dressing over a silicone net dressing.

Regarding the question of prophylactic antibiotic use after surgical repair either in the emergency room (ER) or operation room (OR), no conclusive evidence has been elicited regarding the benefits of prophylactic antibiotic use after surgery [17]. In a large prospective controlled study involving 135 patients with injuries ranging from skin and nail bed lacerations to loss of skin pulp and partial and complete amputations, 69 had no antibiotics and 66 were given cephalexin. Only two infections were reported. One was in the antibiotic group and the other was in

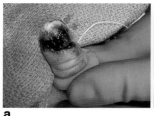 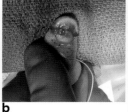 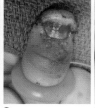 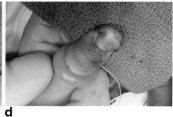

a   b   c   d

Fig. 10.1 a A 3-year-old with a crushing injury to the left thumb from getting her thumb stuck in a bicycle gearshift. **b** Transverse laceration to the nail bed noted after debridement of the edges. **c** Nail bed repaired with 6.0 chromic sutures. **d** Nail plate replaced

the group that received no antibiotics. The authors concluded that no antibiotics are needed to treat acute fingertip injuries as long as the wounds were thoroughly cleaned and debrided [18]. In another study, infections that did result following surgery were related to more severe injuries (partial amputation), requiring a larger than average number of sutures [17].

Comparison of silicone net dressings with paraffin gauze dressings after surgical or conservative management of fingertip injuries reveals a lack of quality evidence of support of one practice over another, with regard to healing time, wound infection, or skin necrosis [17, 19]. Low-quality evidence does not allow firm conclusions to be drawn regarding the superiority of a specific dressing on healing time or complications. However, silicone dressings may be less likely to adhere to wounds, thereby making their eventual removal less distressing to the child [19]. No evidence exists regarding longer-term outcomes on fingertip function, nail growth, or nail deformity.

Fingertip Amputations

In the past, fingertip amputations in children were treated by composite grafting, a euphemism for nonvascular reattachment of the tip [20], local flap coverage, or conservative dressing change. In a study by Moiemen, the outcome of composite graft replacement of 50 amputated digital tips in 50 children over a period of 3 years and 6 months was investigated [21]. Eleven of 18 tips (61%) which were replaced within 5 h survived completely while none of 32 digital tips replaced after 5 h survived completely. This difference was highly significant. For those children who fail this technique and have to rely on secondary reconstruction often end up with a shortened, deformed finger. This may result in negative psychological effects for the child as they enter school age. Thus, replantation of amputated digits in the pediatric hand has gained popularity over the past 20 years. However, studies have shown that it has lower rates of success than in the adult population at 69% [22] as compared to adults at 90% [23]. This is supposedly due to the

increased frequency of crush and avulsion injuries in children and the smaller size of the vessels [24]. Children tend to heal quickly and adapt more effectively to traumatic events. Many of the injuries contraindicated for replantation in adults can be surgically repaired in children. Amputations distal to the lunula of the fingernail may be treated with primary suturing and microsurgical techniques. There are very few contraindications for replantation in the pediatric population due to improved tissue resiliency [24].

However, replantation at a level distal to the distal-interphalangeal joint is technically difficult. Skills proficient with microsurgical techniques are required, as is experience with pediatric patients. The diameter of the terminal arteries might be less than 0.5 mm in children. Veins are even smaller at 0.2 mm [25]. Anastomosis of such small vessels is technically demanding, and requires high-power microscopic magnification. In their series, Shi et al. used 11-0 or 12-0 suture under 25–30x magnification. They used three to four stitches for vascular anastomoses, suggesting that additional sutures were unnecessary and may add damage to the vessel intima, thus increase risk of thrombosis [26].

Despite the fact that good results have been obtained in fingertip replantations of children, it is mandatory to point out that the candidacy for replantation should be carefully assessed before surgery. Yamano classified amputations into four types according to the extent and severity of the injury: clean-cut, blunt-cut, avulsion, or crush [27]. Although replantation of clean-cut amputations has a higher survival rate, crush-amputated replantation is more liable to fail [28]. This may be due to the significant intimal and surrounding soft tissue damage incurred with crush mechanisms of injury. Shi et al. suggest that amputations involving a crush mechanism of injury should be contraindicated for replantation [26].

Apart from the difficulty of repairing small arteries, reestablishing venous outflow poses its own set of challenges. Dorsal veins have been demonstrated difficult to retrieve in some series [29]. With such cases, an artery- only technique of repair, where only one artery is repaired and venous drainage is provided by bloodletting technique, has been used for reperfusion. The bloodletting technique involves excision of a small square of skin from the distal fingertip or a transverse or oblique fish-mouth incision at the pulp tip limited to the dermis layer. The fingertip is evaluated frequently on the basis of its color. If the replant is blue or cyanotic, bloodletting is enhanced. If the tip is pink in color, it is reduced. It is altogether discontinued when the replanted tip takes on a constant pink color that indicates establishment of balanced arterial inflow and venous outflow. Generally, this takes 4–6 days to reestablish venous circulation [26]. Many of these children will require blood transfusions during the early stages of bloodletting, especially if anticoagulants such as heparin, dextran, or aspirin are used [30].

Sensory recovery is another parameter to consider efficacy of digital replantation. Sensory return has been reported in fingertip replantations without nerve repair [31]. Good restoration of nerve function as measured by sharp/dull perception, static two-point discrimination, "skin wrinkle" test, and Semms–Weinstein monofilament testing is related to spontaneous neurotization in children [32]. Factors such as younger age, more distal amputations, and generally good health and tissue resiliency of children contribute to overall good final outcomes [26].

In general, there are factors that have been shown to predict success or failure in replantation in children. Replants that showed poor reflow did not have a successful venous repair or involved an avulsion injury as opposed to a clean-cut were more likely to fail despite local or systemic anticoagulation therapy. One must also take into account that bone growth after replantation is critical to long-term success in restoring function. The physis of the distal phalanx retains an ability to function up to 80 % normal but outcomes are unpredictable [33]. In addition, rehabilitation improved range of motion, decreased stiffness, and indirectly improved functional sensibility [31].

Pediatric Shaft Fractures of the Distal Phalanx (Seymour Fracture)

Suspicion of fracture involving the distal phalanx should be considered with the mechanism of injury, typically a crush mechanism. Seymour fracture involves disruption of the growth plate of the distal phalanx. Detection of this injury can be difficult, as the initial radiographs may be unremarkable. Follow-up films may demonstrate displacement of the distal portion of the phalanx in a flexed position.

A hyperflexion deformity to the fingertip in a child is frequently mistaken for a mallet finger. In reality, the extensor tendon is still attached to the proximal dorsal metaphysis of the distal phalanx, as the flexor digitorum profundus tendon insertion is more distal [34]. Thus, with disruption of the cartilaginous physeal plate, the proximal fragment will be forced into extension and the distal fragment will flex causing an "open-book" flexion fracture of the physis at the proximal end of the distal phalanx. In preadolescents, the fracture is either a Salter–Harris type 1 or 2 (Fig. 10.2), and in adolescents it is generally a type-3 pattern. The diagnosis can be tricky in very small children, under 3 years old, whose epiphysis may not be calcified.

One must carefully examine the nail bed for a transverse laceration and that can only be done

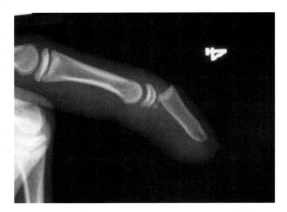

Fig. 10.2 Lateral radiograph of Seymour fracture. Note preservation of articular alignment with displacement of physis. FDP insertion provides deforming force. *FDP* flexor digitorum profundus

by removing the nail plate. In many cases, the nail plate is already avulsed out of the eponychial fold. The nail bed is usually interposed into the fractured physis. This interposition has several ramifications. Firstly, this injury needs to be treated as an open fracture that should be thoroughly cleaned or an infection will result that will destroy the growth plate. In addition, leaving the tissue interposed will result in malunion resulting in a pseudo-mallet deformity (Fig. 10.3).

Thus, if left untreated, growth arrest at the distal phalanx is virtually inevitable and in young children it will result in a shortened distal phalanx with stiffness in the distal-interphalangeal joint (DIPJ) as well as a permanent nail deformity or even absence of the nail plate. These injuries, if closed, can be treated with simple reduction with or without K-wire fixation. However, most of these injuries are open with the physis herniated through the nail bed (Fig. 10.4a, b, c).

Rogers and Labow described a 6-year-old child who was 3 years after a crush injury to the fingertip which was treated expectantly [35]. At 3 years, there was gross nail plate deformity over a nonunion at the distal phalanx. The idea that a small child's fingertips "do fine" regardless of what is done has no basis in fact. Treatment must include removal of the nail plate, careful debridement of the physis, removal of the soft tissue, irrigation, fracture reduction, repair of the nail bed, and replacement of the cleaned nail plate under the eponychial fold to act as a stent to help hold the reduction. A longitudinal K-wire is placed across the fracture, if needed. Good results can be obtained even with delayed presentation up to 1 month. Beyond that time, healing may be too definitive, and resultant deformity may adversely affect function and appearance [34] (Fig. 10.5).

Pediatric Middle Phalanx Fractures

Fractures of the distal portion of the middle phalanx may also be involved with the crush mecha-

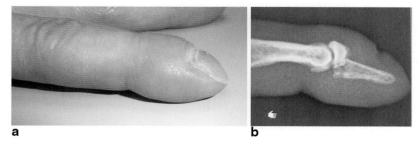

Fig. 10.3 a Pseudo-mallet deformity from an old untreated Seymour fracture. **b**. Lateral X-ray of a pseudo mallet deformity due to a malunion of the proximal metaphysic

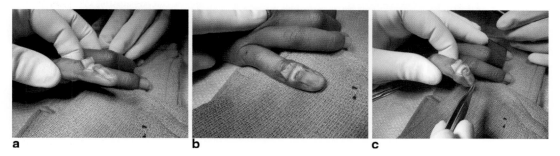

Fig. 10.4 a Seymour fracture with herniation of physis. Nail plate is removed to identify pathology. **b** Herniation of physis noted after removal of nail plate. **c** Seymour fracture deformity accentuation to emphasize physeal instability

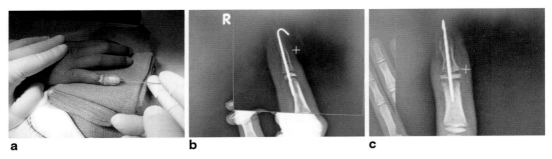

a   b   c

Fig. 10.5 a Appearance after open reduction of physis with retrograde percutaneous pin application. **b** Lateral radiograph after open reduction percutaneous pinning.

c Anteroposterior radiograph with reduced physis after open reduction percutaneous pinning

nism of injury. These can present themselves initially as rather benign injuries, as often neither nail plate, nail bed nor physeal plate are involved (Fig. 10.6). However, close inspection of the radiographs of the distal portion of the middle pha-

lanx and its articular condyle may reveal joint disruption and inherent instability or malalignment of the joint (Fig. 10.7). These fractures, if not managed in a timely fashion, may become difficult to reduce via closed reduction methods

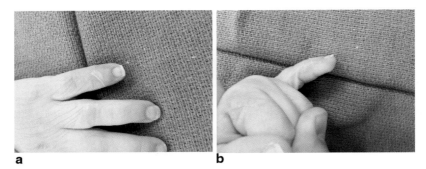

a   b

Fig. 10.6 a Appearance of crush injury to small finger in a 3-year-old. **b** Appearance of crush injury to small finger in a 3-year-old

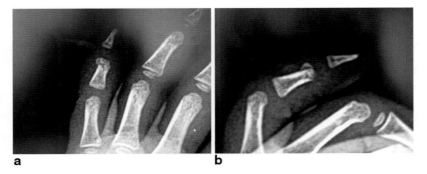

a   b

Fig. 10.7 a AP radiographs show subtle disruption of distal portion of middle phalanx. **b** Lateral radiograph with more profound deformity of distal middle phalanx

condyle with clearly identified malalignment of the distal interphalangeal joint. *AP* anteroposterior

due to the healing capacity of a healthy child. In addition, due to external forces surrounding the joint in the way of tendinous insertions, it may be difficult to maintain any reduction of these injuries without internal fixation. Open reduction of the small fragments with judicious use of internal fixation may provide sufficient positioning of the fracture fragments and stabilization to allow for satisfactory healing and minimization of functional limitations due to malunion or instability.

Classification

Fingertip injuries involve three basic structures: soft tissue, nail and its supporting tissues, and the distal phalanx. Any one of these or a combination of all these structures may be involved in injury to the fingertip in a child. However, due to the varied involvement of injured tissues, wordy descriptions can prevent succinct communication and description of the injury at hand. Classification systems should concisely convey the description of the injury details, they should help determine the injury severity, and provide for treatment recommendations on the basis of injury severity.

Evans and Bernadis (2000) presented a fingertip injury classification system that described the injury on the basis of "pulp, nail, bone" (PNB), as often is the case, all three components may be involved. Each of these structures was given a numeric value depending on its level of injury [36]. These subdivisions of injury level for the given structure started at 0, indicating no damage, to the highest number (7 for pulp; 8 for nail and bone), indicating total loss of that structure (Table 10.1). For any given fingertip injury, the three tissues are graded and a three-digit number is elicited that should accurately define the injury. Validity and applicability of this system remain to be determined. However, it has promise for a number of uses including injury description, standardization of treatment parameters, and may provide a basis for comparative studies of the result of treatment with readily available data derived from the numeric nature of the system.

Table 10.1 The "pulp, nail, bone" (PNB) classification of fingertip injuries

Pulp level	
0	Intact
1	Laceration
2	Crush
3	Distal traverse
4	Palmar oblique
5	Dorsal oblique
6	Lateral
7	Complete
Nail level	
0	Intact
1	Sterile matrix laceration
2	Germinal and sterile matrix laceration
3	Crush
4	Proximal nail bed avulsion
5	Distal third
6	Distal two thirds
7	Lateral
8	Complete
Bone level	
0	Intact
1	Tuft loss
2	Comminuted nonarticular fracture
3	Articular fracture
4	Displaced metaphaseal fracture
5	Bone exposed
6	Distal half loss
7	Subtotal
8	Complete

Sebastin and Chung proposed a classification system for distal amputations that separates the amputations at the level of involvement of sterile matrix or level of germinal matrix [37]. In this classification, zone 1A is distal to the lunula, including all the amputations through the sterile matrix. Zone 1B is between the root of the nail bed and the lunula, including amputations through the germinal matrix. Zone 1C lies between the neck of the middle phalanx and the flexor digitorum profundus insertion, and includes all periarticular amputations. Zone 1D is between the flexor digitorum superficialis insertion and the neck of the middle phalanx (Fig. 10.8).

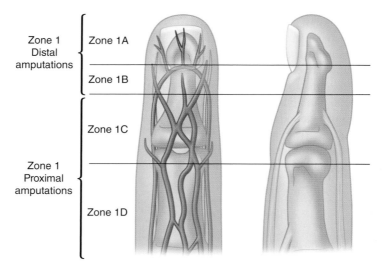

Fig. 10.8 Sebastin and Chung's classification system for distal amputations

Techniques

Reconstructive surgery of soft tissue defects of the hand has been revolutionized by introduction of flap surgery. Coverage is crucial. Even simple defects can expose important structures, including tendon, nerve, and bone. Ideal skin coverage should permit coverage of the associated lesions, and allow for early mobilization. Coverage of digital defects in pediatric patients can be achieved by a variety of methods.

Skin Grafting

The simplest of these is skin grafting. Skin grafting requires a well-vascularized bed of tissue. Palmar skin is well vascularized, but not well mobilized. Conversely, dorsal skin is quite mobile and pliable, but is poorly vascularized. In addition, placement of skin grafts over tendon or bone is prohibited unless the epitenon or periosteum is intact. Skin grafting (either full or split-thickness) is sometimes of limited utility in the coverage of tissue defects. This is dependent upon the area requiring coverage. These take several weeks to incorporate and involve a certain degree of contracture of the tissue, particularly with split-thickness grafting. For this reason, skin grafts at the hand are mostly full-thickness grafts. They are usually more durable than split-thickness grafts, and have better-tolerated donor sites. Full-thickness grafts for the hand may be harvested from the medial forearm, antecubital fossa, or hypothenar eminence.

Drawbacks to skin grafting include requirements of immobilization to allow the graft to incorporate, which may delay rehabilitation of the finger. There have also been demonstrated higher incidences of diminished sensation, cold intolerance, and dysesthesia [38]. Schenck et al. reported a return of less than 6 mm of two-point discrimination in about half of the patients they studied [39].

Skin grafting provides rapid definitive closure of the defect, which may prove beneficial in children who may not cooperate or tolerate complicated wound dressing changes or allowing skin to heal by secondary intention. In lieu of skin grafting defects that require coverage, application of a bilaminate dressing matrix (Integra) has been shown to allow reepithelialization within 3–6 weeks.

Secondary Intention

Fingertip amputations that involve the volar or lateral pad of the finger and do not involve nail bed or exposed bone may achieve the best results cosmetically and functionally with nonoperative management and regular wound care, provided the wound bed is clean and appropriately debrided.

Healing by secondary intention involves gradual phagocytosis of the necrotic tissue with local blood vessel dilation. This creates the formation of an exudate of fibrin and inflammatory cells that cover the wound, seemingly "covering" the defect. Phagocytes clean the necrotic tissue to make way for fibroblasts to begin laying down bridging scar tissue. Peripheral epithelial cells grow inward, covering the defect. New nerve endings grow into the subdermal layers of tissue as specialized sense organs begin to repopulate the newly covered area [40].

This method requires meticulous, regular wound care and appropriate management. Wet-to-dry dressings applied twice daily are typical for the first 10–14 days, but may not be well tolerated in the young child. New epithelium gradually covers the defect in 3 weeks. This treatment method is relatively inexpensive, does not require surgical expertise, and is free of donor-site morbidity. However, it may prove difficult in some young patients. But appropriate instruction of the caregiver and perhaps initial dressing applications in the office may enable better tolerance from the patient. Encouragement of the caregiver is very important, and ensures that proper wound care will be provided.

Treatment of fingertip injuries via secondary intention has demonstrated excellent return of cosmetic appearance and pain-free sensation in the fingertip with two-point discrimination approaching 2.5 mm at 3 months post injury [41].

Composite Grafting

Composite tissue replantation offers the possibility of maintaining digital length and function

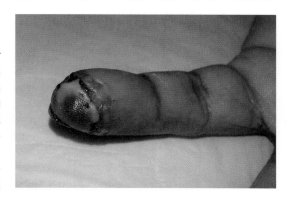

Fig. 10.9 Secondary necrosis of a non-vascularized composite graft in a 3-year-old with a distal complete amputation at 4 weeks

with the patient's own fingertip skin, in an effort to achieve a painless, minimally shortened digit with sensate and durable skin at the tip. This method of treatment has been derived as an alternative to microscopic revascularization, for injuries too far distal for microsurgery (distal to the DIP joint), given the distal fingertip vasculature's diminutive size and the fact that successful microvascular anastomosis of vessels smaller than 0.3 mm in diameter is very difficult.

Composite grafting as a means of defect coverage can be useful in children and adolescents, particularly if the defect accompanies the patient to the emergency room with the amputated part properly protected and preserved "on ice." This method is less effective in older adults, and especially smokers and those with peripheral vascular disease. The tip in these patients has a tendency to become necrotic, thus requiring secondary debridement and coverage procedures (Fig. 10.9). In a prospective study of patients <18 years of age, composite grafting showed survival rates of 77 %. This may be diminished in crush-type injuries and in diabetic patients [42]. In the event of graft failure, this method of coverage may serve as a suitable biological dressing, protecting the underlying tissue as it heals. Secondary intention techniques may then be employed for definitive healing, or additional procedures for coverage may be attempted.

V–Y Advancement Flaps

Amputations at the level of the distal half of the nail bed that are perpendicular to the long axis of the finger may be best managed with advancement of local, triangular vascularized pedicles. These can be achieved with use of tissue from either the volar pad or sides of the fingers, in an effort to provide durable, padded fingertip defect coverage, particularly in the event of exposed bone. These flaps are classified as random flaps, receiving their blood supply from the tiny vessels within the subcutaneous tissues. These are advanced along their neurovascular pedicles. The volar flap of Atasoy et al. [43] and the lateral flaps of Kutler [44] are triangular flaps that are elevated subperiosteally with the apex proximal. These must be mobilized sufficiently in order to allow up to 8 mm of advancement (for volar flaps) and up to 5 mm of advancement (for lateral flaps), without compromising the vascular pedicles supplying the flap. Gentle blunt dissection and cutting of fibrous tissue tethering the flap proximally will allow for adequate mobilization without injury to the nerves and vessels. The angle of the apex for the volar flap should not be less than 45°, but may be safely extended proximal to the volar distal interphalangeal joint crease without creation of a contracture. The angle of apex for the lateral flaps is much sharper than the single volar flap, and as such, a decreased length of advancement can be anticipated (Fig. 10.10).

Once the flaps are advanced, these are sutured into the dorsal end of the defect to provide adequate coverage of the defect, and particularly of any exposed bone. A durable, sensate, painless tip is the ultimate goal. Some studies report dysesthesia and cold intolerance with advancement flaps, but this diminishes with time [45]. An average difference of 3 mm of two-point discrimination in digits covered via volar V–Y flaps compared to normal controls has been demonstrated [46].

Although nicotine use is not often an issue in the pediatric population, great care must be exercised if these flaps are used in smokers or patients who use smokeless tobacco. The author has experienced just such an incidence, where a volar advancement flap was compromised by smokeless tobacco use in an adolescent. This individual in particular was concealing his tobacco use by swallowing the juice and secretions. This provided a near-continuous flow of nicotine into his system that compromised the vascularity of a properly prepared flap in an otherwise healthy individual. The patient denied any tobacco use in the social history, but further questioning of the extended family revealed a positive history of smokeless tobacco use. This has prompted the author to be more diligent in acquiring an accurate history of tobacco use, particularly from adolescents.

Moberg Flaps

A Moberg flap is a proximally based axial flap that is used to cover thumb tip defects. It is based on the radial and ulnar digital neurovascular bundles. This flap is capable of considerable

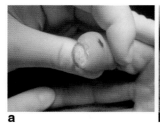 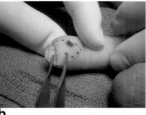 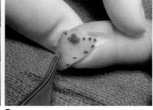 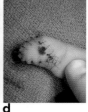

a   b   c   d

Fig. 10.10 a Guillotine amputation of distal tip of the index finger with bone exposed in a 5-year-old. **b** Triangular flap creation for advancement into the terminal defect. **c** Flap mobilization for advancement. Care must be taken to preserve the flaps vascular pedicle incising the retaining septe only. **d** Flap inset. Tourniquet must be deflated in order to check vascularization of the flap

advancement—up to 15 mm. To effect closure distally, however, the interphalangeal joint of the thumb may need to be flexed. The joint may be held in place with a percutaneous pin until healing. This method of coverage sometimes results in flexion contracture of the interphalangeal joint that is correctable in time with splinting and proper therapy. This is a small complication to overcome with the interest of covering large defects of the thumb tip while preserving the maximum possible length of the thumb. This flap is associated with a low incidence of tip dysesthesia and cold intolerance, and normal sensation.

Cross-Finger Flaps

These flaps are random pattern flaps that may be used to cover soft tissue defects on the volar or dorsal aspects of the fingers. The flap involves transfer of adjacent tissue from the dorsum of one finger to the volar aspect of another. The flap is raised on the donor digit, preserving the epitenon, and subsequently sewn in place over the defect site, maintaining its connection to vessels from the donor digit. The donor site is commonly covered with a full-thickness skin graft. The two fingers are "joined" for a period of at least 2 weeks, when the flap is then divided and definitively sewn into place to complete closure of the defect. The blood supply for this flap is from the small vessels of the subdermal and subcutaneous plexus. These plexi are fed by the dorsal digital arteries, originating from the dorsal metacarpal arteries, and from the proper digital arteries. This flap may be used as a direct flap, where elevation of a full-thickness flap from the dorsum of the donor digit is used to cover the volar defect of the adjacent finger. A reverse cross-finger flap consists of the same tissues, but lacks the covering skin. It is also known as a de-epithelialized cross-finger flap. The reverse flap requires turnover of the subcutaneous fascial tissue as well as overlying adipose tissue to cover the defect of the adjacent finger. This preserves the skin, and this is laid back down over the donor defect. The original defect covered by the flap is then covered with full-thickness skin grafting. This flap

has demonstrated excellent return of two-point discrimination.

Author's Preferences

Pediatric fingertip injuries are preferentially handled in the operating theater with sterile instrumentation and general anesthesia. Under the comfort of anesthesia, the child is without anxiety, thus providing a safe, stable work environment for the surgeon. Too often, there is inadequate lighting, instrumentation, sterility, or anesthesia to perform most fingertip procedures in the clinic or emergency department.

In addition, one must respect the complexity of the fingertip injury. The involvement of the numerous tissues with these injuries should prompt the cautious surgeon to be ready for almost anything. This is difficult in the emergency department, and all but impossible in the clinical setting. Having all necessary instrumentation at your disposal will provide you the best possible options for treatment of these complex injuries, and afford your patients the best possible outcomes.

Failure to recognize injured structures or the tendency of some to overlook these injuries as "just a nail bed injury" will lead to long-term disabling outcomes that could be avoided, given adequate anesthesia and time to evaluate all structures appropriately. One should consider any nail bed injury with a concomitant fracture as an open fracture. Given the hematoma that typically forms under the nail plate in these injuries, removal of the nail with evacuation of the hematoma will not only provide pain relief but also allow evaluation and repair of the nail bed with allowance for proper debridement of the fracture, if present. Careful evaluation of the involvement of the growth plate with removal of any interposed soft tissue will prevent growth restrictions or deformity. Internal stabilization of fractures with percutaneous application of Kirchner wires prevents loss of reduction in often-rambunctious patients with inadequate stabilization.

Lacerations to the soft tissues or nail bed are preferentially repaired with small-gauge absorbable suture. The only thing worse than application of suture to an unwilling, uncooperative child is removal of a nonabsorbable suture in the same. Loss of soft tissue may be managed acutely with local soft tissue transfers or coverage procedures, and prevent the need for difficult and anxious dressing changes that may prove uncomfortable for both the patient and caregiver. The definitive dressing placed in the operating room should suffice for at least 2 weeks, provided no infectious process is present. The dressing is applied with the anticipation that it stand up to the most rigorous play and the most curious of patients. Often, minimal dressing is not appropriate with pediatric patients, as they are clever, and often find ways out of the dressing prematurely. As such, preference lies in application of long-arm splinting or casting for younger patients, thus making it difficult for them to squirm out of the dressing and thereby protecting all your hard work. Lacerations to digital nerves and vasculature are probably best handled under the microscope, given the size of the structures in this patient population, and at this level of injury at the tip of the finger. With adequate tissue, microscopic reconstruction of neurovascular structures gives the family and surgeon peace of mind that all was done to ensure as good an outcome as possible. Often, with the crush mechanism of injury, the smallest blood vessels sustain irreparable trauma, and even in spite of your best efforts, vascular repair is fruitless. However, given the amazing healing capacity of children, the necrotic superficial skin may be left in place as a biologic dressing, serving to cover the underlying granulation tissue that will eventually provide the foundation for skin coverage by secondary intention. As the necrotic cap sloughs away, a healthy new skin is revealed.

Complications

Poor alignment of nail bed lacerations may result in scar development and subsequent nail plate deformities. Splits or absence of the nail plate may result from scarring within the germinal matrix. Nonadherence of the nail plate may result if the sterile matrix is damaged [12, 13, 47]. This may result in cosmetic and functional abnormalities, prompting accurate reapproximation of nail bed lacerations [48–49]. Other nonstructural cosmetic abnormalities may result, consisting of transverse white lines (leukonychia) or depression of the nail plate. These are deemed insignificant with regard to function, and may resolve spontaneously within 2–4 months [1]. However, loss of the nail or obliteration of the nail fold may result in lack of new or abnormal nail growth. Infections are always a possibility [1].

Fractures involving the distal phalanx should be properly aligned, to satisfactorily support the nail plate, and prevent nail growth abnormalities. Fractures involving the growth plate should be properly aligned to minimize growth deformity or restriction. Congruency and stability of the DIPJ is also imperative to prevent digit dysfunction, loss of tactile and fine motor skill, and stable pinch-grasp maneuvers.

Infections are possible with nail bed lacerations and concomitant fractures of the distal phalanges. However, definitive support for prophylactic antibiotic use is lacking. One should consider acute administration of intravenous antibiotics and proper irrigation of nail bed lacerations with concomitant fractures. These measures would be employed to manage any other open fracture, and have become standard of care for open fractures in other parts of the body. In spite of appropriate management of the fracture, osteomyelitis is still possible. This is, at times, not preventable given the mechanism of injury that may be complicated by lack of parental involvement in proper follow-up, or improper supervision of the curious child who insists on compromising dressings, fixation pins, wounds, etc. Operative debridement and a referral to infectious disease specialists with proper culture sampling can help to provide the best possible outcomes and avoid disastrous endings.

Summary

Fingertip injuries in the pediatric population are complex injuries that are often overlooked and dismissed as "just a nail bed injury." The fingertip anatomy is complex. Improper management of these injuries can result in deformity, and possibly impairments in function and development. Proper management of these injuries typically results in excellent outcomes due, in part, to the pediatric population's terrific ability to heal and resiliency of tissues. Several treatment techniques are available and well described for managing these injuries. Replantation with artery-only repair yields excellent cosmetic and functional outcomes, even in the absence of vein and nerve repair. Pediatric fingertip injuries are felt to be best managed in the operative suite where proper lighting, equipment, and anesthesia allow for proper exploration of these complex injuries, proper management of these injuries, and afford comfort for the patient and the operating surgeon in an effort to achieve the best outcomes possible.

References

1. Gellman H. Fingertip-nail bed injuries in children: current concepts and controversies of treatment. J Craniofac Surg. 2009;20(4):1033–5.
2. Zook EG, Brown RE. In Operative H and Surgery. In: Green DP, editor. NewYork, NY: Churchill Livingstone, 1993. p. 1283Y1287.
3. Guy RJ. The etiologies and mechanisms of nail bed injuries. Hand Clin. 1990;6:9Y19.
4. Zook EG. Discussion of "Management of acute fingernail injuries." Hand Clin. 1990;6:21.
5. Vouis J, Hadeed J. Evaluation and management of pediatric hand injuries resulting from exercise machines. J Craniofac Surg. 2009;20:1030–2.
6. United States Consumer Product Safety Commission. National electronic injury surveillance system: exercise equipment estimate report, 1999. Washington, DC: United States Consumer Product Safety Commission; 2000.
7. Karim SA. From 'playstation thumb' to 'cellphone thumb': the new epidemic in teenagers. S Afr Med J. 2009;99(3):161–2.
8. Bakos RM, Bakos L. Use of dermoscopy to visualize punctate hemorrhages and oncholysis in "playstation thumb". Arch Dermatol. 2006;142(12):1664–5.
9. Rashkovsky I, Safadi R, Zlotogorski A. Black palmar macules. Arch Dermatol. 1998;134:1020–4.
10. Matthews P. A simple method for the treatment of finger tip injuries involving the nail bed. Hand. 1982;14:30–2.
11. Zook EG, Guy RJ, Russell RC. A study of nail bed injuries: causes, treatment, and prognosis. J Hand Surg Am. 1984;9:247–52.
12. Chudnofsky CR, Sebastian S. Special wounds; nail bed, plantar puncture, and cartilage. Emerg Med Clin. 1992;10:801–22.
13. Verdan CE, Egloff DV. Fingertip injuries. Surg Clin North Am. 1981;61:237–66.
14. Roser SE, Gellman H. Comparison of nail bed repair versus nail trephination for subungual hematomas in children. J Hand Surg Am. 1999;24:1166–70.
15. Baden HP. Regeneration of the nail. Arch Dermatol. 1965;91:619–20.
16. Simon RR, Wolgin M. Subungual hematoma: association with occult laceration requiring repair. Am J Emerg Med. 1987;5:302–4.
17. Capstick R, Giele H. Interventions for treating fingertip entrapment injuries in children. Cochrane Database Syst Rev. 2014;4:CD009808.
18. Altergott C, Garcia FJ, Nager AL. Pediatric fingertip injuries: Do do prophylactic antibiotics alter infection rates? Ped Emer Care. 2008;24(3):148–52.
19. O'Donovan DA, Mehdi SY, Eadie PA. The role of Mepitel silicone net dressins in the management of fingertip injuries in children. J Hand Surg-Br. 1999;24(6):727–30.
20. Cheng GL, Pan DD, Yang ZX, Gong XS. Digital replantation in children. Ann Plast Surg. 1985;15:325–31.
21. Moiemen NS, Eliott D. Composite graft replacement of digit tips: a study in children. J of Hand Surg Br. 1997;22:346–52.
22. Baker GL, Kleinert JM. Digital replantation in infants and young children: determinants of survival. Plast Reconst Surg. 1994;94:139–44.
23. Urbaniak JR. Digital replantation: a twelve year experience. In JR Urbaniak, editor. Microsurgery for major limb reconstruction. St. Louis: Mosby, 1987. p. 12–21.
24. Mohan R, Panthaki Z, Armstrong MB. Replantation in the pediatric hand. J Craniofac Surg. 2009;20:996–8.
25. Gaul JR, Nunley JA. Microvascular replantation in a seven-month old girl: a case report. Microsurgery. 1988;9:204–7.
26. Shi D, Qi J, Li DH, Zhu L, Jin W, Cai, D. Fingertip replantation at or beyond the nail base in children. Microsurgery. 2010;30:380–5.
27. Yamano Y. Replantation of the amputated distal part of the fingers. J Hand Surg Am. 1985;10:211–8.
28. Kim WK, Lim JH, Han SK. Fingertip replantations: clinical evaluation of 135 digits. Plast Reconstr Surg. 1996;98:470–6.
29. Dautel G. Fingertip replantation in children. Hand Clin. 2000;16:541–6.
30. Baker GL, Kleinert JM. Digital replantation in infants and young children: determinants of survival. Plast Reconst Surg. 1994;94:139–44.
31. Ozcelik IB, Tuncer S, Purisa H, Sezer I, Mersa B, Kabakas F, Celikdelen P. Sensory outcome of fingertip replantations without nerve repair. Microsurgery. 2008;28:524–30.
32. Faivre S, Lim A, Dautel G, Duteille F, Merle M. Adjacent and spontaneous neurotization after distal digital replantation in children. Plast Reconstr Surg. 2003;111:159–64.
33. Demiri Em, BakhachJ, Tsakoniatis N, Martin D, Baudet J. Bone growth after replantation in children. J Reconstr Microsurg. 1995;11:113–22.

34. Seymour N. Juxta-epiphyseal fracture of the terminal phalanx of the finger. J Bone Joint Surg. 1966;48B:347–9.

35. Rogers GF, Labow BI. Diaphyseal non-union in the distal phalanx of a child. J Hand Surg. 2007;32E:85–7.

36. Evans DM, Bernardis C. A new classification for fingertip injuries. J Hand Surg Br. 2000;25(1):58–60.

37. Sebastin SJ, Chung KC. A systematic review of the outcomes of replantation of distal digital amputation. Plast Reconstr Surg. 2011;128:723–8.

38. Shores JT, Lee WPA. Fingertip injuries. In: Hand Surgery Update V. Rosemont, IL: American Society for Surgery of the Hand, 2012:365–377.

39. Schenck RR, Cheema TA. Hypothenar skin grafts for fingertip reconstruction. J Hand Surg. 1984;9A:750–3.

40. Goitz RJ, Westkaemper JG, Tomaino MM, Sotereanos DG. Soft-tissue defects of the tissues: coverage considerations. Hand Clin. 1997;2:189–205.

41. Mennen U, Wiese A. Fingertip injuries management with semi-occlusive dressing. J Hand Surg. 1993;18B:416–22.

42. Heistein JB, Cook PA. Factors affecting composite graft survival in digital tip amputations. Ann Plast Surg. 2003;50:299–303.

43. Atasoy E, Ioakimidis E, Kasdan ML, Kutz JE, Kleinert HE. Reconstruction of the amputated finger with a triangular volar flap. A new surgical procedure. J Bone Joint Surg. 1970;52A:921–6.

44. Kutler W. A new method for finger tip amputation. JAMA. 1947;133:29.

45. Frandsen PA.: A V–Y plasty as a treatment of fingertip amputation. Acta Orthop Scand. 1979;49:255–9.

46. Tupper J, Miller G. Sensitivity following volar V-Y plasty for fingertip amputations. J Hand Surg. 1985;10B:183–4.

47. Hart RG, Kleinert HE. Fingertip and nail bed injuries. Emerg Med Clin. 1993;11:755–65

48. Ashbell TS, Kleinert HE, Putcha SM, et al. The deformed fingernail: a frequent result of failure to repair nail bed injuries. J Trauma. 1967;7:177–90.

49. Beasley R. Fingernail injuries. J Hand Surg Am. 1983;5:784–5.

Sandra Lea Austin

Introduction

The protocols suggested are intended to be general guidelines. All treatment plans should be determined based on individual patients, the nature of the injury including concomitant diagnoses, the strength or stability of the operative intervention, and communication with the physician. In all cases, this author looks first to wound care, edema reduction, the need for orthoses to provide protection or stability, and patient education to facilitate a partnership and compliance during the recovery process.

Wound Care and Scar Management

Scar management begins at the initiation of therapy particularly when a wound is present. Promoting wound healing and facilitation of edema reduction both lead to more pliable scar tissue. Although there is less tissue gliding in the fingertip relative to other areas of the hand, it is still important to address scar tissue as excessive, non-pliable scar tissue can have a devastating impact on the sensory abilities of the normally highly sensate fingertips.

Wound healing consists of three histologically distinct yet overlapping phases. The first stage, the inflammation stage, occurs in response to

injury, provides the body with a means of removing debris from the wound, and lasts from injury to day 5. Collagen synthesis, capillary budding, and angiogenesis are the hallmarks of fibroplasia, the second stage of wound healing, and begin 3–5 days post injury and last 2–6 weeks. There is a strong correlation between the tensile strength of the wound and the deposition of collagen during the fibroplasia stage. Maturation is the third phase of healing. It consists of inter- and intramolecular collagen molecule cross-linking and lasts from 2–3 weeks post injury to possibly many years, although most often scar maturation occurs within 2 years [18].

Superficial wounds and suture lines can generally be gently cleansed with soap and water. This author prefers pump antibacterial soap without heavy perfumes. When pins extrude from the skin, daily cleansing with a cotton swab and a 50/50 mixture of saline and hydrogen peroxide is recommended to prevent pin-site infections and possible osteomyelitis. Pin sites are kept dry at all other times.

Dressings that become adherent to the wound bed can damage epithelial buds and retard wound closure. A layer of petroleum-impregnated mesh applied directly over the wound helps prevent adherence. If adherence does occur, the dressing can be soaked with either saline or a 50/50 mixture of saline and hydrogen peroxide until it loosens. For deeper and larger wounds, MIST Therapy (Celleration of Minnesota) is often effective. MIST Therapy is a noncontact, low-frequency ultrasound therapy. Ultrasound energy

S. L. Austin (✉)
Medical College of Virginia, Fairfax, VA 22032, USA
e-mail: saustin@virginiahospitalcenter.com

L. M. Rozmaryn (ed.), *Fingertip Injuries,* DOI 10.1007/978-3-319-13227-3_11,
© Springer International Publishing Switzerland 2015

is delivered via a mist of sterile saline directly to the wound without contact. In a retrospective study, this treatment was noted to reduce healing time by removing debris and bacteria from the wound and by stimulating the healing process [15]. The recommended frequency for MIST Therapy is 3–5 times per week. The treatment time is based on the square centimeter size of the wound; therefore, most fingertips wounds require no more than 10 min of treatment each session. It is important to measure the width, length, and depth of the wound at each session in order to judge the efficacy of the chosen treatment.

The presence of tough slough or eschar in the wound effectively stalls the healing process in the inflammatory stage [27]. This creates a cascade of cellular response that significantly delays wound healing and renders the wound more susceptible to infection. Prompt removal of eschar and slough is necessary. There are multiple removal methods including sharp debridement, surgical debridement, and use of an enzymatic agent. In this author's experience, enzymatic agent use is often quite effective in removing necrotic tissue of the fingertip due to the small surface area involved. Enzymatic agents are also easy to use and cost effective. Once the eschar is removed, use of a dressing containing silver is often recommended. Silver has antibacterial properties and also promotes healing. Foam or sheet dressings containing silver are easy to use and can be left in place for several days if necessary. A common misconception is that range of motion should be delayed until the wound is healed. Waiting for wound closure can result in significantly decreased range of motion. It is important to educate the patient on this fact as it is counterintuitive for patients to move when a wound is present. Reassurance that the wound will heal and that range of motion and function are more likely to be preserved with prompt initiation of active movement is necessary.

Edema reduction techniques should be implemented on the first visit to the clinic in conjunction with wound care. One exception, however, is the use of contrast baths as wounds should not be submerged in water. Elevation above the heart, elevation combined with active range of motion (overhead fisting), compression wrapping, manual lymph drainage, cold application, continuous passive motion, contrast bathes, and electric stimulation are techniques used to reduce edema. In this author's experience with fingertip injuries, wrapping with a self-adhesive tape is usually sufficient to address localized edema. Whenever applying compression to the finger or hand, check capillary refill after application and educate the patient on the signs of blood flow compromise. Begin at the tip of the finger applying a light stretch to the tape and overlap slightly as the tape is wrapped around the finger. End at the base of the proximal phalanx. This tape can be applied directly over dressings. If the edema is more extensive and involves the dorsum of the hand, this author has found that manual lymph drainage in combination with lymphedema wrapping is very effective. Once the edema is reduced, transition from the bulkier lymphedema wraps to self-adhesive tape in order to allow greater ease with active range of motion. It is beyond the scope of this chapter to describe the specific techniques used in manual lymph drainage and lymphedema wrapping; however, there are many good resources readily available. Cold is often used to reduce edema but is often not tolerated well by those with fingertip injuries. Elevation and elevation with active range of motion, which employs the muscle pump action, are both effective, as well. However, it is important to note all precautions. If there has been an arterial repair or range-of-motion limitations are in place due to tendon repair or fracture, these techniques may not be appropriate. Electrical stimulation, continuous passive motion, and contrast baths are typically not necessary for isolated fingertip injuries.

As with joint range of motion and wounds, it is important to accurately and consistently measure the patient's edema in order to determine the effectiveness of the chosen intervention. The literature supports the use of the volumeter and figure-of-eight measurements as reliable methods for assessing edema; however, these techniques are most often used with more extensive edema of the hand. For fingertip injuries, this author's preference is to assess edema presence and response to treatment via circumferential measurements in centimeters with a tape measure. It is important to measure both the affected and unaffected digit each session as size fluctuates dependent on time of day, temperature, level of activity, and intake. Choose a reproducible landmark, such as the base of nail or the distal-interphalangeal joint (DIP), and apply a similar amount of tension to the tape each time measurements are taken.

Scar formation is necessary for wound healing; however, excessive scarring can lead to joint contracture, pain, anxiety, and a decrease in function. It is important to begin scar management before a significant problem presents as it is much easier to prevent excessive scarring than to remodel it after the fact [9]. Fingertip scar management is of particular import due to the high density of sensory receptors and the intrinsic integration of the fingertips in activities from power gripping to the finessing of guitar strings or a needle and thread. After amputation, it is not uncommon for the sutured end to have a "dog-eared" presentation. If allowed to heal in this shape, the end of the digit will tend to be caught, cut, and pinched during daily activities. Reshaping to a rounded, more natural appearance is not difficult to achieve if shaping through gentle compression is begun early. Dress the wound and apply a self-adhering tape over the dressing at a 45° angle to the lateral and medial borders of the sutured portion of the residual digit (see Figs. 11.1 and 11.2). Over time, the gentle pressure of the tape facilitates an aesthetically pleasing and functionally practical result. Once the

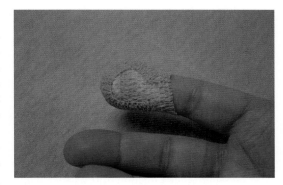

Fig. 11.2 Wrap technique to produce a rounded residual tip

wound is healed, Elastomer Putty® can be used to form a "helmet" over the tip for the circumferential scar management needed after amputation. Silicone gel sheeting is an excellent and routinely used scar-remodeling product that works best on flat surfaces. Scar management products can be used up to 23 h per day with removal only for hygiene purposes; however, the clinician must consider the impact of product use on the integration of the injured digit into functional activities. Daytime use of Elastomer Putty® is not recommended for long periods of time as the rigidity of the product and the lack of sensory input to the tip limit functional use of the hand. Silicone gel sheeting is flexible, allowing unrestricted active range of motion; however, it must be held in place. This author uses self-adherent tape, which limits sensory input. The significance of the scar, the degrees of active range of motion available to the patient, and the stage of rehabilitation should all be considered when establishing the wear time for scar management products.

Scar massage is an adjunctive intervention that is begun promptly upon wound closure. [5] It is performed not only on the frank scar but also on the surrounding tissue when it feels dense, brawny, or hard. Firm pressure is applied to the area followed by one of the following: cross-friction, longitudinal, or circular movements. The clinician and patient should not move their fingers across the skin, but rather, should apply pressure into the deeper tissues changing finger position periodically to cover the entire effected

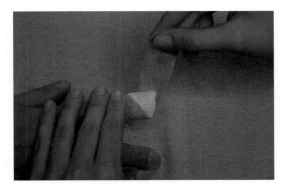

Fig. 11.1 Wrap technique to produce a rounded residual tip

area. The techniques employed in myofascial release provide a three-dimensional approach including applying pressure to the scar tissue through the transverse, sagittal, and coronal planes. Finger pressure is applied straight down into the affected area until resistance is met. Then a longitudinal, or sideways, pressure is applied to the tissue in the direction of scar or tissue resistance. The technique is completed by the third component of either a clockwise or counterclockwise pressure in the direction of resistance while maintaining the previous two directions of pressure. At this point, the scar tissue has been placed on tension in all three planes providing maximum therapeutic deformation forces. Pressure is held at this end point until tissue release is noted after which pressure is slightly increased to take up the slack from release. There are no published studies on the effectiveness of scar massage, but it is this author's experience that tissue is noted to soften and lengthen when these techniques are employed.

Ultrasound may be used as an adjunct modality for the benefit of increasing range of motion and tissue extensibility. It is considered a superficial heating agent, and the literature demonstrates that the 3-MHz sound head may heat tissues to a depth of 2 cm. The literature does not, however, support the effectiveness of the use of ultrasound. Support for this modality is anecdotal. This author has found it effective in the majority of patients with recalcitrant scar tissue particularly when the scar crosses a joint. Putting the tissue on a stretch by passively moving the joint involved increased effectiveness. As with all modalities, it is important to be fully aware of all precautions and contraindications related to ultrasound use.

Distal Phalanx Fractures

Distal phalanx (P3) fractures are the most common fractures in the hand and are, typically, the least difficult to manage due to the relative simplicity of the soft tissue structures about the fingertip [31]. These fractures can be open or closed, may involve tendons, and be part or all of the structures of the nail. When establishing a treatment plan, it is important to consider the type of fracture, any surgical intervention performed, soft tissue structures involved, and fracture stability.

Tuft fractures, the most common P3 fractures, are often the result of crush injuries and usually require no surgical intervention. The hand surgeon may allow active range of motion during the first week with immobilization between exercise sessions. More often, immobilization of the DIP for 2–3 weeks is recommended [29]. A volar or clamshell orthosis with the DIP in neutral extension and the proximal-interphalangeal (PIP) free is recommended. There is no concern for possible development of a swan neck deformity with tuft fractures as the extensor tendon inserts proximal to this fracture sight. Three weeks post injury, the orthosis is discontinued and range of motion is begun. Periodic use of the orthosis during heavier tasks may be useful in preventing discomfort. Progression of therapy is based largely on patient tolerance as crush injuries to the fingertip often result in significant pain. In this author's experience, tuft fractures generally do not require prolonged rehabilitation. Occasionally, the recalcitrant finger will require more aggressive treatment including prolonged stretching via static progressive or dynamic orthosis use to achieve maximal gains (Fig. 11.3). Rarely is a formalized strengthening program warranted. Often the sterile matrix is compromised with tuft fractures due to the congruous nature of the periosteum and the sterile matrix. After surgical repair of the sterile matrix, the surgeon will either reuse the nail plate or suture sterile foil in place for protection. It generally takes two full nail growth cycles to determine the final outcome of the nail. Preservation of the nail is preferred as it gives proprioceptive input to the pulp during manipulation and gripping activities. If the surgeon has not applied the nail or foil over the repaired matrix, pressure must be applied to the nail bed. This can be done by fabricating a dorsal orthosis fabricated from 1/16" thermoplastic material. The orthosis can be applied over a piece of gauze and held in place with self-adhering tape. It should be removed only for exercise and hygiene purposes. The pressure from the orthosis on the healing nail bed helps to facilitate a smoother end result.

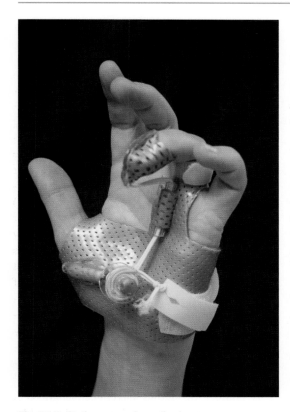

Fig. 11.3 Static progressive orthosis

Both longitudinal and transverse fractures of the distal phalanx have been described, and, are frequently the result of crush injuries [29]. These fractures can be open or closed, involve the perionychium to varying degrees, and may be intra- or extra-articular. Simple, well aligned, closed fractures are typically treated with immobilization for 2–4 weeks based on healing progress and residual pain and swelling. When the orthosis is removed, active range of motion is initiated in the clinic, often two to three times a week, and at home five to six times daily. A desensitization program may need to be initiated at this point as, due to the high density of sensory receptors in the fingertip, hypersensitivity after crush injury is common. This author typically initiates passive range of motion at weeks 5–6 post injury or repair followed by strengthening and work simulation at weeks 7–8. Good communication with the referring physician is essential in determining the time line for rehabilitation based on fracture healing.

Some fractures require pinning to achieve proper alignment and future stability. Typically, a K-wire is used for internal fixation and is left in place for 4–6 weeks [1, 29]. If the DIP is not immobilized, the hand surgeon may allow gentle DIP active range of motion while the pin is in place with immobilization at all other times. If the pin protrudes from the skin, the orthosis should be fabricated to protect the pin from being inadvertently bumped during daily activities. Instruction in pin care is essential to prevent pin-site infection and possible osteomyelitis. Daily cleaning with a cotton swab and a mixture of 50/50 saline and hydrogen peroxide is recommended. The patient is instructed to keep the pin site dry at all other times. Once the pin is pulled, it is important to progress range of motion exercises with an eye toward possible attenuation. Over stretching of the relatively thin terminal extensor tendon can occur after prolonged immobilization, swelling, and scar formation from the initial injury and corrective surgery. If a lag is noted, daytime orthosis use with removal for active range-of-motion exercises, and night time immobilization are recommended. Exercises should be focused on full digit extension as well as flexion. Weaning from the orthosis may be initiated as DIP extension improves. Nighttime orthosis use may continue for several weeks. Passive range-of-motion exercises are initiated 1–2 weeks after pin pulling, dependent on fracture healing and status of DIP extension. These injuries may also require static progressive or dynamic orthoses to increase DIP joint flexion secondary to adaptive shortening of the oblique retinacular ligaments as well as other soft tissue about the joint (Fig. 11.3). As mentioned previously, careful monitoring for signs of attenuation is prudent. Strengthening and work simulation activities are initiated 8 weeks after surgery.

Seymour fractures are distal phalanx fractures that occur in children at the trans-epiphyseal plate. The terminal extensor tendon remains intact; however, the pull of the flexor digitorum profundus on the bone distal to the fracture sight causes the injury to present like a mallet injury. Often there is concomitant nail bed injury. Current literature supports fixation with a K-wire due to the severity of the fracture and potential noncompliance of children with orthosis use. Postoperative orthosis use to support the joint and protect the pin is recommended. Typically, formal therapy is not required.

Mallet Finger

Mallet finger injury is a disruption of the terminal extensor tendon that results in an inability to actively extend the DIP joint. Injury is generally caused by axial loading to an extended digit and may occur during sports, work, and household activities [23]. Mallet finger injuries occur in nearly 10 per 100,000 individuals [3] with a greater incidence in men than in women and they more often occur in the dominant hand. The digit most frequently affected is the long finger followed by the ring, index, small, and thumb, although mallet type injury of the thumb is rare [12]. The result of an untreated mallet finger may include the development of chronic DIP flexion with possible joint contracture, cold intolerance, osteoarthritis, chronic joint pain, and swan neck deformity resulting from the collapse of the extensor system from over pull of the central slip. Several classifications systems have been developed in order to describe the relative severity of the injury, including soft tissue and bony involvement [3]. Doyle's classification describes four subsets of injury ranging from closed to greater than 50 % involvement of the articular surface [3]. Wehbe and Schneider's classification describes three subsets of injury ranging from stable soft tissue injuries without DIP subluxation to unstable with bony involvement greater than two thirds of the articular surface.

There is controversy over whether to treat mallet finger injuries conservatively or surgically; however, it is generally accepted that conservative treatment is most appropriate when there is no bony involvement or when bony involvement does not exceed one third of the articular surface [1, 3, 16]. Furthermore, some studies suggest that, due to the distal phalanx's superior ability to form bony callus, bony involvement with greater than two thirds articular surface

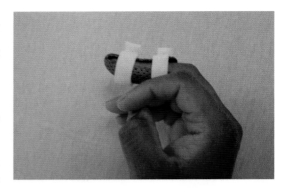

Fig. 11.4 Lever-type thermoplastic orthosis

involvement can be successfully treated conservatively with immobilization [1]. In fact, some prefer conservative treatment even with significant bony involvement due to the possible complications of surgery including pin-site infection and osteomyelitis. The financial cost of surgery can also be a concern. Regardless, as current literature confirms, patient compliance is necessary in order to achieve a successful outcome.

A number of studies have been conducted comparing casting and orthoses use for conservative treatment of mallet finger. Tocco [12] conducted a prospective randomized comparison of 57 closed mallet finger injuries that were treated conservatively with either the Quickcast® finishing tape or custom-made "lever type" thermoplastic orthoses (Fig. 11.4). All participants had either tendonous involvement alone or less than one-third articular surface involvement. Participants were immobilized at all times for 6–8 weeks, followed by 2 weeks of intermittent immobilization and 2 additional weeks of nighttime immobilization. Tocco concluded that DIP joint extension was greater in the continuous immobilization group that was casted than in the thermoplastic orthosis group. There were also a higher number of failures in the group that used an orthosis. However, there was no difference in pain or discomfort between the two groups [23, 30]. A single blind, prospective, randomized controlled trial was conducted comparing Stack® (Fig. 11.5), dorsal aluminum, and custom thermoplastic orthoses in 64 participants with terminal tendon involvement only or a small bony

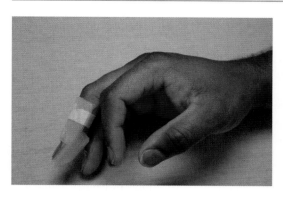

Fig. 11.5 Stack (registered) splint

avulsion without DIP joint subluxation. [23] This study concluded that there was no significant difference in extensor lag no matter the form of immobilization. However, there were fewer complications with skin irritation and maceration with the use of the custom thermoplastic orthosis.

In keeping with the basic principles of hand therapy, the clinician must always be mindful of potential complications that may occur with orthosis and cast use. The epidermis may be compromised by maceration, pressure points, skin ulceration, ischemia, and skin necrosis. Ineffective protection of injured structures is also primary concern. Patient education and compliance are of paramount importance when conservative treatment is employed. A Cochran review in 2004 found that patient compliance is the most important factor when treating mallet finger injuries with orthosis immobilization [2]. The patient must have a clear understanding that fingertip immobilization in extension must be maintained for 6–8 weeks. If at any point during that time the DIP joint is allowed to flex, the timeframe for repair and immobilization essentially begins again. The DIP is positioned in slight hyperextension. Blanching should be avoided as it is an indicator of ischemia. The PIP joint is not immobilized. [28] However, if a swan neck deformity is noted, the PIP joint is positioned to prevent extension beyond 30° to lessen the pull of the lateral bands on the DIP joint. [13] Immobilization is continued for a period of 6–8 weeks. The orthosis is removed minimally. Once daily for hygiene purposes is recommended. The patient

must maintain full DIP joint extension during orthosis removal. This author recommends practicing daily hygiene techniques in the clinic during the first visit to facilitate a clear understanding of tendon protection. At 6 weeks post immobilization, the tendon is "tested" with full extension place and hold. If the patient is unable to maintain DIP joint extension, the orthosis is continued for another week. If healing is sufficient to maintain full extension, gentle active flexion exercises are initiated. Best practice is to move forward gradually with gentle active range of motion. If attenuation occurs, it is very difficult to remedy, and most patients are left with some degree of extensor lag. If extensor lag is in excess of 30°, there is noted impact on function. There is a delicate balance between progressing flexion while maintaining extension versus progressing beyond tissue tolerance thus increasing extension lag. Thorough documentation including analysis of goniometric measurements at every therapy session is required. The savvy patient is able to progress orthosis weaning between therapy sessions based on observation of his or her ability to maintain DIP joint extension. With most patients, however, advance weaning only after careful observation and measurement in the clinic. If, after 2–3 days of active flexion during exercise sessions, DIP joint extension is maintained, the patient is instructed to advance orthosis weaning. Continue to progressively increase time-out of the orthosis as the patient is able to maintain joint extension. Typically, full transition to nighttime-only orthosis use occurs within 2–3 weeks of initiation of weaning. The patient may need to continue with nighttime splinting for 2–4 weeks after daytime orthosis use has been discontinued. Protection during contact sports is recommended through week 12. Typically, patients who sustain mallet finger injuries do not require formalized strengthening, desensitization, or work conditioning activities and rarely even require passive range of motion in order to gain functional flexion without a significant lag.

Mallet thumb injuries are much less common than mallet finger injuries and are typically open [29]. These injuries are managed in the same fashion as mallet finger injuries.

Extensor Pollicis Longus Zone I Repair

Extensor pollicis longus (EPL) injuries usually occur as the result of a laceration over the dorsum of the thumb; however, associated crush injuries are not uncommon and result in an inability to fully extend the IP joint. The literature lacks in studies of EPL repair with the vast majority being conducted on the extensor system of the fingers [5]. Typically, zone I EPL injuries are managed in the same fashion as mallet finger injuries, with continuous extension immobilization of the inter-phalangeal (IP) joint in slight hyperextension for 6 weeks. [11]. Refer to the section "Mallet Finger Injuries" for treatment recommendations and considerations. Zone I EPL repairs often require a focus on scar management and efforts to increase IP flexion once the tendon is sufficiently healed. Generally, active range of motion is begun 4 weeks post repair followed by passive range of motion and discharge of orthosis 6 weeks post repair. Static progressive or dynamic orthosis use may be necessary in order to gain full IP flexion. Strengthening is initiated at 8 weeks post repair. As with mallet finger, careful monitoring for extension lag and appropriate adjustment of the therapeutic program is required.

Zone I Flexor Pollicis Longus Injuries

Zone I flexor pollicis longus (FPL) injuries can be the result of a laceration, crush, or avulsion, and they require surgical repair. The FPL retracts further than other digit flexors and the muscle itself has a tendency to adaptively shorten quickly [1] which may lead to a repair under tension. Additional special considerations include gap formation and A4 pulley involvement. Clear communication with the surgeon is essential to successful rehabilitation. As is the case with EPL injuries, there is a scarcity of published research on the rehabilitation of FPL repairs. Conservative treatment is typically employed via static immobilization and early passive range of motion. The patient is seen 2 days post repair for removal of the bulky dressing, wound care, edema reduction efforts, and orthosis fabrication. There are several approaches to joint position within the static, forearm-based orthosis. One approach recommends the orthosis be fabricated with the wrist in comfortable flexion (20°), the thumb midway between radial and palmar abduction, the metacarpal-interphalengeal (MIP) joint in comfortable flexion (20°), and the IP in neutral extension [1]. Cannon suggests positioning the wrist in 20° of flexion, MIP joint in 15° of flexion, the IP joint in 30° of flexion, and the car-pometacarpal (CMC) joint in palmar abduction. Both protocols recommend isolated and composite passive flexion of the IP and MIP joints upon initial treatment. Passive flexion of the IP and the MIP are initiated five to six times per day. Isolated IP passive flexion and extension with the MIP joint immobilized increases the glide of the FPL over the proximal phalanx, according to Brown and McGouther. [1] Cannon further recommends initiating gentle active range-of-motion exercises within the confines of the splint six to eight times per day at 3 ½ weeks post repair. Gentle active range of motion outside of the orthosis begins at 4 ½ weeks followed by orthosis discontinuation at 5 ½ weeks. Six weeks post repair, coordination and light prehensile activities are initiated as well as static or dynamic extension orthosis use to address IP joint stiffness and extrinsic tightness. Extrinsic flexor tightness is often present but usually responds well to static, progressive orthosis use. Gentle strengthening is initiated at 8 weeks post repair.

Zone I Flexor Digitorum Profundus Injuries

Zone I of the flexor tendon system extends from the insertion of the flexor digitorum superficialis (FDS) to the insertion of the flexor digitorum profundus (FDP) on the volar distal phalanx. Flexion of the DIP joint is performed by a single tendon with a short moment arm resulting in decreased tendon excursion. The tensile strength of repairs in this zone is decreased due to decreased tendon diameter size and anatomic limitations preventing a circumferential repair [11]. Gap formation is a primary concern.

The advancement of suture materials, improved surgical technique, and an increased knowledge of tendon healing and tensile strength have led to significant changes in the therapeutic management of flexor tendon repairs. [25] Historically, very little tension was applied to the healing tendon for the first 4 weeks post repair with either the Klienert protocol of flexion traction to the digits or the Duran protocol, both allowing only passive flexion, protected digit extension and significant wrist and metacarpal phalangeal (MP) joint flexion within the dorsal blocking orthosis. Reliable studies have concluded that controlled, early tension to the repaired flexor tendon promotes superior tendon healing, decreased adhesion formation, and improved outcomes [11].

Evans [11] promotes a technique of limited extension and active flexion (LEAF) in which the DIP is blocked to prevent extension beyond 35–45°, thus decreasing gap formation and preventing the oblique retinacular ligaments from imparting extension forces on the DIP joint during PIP extension. [10] Within the dorsal blocking orthosis, the wrist is positioned in 20–30° of flexion, the MPs in 30° of flexion, and the IPs are allowed full extension. Exercise consists of passive digit flexion, place and hold of the FDS with the wrist in flexion, wrist tenodesis, and modified-position composite flexion place and hold. During place and hold, passively place the wrist in 20° of extension, the MPs in 80° of flexion, the PIPs in 70° of flexion, and the DIPs in 40° of flexion. The patient gently holds his or her hand in this position for several seconds.

This author has had good success following Evans' protocol with the following changes: The dorsal blocking orthosis is fabricated with the wrist in neutral to 10° of flexion, the MPs are positioned in 45–55° of flexion, and modified-position composite flexion place and hold is performed with the wrist in neutral (Figs. 11.6 and 11.7). Gentle active flexion and discontinuation of dorsal DIP flexion orthosis begin at 4 weeks post repair with forearm-based orthosis use continued between exercise sessions for 2 additional weeks. Orthosis use is discontinued at 6 weeks post repair and gentle composite extension and

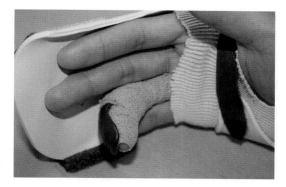

Fig. 11.6 DIP extension blocking orthosis with extension blocked at 35–45° extension

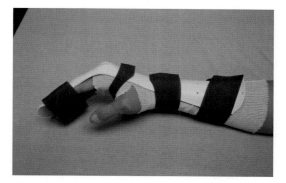

Fig. 11.7 Dorsal blocking orthosis

FDP blocking exercises are initiated. Gentle strengthening begins at 8 weeks post repair. Typically, unrestricted return to activities is allowed at 12 weeks post repair.

Sensory Testing

Assessing both slowly and quickly adapting fibers in the fingertips is essential for establishing a baseline for sensation and developing a logical, sequential treatment plan for sensory reeducation. It has been well established in the literature that there is no one sensory test that accurately assesses all sensation or accurately predicts overall function. Standard practice in many hand clinics is to use several forms of testing in order to understand localization, acuity, threshold, discrimination, and protective sensation.

Touch Threshold: Light Touch to Deep Pressure

The Weinstein Enhanced Sensory Test (WEST) (Bioinstruments, Connecticut, USA) is the latest in a series of monofilament-type pressure tests that began with Von Frey's use of hair of varying diameters to determine pressure thresholds more than half a century ago. [20] The WEST is easy to use, quickly administered, and has good inter- and intra-tester reliability [14]; however, care must be taken to ensure consistency in the administration of the test. The number associated with each monofilament represents grams of force needed to bow the monofilament. Administer in a quiet room with the patient's vision occluded. The smallest-diameter monofilament, 2.83, representative of normal light touch, is the first used with a progression from the smallest to largest monofilament. When applying the stimulus, position the monofilament perpendicular to the tissue, apply pressure until it bows, and hold for 1–1.5 s (Fig. 11.8). The largest monofilament, 6.65, will not bow but will bend slightly. [1] The stimulus is applied three times. One correct response indicates a positive response. If a positive response is not evoked, move to the next larger monofilament 3.61. Repeat until either all monofilaments have been exhausted or positive responses were elicited in all areas tested (Table 11.1).

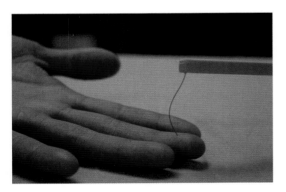

Fig. 11.8 WEST light touch testing

Table 11.1 WEST

2.83	Within normal limits: light touch and deep pressure intact
3.61	Diminished light touch: pain and temperature intact; dropping of objects, decreased coordination and decreased use of the hand
4.31	Loss of protective sensation: significantly decreased use of the hand; vision used as compensatory technique for gross manipulation of objects; risk for injury
6.65	Deep pressure sensation: minimal use of hand; discrimination is lost; significant risk for injury
No response	Minimal to no use of hand; significant risk for injury [1]

WEST Weinstein Enhanced Sensory Test

Tactile Discrimination

Two-Point Discrimination: Static and Moving

Two-point discrimination has long been the mainstay for physicians when attempting to isolate and identify the progression of reinnervation after nerve injury or repair. It is thought to be a good indicator of the quantity or density of innervated sensory receptors as well as return of object identification [1, 7, 17, 22]. Initially, a bent paperclip was the commonplace tool; however, the Disk-Criminator (Neuroregen, Baltimore, Maryland) and the Two-point Aesthesiometer (Smith + Nephew, Germantown, Wisconsin), both widely available, provide significantly greater accuracy. As with monofilament testing, administer in a quiet environment with the patient's vision occluded. In assessing static two-point discrimination, begin with the 5-mm distance probes. Randomly apply either one or two probes, holding for 5 s, with enough pressure to note minimal tissue deformation without blanching [14]. Increase the probe distance in 1 mm increments until the patient identifies seven out of ten responses correctly. When testing two-point discrimination, position the instrument in a longitudinal fashion to avoid crossing into a separate innervation (Fig. 11.9; Table 11.2).

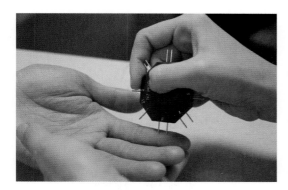

Fig. 11.9 Static two-point discrimination

Table 11.2 Static two-point discrimination

Normal:	Less than 6 mm
Fair:	6–10 mm
Poor:	11–15 mm

Moving two-point discrimination is tested in a similar fashion but with a moving stimulus of either one or two probes applied proximally to distally in a parallel fashion (Fig. 11.10). The smallest distance that the patient correctly identifies between one and two probes, seven out of ten times, is considered the patient's moving two-point discrimination. Two millimeters is considered normal.

Localization

Decreased ability to localize touch is not unexpected post nerve injury, as regenerating axons

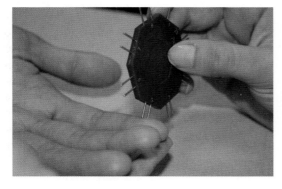

Fig. 11.10 Moving two-point discrimination

often do not reconnect with their original mechanoreceptors no matter how accurate the nerve repair is. [17, 24] This results in altered representation of sensation within the hand. Patients often can "feel" a sensation but report that the stimulus is in a different finger or they can localize only to a generalized area and not a focal one. [24] Localization mapping is useful in providing information regarding degree of regeneration and associated functional use of the hand. Localization testing: A hand chart is divided into sections using median and ulnar nerve innervation as a guide. The heaviest monofilament in the WEST, 6.65, is used as the stimulus. Slight pressure is applied to a specific area. The patient is asked to point, using the other hand, to the specific spot stimulated. If the patient identifies the stimulus correctly, a mark is placed on the hand chart. If the sensation was referred to another area, an arrow is drawn on the chart from the point of application to the point sensation was reported. As nerve regeneration improves, localization usually improves.

The Ten Test

The ten test evaluates light moving touch. It is a screening tool that allows the patient to compare a stimulus applied to the affected side with the unaffected side. The examiner's finger is used to provide a light moving stimulus to an unaffected area on the patient's uninjured side, thus establishing a baseline of 10/10 or normal light touch for that particular patient. The patient is then touched in the same fashion simultaneously on the affected and unaffected sides and asked to grade the stimulus on the affected side between 0 (no sensation) and 10 (normal sensation). This therapist uses the ten test as a quick screening tool to determine if more specific testing is warranted.

Vibration Thresholds

Perception of vibration is one of the first indicators of sensory reinnervation. Low-frequency vibration (30 cps) is used post nerve injury to assess for the presence of reinnervation. [7] The instrument is tapped on a firm surface then applied to the area being evaluated. If the patient feels the vibration, a degree of reinnervation of slowly adapting fibers is indicated.

Sensory Reeducation

Sensory reeducation is the process of reclaiming lost somatosensory representation as well as improving the patient's ability to perceive and discriminate touch through cognitive behavioral techniques. [26] While more research is needed, sensory reeducation has been observed in the clinical setting to have a positive effect on improved localization, discrimination, stereognosis, and fine motor coordination. [4] Improved function is a result of a combination of nerve healing and regeneration and of changes in the somatosensory cortex via neural plasticity. The literature divides sensory reeducation into two phases: [19] Phase I begins with the injury or repair, and phase II begins when the patient is able to perceive touch. Historically, sensory reeducation has been initiated during phase II when some perception of sensation has returned. More recently, evidence has been provided via positron emission tomography (PET) scan and magnetic resonance imaging (MRI), that initiation of reeducation during phase I is beneficial in reestablishing cortical territory that is lost immediately upon peripheral nerve injury. [8, 21] Therefore, sensory reeducation involves not only stimulation of tissue but focus, cognition, perceptual abilities, and memory as well. A quiet environment and a concerted, consistent effort on the patient's part are both necessary during sensory reeducation.

Phase I sensory reeducation with a multisensory approach is initiated immediately upon injury or repair with the intent of minimizing the amount of cortical territory lost. [8] Several different techniques are recommended for inclusion in a home program which is performed in 10-min sessions, four to five times per day. Visual imagery has been shown to stimulate the sensory cortex [1]. The patient is asked to simply imagine the affected area being touched. Mirror box use has resulted in some perceiving touch in the injured area while watching the unaffected hand receive

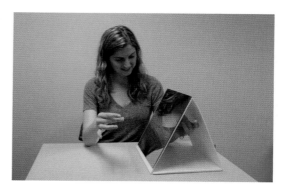

Fig. 11.11 Mirror box therapy

stimuli. [3, 21]. A mirror is placed on a tabletop perpendicular to the patient. The injured hand is placed behind the mirror, out of sight, while the unaffected hand rests in front of the mirror and is reflected in it (Fig. 11.11). In this form of "trickery," the patient looks into the mirror and watches the unaffected hand receive stimuli via tapping or rubbing, but, because the patient is looking in a mirror, the brain perceives the stimuli as being provided to and perceived by the injured hand. Additionally, direct observation of the affected hand being touched has been shown to stimulate the somatosensory cortex. [1]

Phase II sensory reeducation is initiated once touch is perceived in the affected area. Begin with efforts aimed at improving localization. The patient is asked to watch point stimulation to the affected area provided by a small dowel or the eraser end of pencil. The stimulus is then repeated in the same location with eyes closed; the stimulus is then applied for a third time while the patient watches. During the activity, the patient should focus on what is seen and felt. It may be helpful to begin with those areas closest to the periphery of the injury. Once localization has improved, a focus on tactile gnosis, or the recognition of shapes and textures, begins. Incorporating the unaffected hand is often recommended. The patient is asked to touch or trace an obscured shape, then to touch the same shape with the unaffected hand. If there is a perceived discrepancy, the patient is asked to touch the shape again with the affected hand while watching and then again

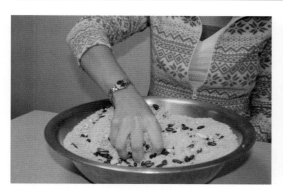

Fig. 11.12 Sensory reeducation

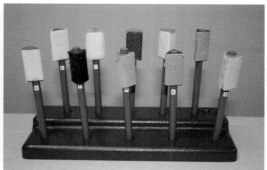

Fig. 11.13 Rolyan sensory reeducation wands

with vision occluded. Asking the patient to locate objects hidden in items of a different texture, such as blocks or beads hidden in dried beans, with vision occluded is also an effective technique as the patient must differentiate between different stimuli to locate the sought-after item (Fig. 11.12). As gross shape identification improves, progress toward smaller and more complex items such as buttons, keys, screws, and other everyday items. Encourage the patient to touch and explore commonplace items in the environment as much as possible.

Fingertip Hypersensitivity

After a fingertip injury, patients will often go to extreme lengths to "protect" the injured area from as much sensory input as possible. These patients are usually seen with the affected digit or digits sticking straight out while the other digits attempt the necessary manipulation. Persuading patients to participate in a desensitization program and to integrate the affected digit into functional activities is often met with much resistance. It is important to present a graded desensitization program in order to ease anxiety and facilitate compliance.

As supported in the literature, it is not uncommon for hypersensitivity to persist after a fingertip injury. Hypersensitivity limits functional use and can cause a significant delay in return to work. A desensitization program should begin as

soon as wound closure is noted and skin stability is present. Rendall [6] proposed the three-phase desensitization treatment protocol: phase I, dowel textures; phase 2, contact particles; and phase 3, vibration. In phase 1, the patient is instructed to use a series of ten dowels overlaid with varying textures ranging from smooth to very rough by rolling, rubbing, or tapping the dowel on the affected area for a duration of 10 min (Fig. 11.13). The patient begins with the dowel texture that he or she identifies as noxious. Dowel use is advanced as the stimulus becomes nonirritating. Contact particles are used in the same manner and progress from soft to hard. The patient digs his or her hand into the appropriate particle for 10 min. In phase 3, a MiniMassager (Hitachi) with three different heads (flat, round, and spot) is used for a 10-min period. [6] Graded putty is also used for both desensitization and strengthening. Coordination activities involving fingertip precision and ulnar translation should also be included in the rehabilitation process.

Careful review of the patient's work demands is required in order to provide work simulation activities. The BTe Primus (Baltimore, MD) is an excellent tool for work simulation, strengthening, and desensitization. Several of the smaller tools have removable smooth caps that reveal a rigged surface to which the patient can progress as hypersensitivity decreases. The use of actual work tools such as nuts, bolts, hammers, and nails is incorporated whenever possible.

References

1. Abzug J, Adams J, Alter S, Altman E, Amadio P, Armstrong T, et al. Rehabilitation of the hand and upper extremity sixth edition. Philadelphia: Mosby Inc.; 2011.
2. Anderson D. Mallet finger: management and patient compliance. Aust Fam Physician. 2011;40:47–8.
3. Bloom J, Khouri J, Hammert W. Current concepts in the evaluation and treatment of mallet finger injury. Plat Reconstr Surg. 2013;132:560–6.
4. Byl N, Leano J, Cheney L. The bly-cheney-boczai sensory discriminator: reliability, validity, and responsiveness for testing stereognosis. J Hand Ther. 2002;15(4):315–30.
5. Cannon NM. Rehabilitation approaches for distal and middle phalanx fractures of the hand. J Hand Ther. 2003;16(2):105–116.
6. Chu M, Chan R, Leung Y, Fung Y. Desensitization of finger tip injury. Tech Hand Up Extrem Surg. 2001;5(1):63–70.
7. Dellon AL, Kallman C. Evaluation of functional sensation in the hand. J Hand Surg Am. 1982;8(6):865–70.
8. Duff SV. Impact of peripheral nerve injury on sensorimotor control. J Hand Ther. 2005;18(2):277–91.
9. Edward J. Scar management. Nurs Stand. 2003; 17(52):39–42.
10. Evans R. Zone I flexor tendon rehabilitation with limited extension and active flexion. J Hand Ther. 2005;18:120–40.
11. Evans R. Managing the injured tendon: current concepts. J Hand Ther. 2012;25:173–90.
12. Geyman J, Fink K, Sullivan S. Conservative versus surgical treatment of mallet finger: a pooled quantitative literature evaluation. J Am Board Fam Pract. 1998;11:382–90.
13. Hart R, Kleinert H, Lyons K. The kleinert modified dorsal finger splint for mallet finger fracture. Am J Emerg Med. 2004;23(2):145–8.
14. Jerosch-Herold C, Sheptone L, Miller L, Chapman P. The responsiveness of sensibility and strength tests in patients undergoing carpal tunnel decompression. BMC Musculoskelet Disord. 2011;12:244
15. Kavros SJ, Liedl DA, Boon AJ. Expedited wound healing with noncontact, low frequency ultrasound therapy in chronic wounds: a retrospective analysis. Adv Skin Wound Care. 2008;21:4116–23.
16. Leinberry C. Mallet finger injuries. J Hand Surg. 2009;34:1715–17.
17. Lundbor G, Rosen B. Hand function after nerve repair. Acta Physiol Scand. 2007;189(2):201–17.
18. McOwan CG, MacDermid JC, Wilton J. Outcome measures for evaluation of scar: a literature review. J Hand Ther. 2001;14(2):77–85.
19. Miller LK, Chester R, Jerosch-Herold C. Effects of sensory reeducation programs on functional hand sensibility after median and ulnar repair: a systematic review. J Hand Ther. 2012;25(3) 297–306.
20. Novak CB. Evaluation of hand sensibility: a review. J Hand Ther. 2001;14(4):266–72.
21. Novak CB. Clinical commentary in response to: sensory relearning in peripheral nerve disorders of the hand: a web-based survey and Delphi consensus method. J Hand Ther. 2011;24(4):300–2.
22. Novak C, Mackinnon S. Evaluation of nerve injury and nerve compression in the upper quadrant. J Hand Ther. 2003;30:127–38.
23. O'Brien L, Bailey M. Single blind, prospective, randomized controlled trial comparing dorsal aluminum and custom thermoplastic splints to stack splint for acute mallet finger. Arch Phys Med Rehabil. 2011;92:191–8.
24. Oud T, Beelen A, Eijffinger E, Nollet F. Sensory reeducation after nerve injury of the upper limb: a systematic review. Clin Rehabil. 2006;21(6):483–94.
25. Pettengill K. The evolution of early mobilization of the repaired flexor tendon. J Hand Ther. 2005;18:157–68.
26. Phillips C, Blakey III G, Essick G. Sensory retraining: a cognitive behavioral therapy for altered sensation. Atlas Oral Maxillofac Surg Cliin North Am. 2010;19(1):109–18.
27. Ramundo J, Gray M. Enzymatic wound debridement. J Wound Ostomy Cont Nurs. 2008;35(3):273–280.
28. Rees E, Warwick K. Hand therapist-led management of mallet finger. Br J H and Ther. 2005;10:17–20.
29. Seitz Jr. William H. Fractures and Dislocations of the Hand and Fingers. Chicago: American Society for Surgery of the Hand; 2013.
30. Tocco S. Effectiveness of cast immobilization in closed mallet finger injury: a prospective randomized comparison with thermoplastic splinting. J Hand Ther. 2007;20(4):362–63.
31. Bowers, Wh, Putnam MD, Firn Z, Brehmer JL, Rozmaryn LM, Menge TJ. Fractures and Dislocations of the Hand and Fingers, Chicago, IL. ASSH. 2013.

Index

L. M. Rozmaryn (ed.), *Fingertip Injuries,* DOI 10.1007/978-3-319-13227-3
© Springer International Publishing Switzerland 2015

Printed in the United States of America